Omega Balance

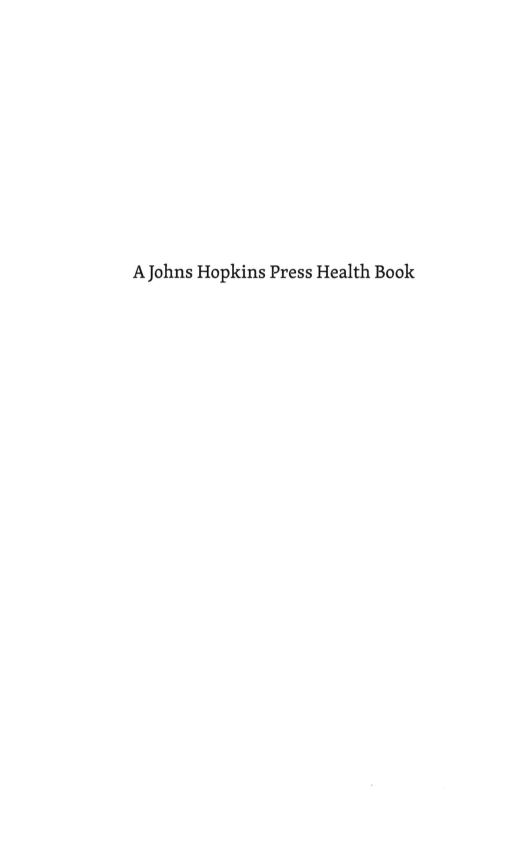

A Johns Hopkins Press Health Book

OMEGA
BALANCE

Nutritional Power
for a Happier, Healthier Life

ANTHONY JOHN HULBERT

JOHNS HOPKINS UNIVERSITY PRESS
Baltimore

Note to the reader: This book is not meant to substitute for medical care, and treatment should not be based solely on its contents. Instead, treatment must be developed in a dialogue between the individual and their physician. The book has been written to help with that dialogue.

Johns Hopkins University Press
2715 North Charles Street
Baltimore, Maryland 21218
www.press.jhu.edu

Cataloging-in-Publication Data is available from the Library of Congress.
A catalog record for this book is available from the British Library.
ISBN: 978-1-4214-4577-9 (hardcover)
ISBN: 978-1-4214-4578-6 (ebook)

IIllustrations by Jane Whitney

Special discounts are available for bulk purchases of this book. For more information, please contact Special Sales at specialsales@jh.edu.

To
Ralph T. Holman
(1918–2012)
and
Leonard H. Storlien
(1947–2022)

Contents

Preface

Fats, lipids, and oils are all essentially the same thing, and this is a book about fats, specifically polyunsaturated fats. It is not a "diet book," but diet and food are central to the book. There are two types of polyunsaturated fats: omega-3 and omega-6 fats, and *both* are essential in the human diet. In this respect, they differ from the other fats (saturated and monounsaturated), which are not essential requirements. I will tell you a story about how the balance between omega-3 and omega-6 in the human food chain has changed over the last half-century, favoring omega-6 over omega-3, and how this has had several serious consequences. I hope to convince you that this change, relatively unknown by the general public, is a major contributor to many modern epidemics.

I come to the task trained not as a nutritionist but as a zoologist (a zoo-physiologist to be precise) who developed an interest in membranes (the "skin" around every cell). My understanding thus stems from an evolutionary perspective. The twentieth-century biologist Theodosius Dobzhansky famously said, "Nothing in biology makes sense except in the light of evolution." This also applies to understanding nutrition, which unfortunately is generally not situated in an evolutionary context but instead is taught as a list of almost secret ingredients.

My path started with a sense of wonder and awe when, as an undergraduate, I learned that the breath a bird inhales does not leave the bird in the next exhalation but rather in the second exhalation after it was first breathed in. I was curious as to why and how, and I developed a desire to understand how animals work. My early studies concentrated on metabolism, specifically the rate of metabolism of Australian marsupials. After earning my PhD in Australia and doing postdoctoral research in the United States, I accepted an academic appointment at the University of Wollongong in Australia, where I continued to investigate the metabolism of various animal species and which specific cell processes use the energy in food. It became obvious that the processes associated with cell membranes are important, and I became interested in the fat molecules that form the basis of these membranes. In the 1980s, Len Storlien, who was researching obesity and appetite, as well as Type 2 diabetes, contacted me. Len, who later also took up a position at the University of Wollongong, was interested in how our findings might be relevant to his own work. He introduced me to the difference between omega-3 and omega-6 fats. He is one of the two scientists to whom I have dedicated this book. Over the years I became fascinated by these fats and their role in cell membranes. I also became aware of the imbalance between omega-6 and omega-3 fats in the modern human food chain.

As scientists, we stand on the shoulders of those who come before us. Sometimes they are dead, leaving their thoughts, findings, and words for us in the literature, while others are living authors or stimulating speakers at scientific meetings. Many have influenced my own path; some I have had the pleasure of meeting in person, while others I have met only through the scientific literature. I will acknowledge a small number of significant contributors to our knowledge of these fats, but there are many others whom I cannot acknowledge because of space limitations, and I apologize in advance to them for their omission.

George and Mildred Burr discovered the essential requirement for polyunsaturated fat in the diet in the 1920s–1930s. I have co-dedicated this book to Ralph Holman, a student of George Burr, whom I regard as the father of omega-6 and omega-3 fatty acids, being responsible for much of our knowledge regarding these fatty acids. He invented the "omega-" naming system, which departed from the chemical naming conventions of the time but was helpful for understanding these fats. The English scientist Michael Crawford was influenced by his experiences in Africa in the 1960s and highlighted the differences between wild and domesticated mammals, as well as the important role of omega-3 fats in brain function. William ("Bill") Lands performed important work, beginning in the 1950s, on the processes determining the fatty acid composition of membranes. He was involved in the early research on inflammation mediators and in the 1970s reported that mediators made from omega-3 were less inflammatory than those made from omega-6 fatty acids. Together with the investigations by Hans Olaf Bang and Jorn Dyerberg into the blood lipids of Greenland Inuit, Bill Lands's findings were important for the emergence of fish oil as a treatment for a variety of conditions. Lands may have been the earliest investigator to realize the importance of the balance between omega-3 and omega-6 in the diet.

A key moment in this history was an international conference in 1985 to consider the health effects of polyunsaturated fatty acids in seafoods. Many of the participants, including the chair, Artemis Simopoulos, recount that they were struck by the realization that although a diet low in omega-3 was connected to many modern diseases, a large part of the problem was that many individuals were awash with omega-6 fats because of its abundance in the modern food chain. Omega-6 and omega-3 are competitors, and it is the balance between the two types of essential fats that is critical. For me, Simopoulos stimulated the generalization that "leaves" are important sources of omega-3 while "seeds" predominantly provide omega-6.

In the 1990s, I felt privileged to be scientifically aware of the increasing imbalance between omega-3 and omega-6 fats in our food chain and its possible ill-health consequences. I was expecting this knowledge to permeate society and have beneficial consequences. By the 2000s, I became disappointed that this was not happening. Following my retirement from formal teaching duties in 2008, I continued research activities, and in 2009 I decided to write this book.

Initially, I intended to concentrate only on obesity and diabetes as the consequence of the imbalance between omega-3 and omega-6. However, the more I studied the topic, the more I realized that this change in the modern food chain (which I call the omega story) partly explains the increased incidence of a wide variety of modern diseases. An important revelation was that although change in the food chain need not initiate the specific diseases, it amplifies the ill-health associated with disease state and thus might account for the increase in prevalence of many chronic diseases. It can also explain their extensive comorbidities. It is the same fundamental diet problem that underlies the various co-occurring conditions.

I have tried to write for both a scientific audience and interested laypeople, and it has not been an easy task to communicate to both audiences. Professionals will be annoyed by my simplification and lack of precise terms, while the general audience may sometimes be intimidated by the scientific jargon and perceived complexity.

Most nutritional advice is centered around "minimum daily requirements," with the specific nutrient considered individually. This book proposes that this concept is inadequate when we consider the omega-3 and omega-6 fats. These fats compete with each other for their positions in cell membranes; consequently, it is the balance between them that is important. I am often asked, "How much omega-3 should I take?" My answer is, "I can't suggest an amount unless you tell me how much omega-6 you are eating." My emphasis, and the evidence presented, will show that you should not consider these essential fats in isolation.

To counter the inadequacy of the minimum-requirement approach as far as the polyunsaturated fats are concerned, I will introduce the concept of omega balance in chapter 2, and use it throughout the rest of the book. The concept is simple—namely, the percentage of polyunsaturated fats that are omega-3—but it is not the way that omega-3 and omega-6 content is normally presented elsewhere. In reporting the findings of other researchers, I have recalculated their results as well as calculating omega balance from individual values for omega-3 and omega-6 content in various databases and scientific papers. I have used it to simplify what we know about these important fatty acids and also to maintain a simple, single method of expression throughout the book. It is analogous to, but not the same as the ratio of omega-3 to omega-6 fats. It has certain advantages over the use of a ratio and can also be presented visually as a pie chart. I hope that you find it useful.

The change in our food that I describe has been coincident with the rise of ultraprocessed foods, but it is not restricted to it. The omega story is the story of a change in both the production and consumption of our food while ignoring the nutritional and biological importance of these two types of essential fats. It is a warning, and I hope I have done this important story justice.

I

PART I

FOOD
and
DIETS

CHAPTER 1

ESSENTIALS OF NUTRITION

An Evolutionary Perspective

The Discovery That Certain Fats Are Essential in the Human Diet

It's a parent's nightmare. You allow your child to be looked after by a friend, and there's a gun accident. So it was for Dorena Strobel of Morris, Illinois, when she went to work on Halloween in 1978, leaving her 6-year-old daughter Shawna with a friend of the family.[1] Shawna suffered a severe abdominal gunshot wound that necessitated the removal of a large length of her intestines. Shawna then had to be fed intravenously, and a year later, she developed symptoms that nobody could explain. These included blurred vision, numbness, tingling, and weakness in her legs as well as the inability to walk.

While some considered Shawna's problems to be psychological, one of her doctors thought that it might be associated with her intravenous nutrition and asked the biochemist Ralph Holman to analyze her blood. There are two types of polyunsaturated fatty acids: omega-3 and omega-6. Holman found that Shawna's blood had very low levels of omega-3.[2] At the time, two approved intravenous food sources contained fats. In one, the fats came from safflower oil, while the other used soybean oil. Shawna was being fed the one with fats from safflower oil. The polyunsaturated fats in safflower oil are omega-6, but the oil contains *no* omega-3. Soybean oil, by contrast, contains *both* omega-3 and omega-6 fats.

Holman suggested that Shawna's diet be changed to the soybean-based intravenous solution. Over the next few months, her blood omega-3 returned to normal levels, and the unpleasant symptoms she'd had went away. One indication of the effects of her increased omega-3 was that the speed of her nervous impulses had increased compared to when she was on the safflower-based intravenous food.

For the period she was fed the safflower-based solution, Shawna was getting plenty of omega-6 but *no* omega-3. After changing to the soybean-based intravenous food, she recommenced intake of omega-3 as well as continuing to get plenty of omega-6. Shawna Strobel is the first documented case to show that while the requirement for omega-3 by humans is small (from Shawna's experience, it was estimated to be about 0.5 percent of dietary energy), omega-3 fats are an essential component of the human diet, separate from a need for omega-6.

There are four types of fatty acids: (1) saturated, (2) monounsaturated, (3) omega-6 polyunsaturated, and (4) omega-3 polyunsaturated fats. I will explain in chapter 5 why they are given these names. Here, all we need know is that the last two types are *both* essential components of the human diet and furthermore are *separately* essential (they cannot substitute for each other). In contrast, the saturated and monounsaturated fats are *not* essential components of our diet. This is because saturated fats can be synthesized *de novo* from other (non-fat) food molecules, and we can also then make monounsaturated fats from saturated fats. Both saturated and monounsaturated fats are almost always present in our diet, but, unlike omega-6 and omega-3, they are not an essential part of our food.

The reason why both omega-6 and omega-3 are essential in our diet is that we are unable to synthesize them; consequently, we must obtain both types of polyunsaturated fats already preformed in our food. Furthermore, we are also unable to convert omega-6 fats into omega-3 fats (or vice versa), and thus both are independently essential. The thesis of this book is that while both types of polyunsaturated fats are essential, it is the *balance* between these two essential fats in our diet that contributes to good health.

Shawna Strobel's experience provided evidence for the essential requirement of omega-3 fats but not for the essentiality of omega-6 fats, since throughout her ordeal she was receiving adequate amounts of omega-6 fats. Earlier cases of intravenous feeding provided evidence for the essentiality of omega-6 fats in the human diet. The first intravenous feeding solutions were fat-free, because fats and water don't mix very well. It was difficult to include fats in the sterile solutions produced for such emergency feeding, so they were omitted. The introduction of fats into intravenous feeding solutions waited until the development of the technology of nontoxic emulsions. Tragically, Ralph Holman's mother died in 1962 before this event. After abdominal surgery she was intravenously fed a fat-free solution, and at that time neither her doctor nor her son could figure out how to safely and adequately provide her with the fats that Holman knew were important.

In 1969, another elderly woman underwent severe intestinal surgery and was maintained on a fat-free intravenous feeding solution for seven months. In 1970, an infant who also had undergone substantial intestinal surgery, was similarly put on fat-free intravenous feeding. In both cases, skin problems developed within a few months, and Holman was asked to measure their blood. He found that their blood contained plentiful amounts of saturated and monounsaturated fats but was deficient in both omega-6 and omega-3. This showed that although neither patient was provided with any source of fat in their intravenous food, they were still able to make saturated and monounsaturated fats (from non-fat sources) but were incapable of synthesizing either omega-6 or omega-3 fats. Both omega-6 and omega-3 are essential in the human diet, and together these two types of polyunsaturated fats are also called "essential fatty acids."[3]

The concept of dietary essential fats was first identified for rats, but many believed that it did not apply to human nutrition. In 1929, George and Mildred Burr had shown rats to have an essential requirement for fat in their diet. It was the Burrs who first coined the term "essential fatty acids."

After obtaining his PhD, George Burr went to the University of California, Berkeley, where he researched vitamin E. Mildred was in charge of the rat colony. They fell in love and married. During his vitamin E research, Burr used rat diets that were highly purified and fat-free. The rats on these fat-free diets showed deficiency symptoms. Although the head of the laboratory thought that they were dealing with a different, strange new fat-soluble vitamin, Burr suspected that the fats themselves were responsible for the deficiency symptoms. While at Berkeley, he was offered a position in plant physiology at the University of Minnesota. When he said that he wanted to continue his work on rats in a department concerned with plants, the department head replied, "I don't care what you work on, just so it is good." So the Burrs set off for Minnesota in their Model T Ford roadster, with two cages of their rats from Berkeley. On cold nights they would smuggle their rats into their hotel rooms under long overcoats.[4]

At Minnesota, the Burrs continued working together and found that rats fed a diet rigidly excluding all fat grew very slowly and developed scaly skin. Their tails began to swell and die back, their kidneys degenerated, blood appeared in the urine, and they were unable to reproduce. In 1929 the Burrs announced that unsaturated fats were essential in the diet of rats,[5] and in 1930 they narrowed the responsibility for these problems down to a specific omega-6 called linoleic acid (with the possibility that other unsaturated fatty acids might also be involved).[6] Surprisingly, this was regarded as controversial at the time, as it was already known that rats could make fats from carbohydrates, and it was thought that the effects the Burrs reported were due to some as-yet-undescribed fat-soluble vitamin. It wasn't realized at the time that the only fats rats can make from carbohydrates are the saturated and monounsaturated fats, but they are *not* able to synthesize omega-6 or omega-3.

After showing that rats had this essential need for fats in their diet, George Burr decided to test whether this was also the case for humans. A fellow biochemist volunteered to live for six months on a diet extremely low in fat.[7] However, he remained healthy for the whole six months, and consequently many believed that this provided evidence that humans were different from rats and did not have an essential need for fat in their diet. At the time, it was not understood that an average adult human has more than a kilogram (more than two pounds) of omega-6 fats and that it would require *more than* six months to deplete this source.

It is little appreciated that time is relative in different species because the rate of metabolism varies systematically among species. This will be discussed in more detail in chapter 5, but suffice to say here that in a comparative metabolic sense, a six-month diet experiment in a human is equivalent to a four-week diet experiment in a rat. The Burrs had shown that it took about fifteen weeks in a young growing rat before the symptoms of essential fatty acid deficiency became apparent. In hindsight, it is not surprising that the human experiment did not produce symptoms, as one would expect it to take about two years before the symptoms of essential fat deficiency to become manifest in a human. George Burr, many years later, concluded that the dietary requirement for omega-6 is small, being about 1–2 percent of dietary energy.[8]

At the time of George and Mildred Burr's experiments, it was common practice to use a mixture of skim milk and sugar when bottle-feeding babies. Skin problems were often observed in babies fed this fat-reduced diet, and this was a serious medical problem. One of Burr's students found that these eczema-prone infants have very low levels of polyunsaturated fats in their blood.[9] It was shown that such babies were essential fatty acid-deficient and responded positively to provision of the essential fats in their milk.

The two seminal scientists I have mentioned are connected. In 1941, George Burr took on Ralph Holman as a graduate student. Initially, Holman intended to study carbohydrate metabolism, but the secret development of the atom bomb (the Manhattan Project) at the time interfered with his proposed dissertation. The supply of radioactive carbon that he intended to use in his PhD studies dried up, and Holman asked Burr to give him a new research problem on fats. It is to our advantage that Holman took on the task of investigating, isolating, and identifying the wide range of different fatty acids. He can rightly be called one of the fathers of modern lipid biochemistry. He is responsible for introducing the "omega-" naming system, which is the opposite of the normal chemical rules and conventions for naming molecules but is a helpful concept for understanding these important fats.

Since this early work on rats and humans, we have become aware that omega-6 and omega-3 are also essential in the diet of many other animals. For example, in view of the common knowledge that fish are a good dietary source of omega-3 fats, many are surprised to find out that fish have long been known to have an essential dietary requirement for omega-3. That's right: fish do not make omega-3 fats; just like us, they need to obtain them pre-formed, as essential components, in their diet. During the aquaculture boom of the 1960s, corn and corn oil were tried as a substitute for the normal food of trout; unfortunately, this resulted in a lethal condition known as "transport shock." It was discovered this lethal condition was due to an omega-3 deficiency. While corn oil was able to provide plenty of omega-6 to the trout, it did not provide omega-3, which was essential to avoid the lethal shock syndrome, as well as to avoid heart myopathy and fin erosion.[10] This discovery preceded, by a decade, the discovery that humans also have an essential requirement for omega-3.

In a later chapter I will explain why omega-3 and omega-6 are given these names and describe the different fatty acids that belong to these types of fat. It will explain that all types of unsaturated fats can be classified into a specific "omega-X" group. For example, it will explain why the most common monounsaturated fatty acid is an omega-9 fat. We can make omega-9 (and omega-7) fats, and thus they are *not* essential components of our diet. These will not concern me in the rest of this book. Only omega-3 and omega-6 are dietary essential fats.

How Nutrients Become Essential Components of the Diet

Vitamins: Ascorbic Acid as an Example

The basic reason that some molecules are essential nutrients is that we don't have the cellular machinery to manufacture them. We don't have the specific enzymes in our cells to make such molecules,[11] and consequently we must obtain them pre-formed in our food. In order to more fully understand this concept, let's consider ascorbic acid.

Ascorbic acid, or vitamin C, is also an essential component of the human diet. Yet your cat, your dog or your sheep, goat, or pet rat don't have the same need to consume it in their food. They can make it themselves, having the necessary enzymes to synthesize it. The reason why it is a vitamin for humans is that, sometime in our primate past, our ancestors lost the enzyme required to synthesize ascorbic acid. This ancestor wasn't careless; it didn't actually *lose* the enzyme. Rather, there was a mutation in the gene for the particular enzyme, and this change in the gene altered the enzyme's structure, such that it was no longer able to do its job of making ascorbic acid molecules. However, although it could no longer make ascorbic acid molecules, there was no disadvantage to this ancestor because it was already consuming plenty of ascorbic acid in its food. At that particular time, ascorbic acid went from being an optional component of this animal's diet to being an essential component. This was the moment that ascorbic acid became vitamin C.

At first, it might be presumed that this ancestor was a fruit-eater and that it was the fruit in the diet that provided the ascorbic acid that the ancestor was no longer able to synthesize. However, this need not be the case; this ancestor may have been a carnivore. Although citrus fruits are a well-known source of vitamin C (oranges and lemons have 53mg per 100g), some meats also provide significant amounts of vitamin C (thymus and spleen from cattle have 34–46mg per 100g).[12]

Most mammals can make their own ascorbic acid, but the species unable to do so include a number of higher primate species, the guinea pig, and the fruit bat. For these species, like humans, ascorbic acid is a vitamin.

Vitamins are small organic molecules that are essential for our biochemistry,[13] but somewhere in our ancestry we "lost" the enzymes to synthesize them, and they became essential dietary components. Our inability to synthesize them is the only thing common to vitamins: They have no common chemical structure. The evolutionary sequence is: an animal loses the ability to synthesize a particular molecule; it does not experience any selective disadvantage as long as the particular molecule is part of its food; and the particular molecule becomes an essential nutrient.

The Building Blocks of Proteins: Amino Acids

Back in our evolutionary past, there were mutations in the enzymes responsible for synthesizing various amino acids. This early ancestor could thus no longer make some of the amino acids that, when linked together, make up proteins. No problem: this ancestor used the proteins of the organisms it was eating to obtain the amino acids needed to make its own proteins. Consequently, protein became an essential component of our diet. To be more precise, about half of the twenty amino acids that make up proteins are essential in our diet. We still have enzymes that can modify these essential amino acids to make the nonessential amino acids. (When we use the word *essential* in this context we are referring solely to the diet.) All twenty amino acids are essential for making up the proteins we need for the normal functioning of our body cells, but about half have to be obtained already preformed in the diet; only these are the dietary essential amino acids. The list of essential amino acids will vary between species, being dependent on their specific evolutionary history and which enzymes they have "lost."

There are consequences from this evolutionary process, and our dietary protein can be labeled either "high-quality" protein or "low-quality" protein. What do we mean by these tags? The source of the protein will determine whether it is "high quality" or "low quality." High-quality proteins are those that have the twenty amino acids we require in just the right proportions that we need in order to make our own proteins. Low-quality proteins are those that, with respect to our requirements, are deficient in one or more of the essential amino acids. Thus, it makes sense that high-quality proteins come from organisms closest to us, in an evolutionary sense. High-quality protein sources include meat, poultry, eggs, dairy products, and fish. Plants are further away from us, in an evolutionary sense, and consequently some plant proteins are deficient in one or more of the amino acids that we need to make our own proteins. They don't have the right balance of the different amino acids we require. The unused amino acids—the ones in excess of our requirements—cannot be stored in our body, and consequently we are unable to efficiently use *all* of the amino acids that make up these "low-quality" proteins. They are incomplete for us as a protein source.

An example is corn (maize). Corn has just the right amount of lysine (an amino acid) for its own proteins to function properly, but when we humans digest the proteins of corn to make a mixture of amino acids to manufacture our own specific proteins, the mixture is deficient in lysine. We will not be able to use the complete amino acid mixture from the corn—it will be incomplete or of "low quality" for our purposes.

Beans are low in methionine (another amino acid), and for humans, beans can also be regarded as a low-quality source of protein. However, beans have an excess of lysine for our purposes, and corn has an excess of methionine. Thus, by combining corn and beans in one meal (a common practice in Central America), these two low-quality sources of protein can compensate each other's deficiency and produce a higher-quality source of protein for us than either can by itself. This is called *protein complementarity*. Many societies from the past, without knowing anything about proteins or amino acids, have combined different foods to achieve protein complementarity.

Another consequence of the evolutionary process that makes certain things essential in food is that the types of essential nutrients differ among different species. Whether something is essential will depend on the particular animal's specific evolutionary past. For example, while humans have the ability to synthesize cholesterol, many insects do not, and consequently cholesterol is a vitamin for these insects. We know little of the essential nutrient requirements for many animal species.

Being an Animal

A prime requirement for all life is a source of energy. Plants, algae, and some microbes use light energy to combine atoms to make the complex organic molecules they need to function. Animals, fungi, and other microbes obtain their energy by breaking down the complex organic molecules that make up other organisms and using the chemical energy in these molecules. Humans are descended from those microbes that ate other microbes, and consequently we are still obliged to eat other organisms (or their products) in order to obtain our energy and essential nutrients.

The most abundant organic molecule on the planet is cellulose, a complex carbohydrate synthesized by plants to make their cell walls, which function as their skeletons. Because they don't have the medium of water to support their weight, terrestrial plants, especially, have lots of cellulose. An interesting nutritional aspect of cellulose is that, being the most abundant organic molecule on the planet, it would theoretically be a great source of energy for animals. Yet as far as we know, no higher animals have an enzyme to break down cellulose, and they are thus unable to use the chemical energy locked up in this abundant molecule. In our diet, we call the cellulose we consume fiber (or roughage).

Herbivorous mammals, such as sheep, cattle, and goats, that eat plant material (such as grass or other leaves) are similar to us in that they can't synthesize an enzyme to break down cellulose. Not even those inveterate wood-eaters, the termites, make the enzyme to breakdown the cellulose molecules that make up wood. So how do they get their energy? They do it through a mutually beneficial relationship, a symbiosis, with organisms that can make the required enzyme. They have evolved an expanded part of their gut in which they grow large numbers of cellulose-digesting microbes and provide these microbes with both the environment and the plant food the microbes need to reproduce. The microbes in this expanded gut (essentially a large fermentation vat) use the cellulose in the plant cell walls provided by their host as their primary source of energy; they reproduce and make lots of copies of themselves, and they also produce wastes. The herbivore absorbs the waste products and uses this waste as a source of energy. More importantly, as the newly produced microbes pass further down the gut, the herbivore digests the microbes themselves and consequently absorbs all the amino acids and vitamins made by the microbes.

In some herbivores (for example, sheep, cattle, goats, and kangaroos), this large fermentation vat comes before the stomach and is a very efficient system. Some of these animals even regurgitate the contents of the fermentation vat and further chew the contents, which makes the plant cell walls more available for digestion by the microbes. This is called "chewing the cud."

Some herbivores provide the gut microbes with a source of nitrogen, which the microbes can use to synthesize new microbial proteins. Rather than excrete all their nitrogenous waste (from protein breakdown) in their urine, as we do, these herbivores excrete some of the nitrogenous waste in their saliva, sending it directly to the microbes in their gut. They effectively "recycle" nitrogen. This and other tricks allow these herbivores to live on low-quality food such as grass. No wonder these herbivorous mammals are the major species that we domesticated, completing a tripartite deal. We humans provide the herbivores with protection and pasture. The herbivores provide their gut microbes with a comfortable environment and the food and nutrients they need to grow. The gut microbes provide the herbivore with both energy and themselves (and thus the essential amino acids and vitamins needed by their host). In turn, the herbivore hosts provide us with the food and essential nutrients we need; in the form of either milk or meat. It's a good deal.

Even though we sometimes obtain our essential nutrients from eating other animals, most often these essential nutrients have originally been synthesized by plants, algae, or microbes at the base of the food chain. This is the case for the essential amino acids we need to make our proteins, and it also true for the essential fats: the omega-6 and omega-3.

Another difference between plants and animals is that plants make omega-3 from omega-6. The reason why omega-3 and omega-6 are *separate* essential fats is that animals don't have the necessary enzyme to make omega-3 from omega-6. Actually, that's not completely true, for when I use the word *animals* in this book, I am normally referring to the "higher" animals, such mammals, birds, or fish. The lowly nematode worm (*Caenorhabditis elegans*), the first animal to have its DNA completely sequenced, has the genetic information to make the appropriate enzyme and consequently can convert omega-6 to omega-3. However, the fruit-fly (*Drosophila melanogaster*), the second animal to have its DNA completely sequenced, does not have the gene for this enzyme. Consequently, like ourselves and other higher animals, the fruit-fly cannot convert omega-6 into omega-3, and these two fats will also be separate essential nutrients for fruit-flies.[14] Thus we can deduce a time in our evolutionary past when omega-3 became independent essential nutrients: sometime between the evolution of the ancestors of nematode worms and fruit-flies.

A small detour is worthwhile in a chapter that has been devoted to an evolutionary perspective on which nutrients are essential. In later chapters I will describe how different omega-3 and omega-6 fats of plants are generally 16 to 18 carbon atoms in length, while those of animals are 16 to 22 carbon atoms in length. I will describe how higher animals (including mammals) can convert the shorter-chain to the longer-chain polyunsaturated fatty acids (PUFA).

Well, that is not completely true either, because not all mammals can do this. Early in his career, a young Australian biochemist, Andrew Sinclair, along with colleagues began investigating the role of essential fats in the nutrition of a wide variety of mammals. His contributions include the first report of omega-6 deficiency in an adult human,[15] as well as the first report of omega-3 essential requirements in a primate, the Capuchin monkey.[16] Both of these species are able to convert 18-carbon PUFA into longer-chain PUFA. However, when they fed domestic cats diets that in other respects were complete but contained only 18-carbon PUFA, the cats exhibited severe deficiency symptoms. They were listless, grew poorly, had poor skin and fur, became infertile, and developed a fatty liver. After longer-chain PUFA were added to the diet, these symptoms went away.[17] The conclusion is that cats *lack* the ability to convert 18-carbon PUFA to the longer-chain PUFA. It is likely that felids in general have lost this enzymatic capacity. No problem: being carnivores, they were already eating other animals that contained these longer-chain PUFA. Whenever this happened in their evolutionary past was the time that "animal flesh" became an essential part of the felid diet. The longer-chain PUFA and the shorter-chain PUFA have become separate essential components of the diet of felids. Unlike humans, felids are *obligate* carnivores, in that they *must* eat meat because plants would not provide them with all the essential fats required for normal body function.

This has been only a brief overview of some aspects of nutrition. Having an evolutionary perspective explains why some things have become essential in our diet. It helps to understand nutrition and not just learn it. This is an important distinction. We can learn lots of things, and once learned they can be easily forgotten, but once you understand something it is almost impossible to forget it. To my knowledge, we don't even have a word for it. Dis-understand? I don't think so.

It is the premise of this book that omega-3 and omega-6 fats are important and independent essential nutrients, and that it is the *balance* between these two types of essential fats in the diet that is a relatively little understood but a very significant factor for good health. In recent times, the intake of these two essential fats has become unbalanced. Before I examine the modern human diet, we should first understand the relative abundance of these two types of essential fats in different food types.

CHAPTER 2

THE OMEGA BALANCE OF FOODS

Seeds, Leaves, and Meats

Various foods have different omega balances, and we can draw some generalizations from the source of the food. The presence of "seeds, leaves, and meats" in the chapter's subtitle is the first lesson. Omega-3 fats are relatively high in "leaves,"[1] while omega-6 fats are dominant in the "seeds" of plants. The omega balance of animal products relates to the relative importance of seeds and leaves in the animal's diet.

The Omega Balance Concept

I am concerned only with the *relative* content of the omega-3 fat and the omega-6 fat in food and *not* with saturated or monounsaturated fats as neither of these are essential nutrients. The reputation of saturated fat as "bad fat" is undeserved and will be discussed in later chapters. The history of the misunderstanding about the connection between dietary saturated fat and health is well covered in two books: Gary Taubes's *Good Calories, Bad Calories,* and Nina Teicholz's *The Big Fat Surprise.*[2]

Omega balance is a simple concept: It is the percentage of polyunsaturated fats that are omega-3, with the remaining percentage being omega-6 fats. Despite its simplicity, the concept is not commonly used in the scientific literature. Several researchers have examined the relationship between omega-3 and omega-6 fats, but most have used a ratio (either "omega-3/omega-6" ratio, or "omega-6/omega-3" ratio).

While omega balance might appear to be a ratio, it is in fact a proportion. Being a proportion, it has certain advantages over a ratio. Ratios have a specific mathematical nature. For example, ratios of two variables can vary from zero to infinity, with the midpoint value being one. Because of this, they should not be averaged. Let me use a simple example to illustrate: Say, for one week my fruit intake consists of nine oranges and one apple, and for the next week it is one orange and nine apples. Thus, over the fortnight I have eaten an equal number of oranges and apples. Averaging the proportions for weeks 1 and 2 will show that this is the case, while averaging the ratios will not give such a conclusion. The proportion of my fruit intake that was apples was 0.1 in the first week and was 0.9 for the second week, giving an average of 0.5 for the fortnight. The ratio of apples to oranges was 1/9 (0.11) in the first week, while for the second week it was 9/1 (9.00). The average of the apple/orange ratios for the fortnight is 4.55, which is very different from my actual consumption of ten apples and ten oranges over the fortnight (a ratio of 1). The concept of omega balance is a proportion expressed as a percentage. Together with the total PUFA content, it can also be used to calculate both the omega-3 and the omega-6 content of the particular food.

The omega balance (as well as the total PUFA content) of a wide range of foods is presented in appendix 1. The omega balance of a selection of these foods is illustrated as pie charts in figure 2.1 (plant-based foods) and figure 2.2 (animal-based foods). I have primarily used two food composition databases for calculation of omega balance values.[3] Both databases provide the "total polyunsaturated fat" content of the specific food, together with content of individual fatty acids, but neither give the *total* omega-3 or *total* omega-6 content. I have calculated the omega balance for each food type by combining the values for individual fatty acids. The lack of information about *total* omega-3 and *total* omega-6 in foods is a significant inadequacy of these databases that I will cover in the final chapter.

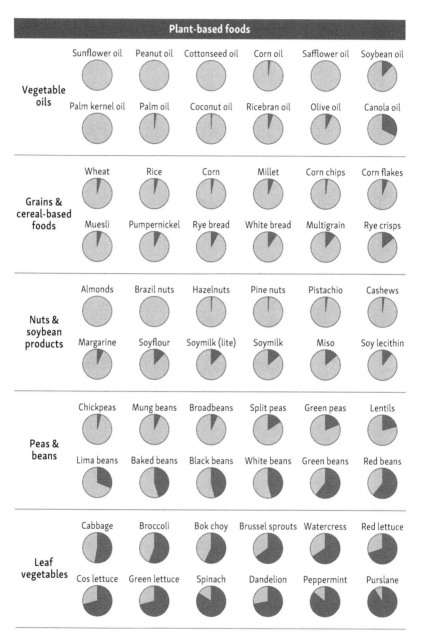

Figure 2.1 Omega balance of selected plant-based foods. In each pie chart, the dark sector represents omega-3 PUFA, while the light sector represents omega-6 PUFA. For actual values and sources, see appendix 1.

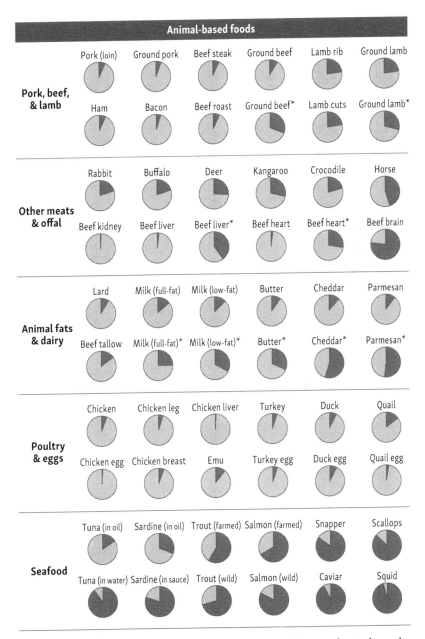

Figure 2.2 Omega balance of selected animal-based foods. In each pie chart, the dark sector represents omega-3 PUFA, while the light sector represents omega-6 PUFA. All values are for US foods, except those marked with * are foods from "grass-fed" livestock from Australia or New Zealand. For values and sources, see appendix 1.

Vegetable Oils and Their Products
Are the Dominant Source of Omega-6

Vegetable oils are the most significant source of fats in the modern human food chain. The Food and Agricultural Organization of the United Nations collects data each year from almost all of the world's nations and from this data constructs "Food Balance Sheets." This information is available from the FAOSTAT database,[4] and it includes calculated values (both for the whole world and for individual countries) for the "per capita" daily provision of fat from a number of food categories.

In 2018 (the most recent year for which data are available at the time of writing), the world food supply provided an average 86g fat per person per day. For the United States, the value is 170g fat per person per day; for Australia it is 158g. The largest single contributor to this fat supply were the "vegetable oils," which provided, for the world, 38 percent of total fat in the food supply, compared to 48 percent of the US food supply and 43 percent of the Australian food supply.

The omega balance values for twelve vegetable oils are illustrated in figure 2.1.[5] Together, these oils provide 95 percent of the total "vegetable oils" contribution to fat in the global food supply.[6] The polyunsaturated fats of most vegetable oils are overwhelmingly omega-6 fats, and most oils either have no, or negligible, omega-3 fats. Safflower oil, while not a common vegetable oil in the human food chain, is included because it was the source of fats in the intravenous food initially given to young Shawna Strobel (see chapter 1). It is essentially devoid of omega-3 fats. The omega-3 deficiency experienced by Shawna Strobel was remedied when soybean oil became the source of fat in her intravenous food. Soybean oil, the most prevalent vegetable oil in the modern human food chain, providing 11 percent of the world's total fat supply (36 percent in United States), has an omega balance of 12 percent.

Rapeseed and mustard are related plants that provide oils with a relatively high omega-3 content. However, rapeseed also has a high content of a monounsaturated fat, erucic acid, that damages cardiac muscle. In the early 1970s, Canadian agricultural scientists produced a rapeseed cultivar low in this toxic fatty acid. They named it "canola" (from "*Canadian oil, low acid*"), which has become the generic term for edible rapeseed. The omega balance of canola oil is 32 percent, while the value for mustard oil is 28 percent.

Many vegetable oils used in food are not included in figure 2.1 because they are not quantitatively important contributors of fat to the food supply. Those with no omega-3 include grapeseed oil, almond oil, hazelnut oil, poppyseed oil, and macadamia oil. Those oils containing predominantly omega-6 but with small amounts of omega-3 include sesame oil, palm oil, corn oil, and coconut oil (omega balance of 1–2 percent). Other oils with slightly more omega-3 include; olive oil (7 percent), walnut oil (16 percent), and hempseed oil (25 percent). Unusually, oils from flaxseed (also known as linseed) and chia seeds have more omega-3 than omega-6 (both have an omega balance of 79 percent), which is similar to many seafoods, but whereas the omega-3 in seafood includes substantial 20- and 22-carbon omega-3, the omega-3 in flaxseed and chia seed are 18-carbon fats.

Vegetable oils also vary in the total amount of PUFA they contain, from very high, where the majority of fats in the food are polyunsaturated (safflower, sunflower, soybean, corn oil, and cottonseed oils), to very low, where the majority of fats are either saturated (coconut, palm kernel, and palm oils) or monounsaturated (olive and canola oils). Using both the total PUFA content and omega balance for each oil, combined with their contribution to global fat supply, we can calculate that only two oils contribute substantial amounts of omega-3 fats to the human food chain. Soybean oil provides 0.65g per person per day (largely because of its quantitative importance in the food chain). Canola oil contributes 0.35g (largely because of its relatively high omega balance) while all the other vegetable oils (in figure 2.1) combined provide only 0.04g. The total provision of omega-3 from all the vegetable oils in figure 2.1 (which represent 95 percent of all vegetable oils in the food chain) is approximately 1g per person per day.

The equivalent omega-6 provision from these oils is approximately 11g per person per day.

Margarine was developed in the late 1800s following a challenge by Napoleon III to find a spreadable butter substitute suitable for use by the armed forces and the lower classes. It is a water-in-fat emulsion, and although animal fat was used in the original margarine, it is nowadays generally made from vegetable oils. The total content of polyunsaturated fats in margarines can vary quite widely but is generally lower than in the particular oil from which it is made. The process of "hydrogenation" (covered in more detail later) is responsible for this reduced PUFA content and made these products spreadable. Unfortunately, "partial hydrogenation" had two unforeseen consequences, (1) producing "trans fats" (see chapter 12), and (2) lowering the omega balance of the vegetable oil (because omega-3 are preferentially hydrogenated compared to omega-6). For example, partially hydrogenated soybean oil has an omega balance of 7 percent compared to 12 percent for normal soybean oil (appendix 1).

Vegetable oils are obtained from the seeds of various plants either by cold-pressing or solvent extraction. The seeds themselves, separate from their oils, are also a significant food source for humans, but their contribution is considerably less than that of vegetable oils. The FAOSTAT database shows that, worldwide, the supply of fat from "oilseed" foods was only 37 percent of that from "vegetable oils" in 2018 (and 17 percent for the United States and 15 percent for Australia).[7]

The omega balance is the same whether the oil or the whole seed is the food source. For example, peanuts have the same omega balance value as peanut oil (both 0 percent). Similarly, soybean-derived foods such as miso, soy milk, soy flour, and soy lecithin all have essentially the same omega balance as soybean oil (see figure 2.1).

Lecithin is a type of fat (a phospholipid), and while the most common lecithin used in food production is derived from soybeans, lecithins can also be derived from other sources. Lecithins have the distinctive property of one end of the molecule being water-loving (hydrophilic) while the other end is fat-loving (lipophilic). This property is ideal for mixing fats and water. The lecithin in milk (1 percent of total fat) is what ensures that milk fat globules and the water in the milk don't separate from each other. This is why lecithins are used as emulsifiers in many food products. They maintain stable blends of materials that would otherwise not mix. They reduce mixing times, control viscosity, and prevent food sticking to contact surfaces or adhering to each other. They help make chocolate smooth and allow powdered baby formula to dissolve easily in water. Lecithins contain polyunsaturated fats, and their omega balance reflects their source.

Nuts and Grains Provide Omega-6 but Negligible Omega-3 Fats

"Nuts" and "grains" are seeds, and in their polyunsaturated fats, omega-6 fats predominate with very little omega-3 fats being present (see figure 2.1). Walnuts, sometimes highlighted as a source of omega-3, contain predominantly omega-6 as their polyunsaturated fat. In 2018, cereals provided approximately 6g of fat per person per day to the global food supply (see note 4), with two-thirds of this fat coming from just two grains: wheat and corn. Together cereal crops provide nearly half of the world's food calories. Although grains are often only thought of as providing carbohydrates, they also provide about 7 percent of the fat in the world's food supply (but only 2–3 percent in the US and Australian food supply). For cereal crops, 50–60 percent of their fat is polyunsaturated, and, as can be seen from figure 2.1, most of it is omega-6 fat. The products made from cereal crops essentially all retain the same omega balance as their source ingredients. Consequently, they have omega balance values typical of most of the other seed-derived foods.

Unusual Seeds: Some Beans Provide Both Omega-3 and Omega-6 Fats

Pulses (peas and beans) contribute mainly carbohydrate and protein to the human diet but also some fat (less than 1 percent of fat globally). Some, but not all, pulses have relatively high omega balance, with approximately half of their PUFA being omega-3 (figure 2.1). This is especially true for varieties of the common bean, which include green beans, red kidney beans, black beans, cannellini beans, and navy beans (used to make "baked beans").

Green Leaves Are Important Sources of Omega-3

Leaf vegetables are not normally thought of as a source of dietary fat. However, whole foods that contain cells also contain "invisible" fats. This is because all cells have membranes, and all membranes contain fat (see chapter 5). More importantly, the membrane fats in green leaves are particularly high in omega-3 relative to omega-6 fats (see note 1). The average of omega balance values for leaf vegetables in figure 2.1 is 70 percent.

I refer to "green leaf" vegetables rather than "green" vegetables, and there's a reason for this differentiation. While omega balance of leaves is approximately 80 percent, that of "green peas" is 19 percent, and similarly, "green" peppers have an omega balance of only 13 percent (see appendix 1). In deciding whether a plant food might be a good source of omega-3 fat, think "photosynthesis" and not just the color green.

Considering leaf vegetables as a good source of omega-3 fats is surprising to many. The total polyunsaturated fat content of leaf vegetables is approximately 0.2g per 100g food, and this is similar to many animal-based foods, such as low-fat ground beef, lobster, a non-oily fish such as tuna, whole milk, and ice cream (see appendix 1). Animal-based foods will often have more *total fat* content but not necessarily more *total PUFA* than green-leaf food, and very importantly the polyunsaturated fats in green-leaf food are overwhelmingly omega-3 fats. Leaf vegetables are a little-appreciated but very important source of omega-3 fats, especially because they also contribute little omega-6 fat to the diet.

As we shall see later in this chapter, the high omega-3/low omega-6 content of leaves is not only relevant to the human diet but is also important for what we feed livestock. An analysis of the fatty acid composition of thirteen forage crops for livestock shows both that PUFA constitute the majority of total fatty acids and that the omega balance of these forage crops averages approximately 80 percent.[8]

The Difference between Plant-Based and Animal-Based Foods

As is obvious in figure 2.1, the omega balance of plant-based foods is related to from which part of the plant the particular food is derived. There is a relatively small influence from the particular species of plant. Apart from a few exceptions, if the food is derived from "seeds," the omega balance is dominated by omega-6 fats, whereas if the food is from the "leaves" of plants, it is dominated by omega-3 fats.

In the next section, I will consider animal-derived foods, and you will see that because animals are unable to synthesize either type of essential fat, the omega balance of the animal-based food will be strongly influenced by the type of plant food the animal has eaten. Food products made from animals that are "seed" eaters will have a poorer omega balance than the food products made from "leaf" eaters. The shift to grain-feeding of livestock has had a detrimental influence on the omega balance of the modern human diet.

Meats Are Significant but Variable Sources of Both Omega-3 and Omega-6

Globally, in 2018, "meat" provided approximately 19g fat per person per day, which was 22 percent of the total fat in the world food supply (see note 4). More than half of this fat (approximately 11g) came from pork, with poultry responsible for about 4g and beef contributing about 3g fat per person per day. Compared with the global average, meat provided much more fat to the US and Australian food supply, whereas poultry contributed 15g and 14g fat respectively, pork provided about 10g, and beef provided about 5g per person per day. Lamb (mutton and goatmeat) contributed less than 1g fat per person per day both globally and in the United States but accounted for more than 5g fat per person per day in Australia.

I'll use my prerogative as author and my predilection for it to start with lamb. I was shocked when researching for this book to find that a dramatic change has taken place in Australia over the last half-century. In 1961, lamb supplied 27g fat per Australian per day, beef supplied 7g fat, pork supplied 5g fat, and poultry supplied 1g fat per day. However, by 2018 these contributions had changed dramatically. Lamb and beef each now supplied only 5g fat, pork supplied 10g fat, and poultry supplied 14g fat per day per Australian (see note 4). These numbers represent a fourteen-fold increase in poultry, a doubling of pork, an 18 percent decrease in beef, coupled with a four-fold decrease in lamb's contribution to fat supply. Lamb had gone from first to last. The omega balance of a wide variety of animal-based foods is presented in figure 2.2.[9]

I have used two online databases to calculate the omega balance of different foods; the main one I have used is American (USDA Food-Data Central), while the other is Australian (FSANZ Food Composition Database) (see note 3). For all the plant-based foods (see figure 2.1), the omega balance values calculated from both databases are essentially the same. However, this is not so for the meats. For lamb, the values calculated from both databases are similar, but the omega balance of various beef-based meats calculated from the USDA database are generally low compared with the values calculated from the Australian database. For example, ground beef from the United States has an omega balance of 9 percent compared with 31 percent for ground beef from Australia (see figure 2.2). Similar differences were observed for other cuts of beef. A porterhouse steak from the United States has an omega balance of 7 percent, compared with 24 percent for an Australian porterhouse steak (see appendix 1). This difference is quite dramatic, and as I will discuss later in this chapter, it is likely due to different methods of feeding cattle in the two countries, being primarily grain-fed (seeds) in the United States compared to grass-fed (leaves) in Australia. In figure 2.2, the animal-based foods marked with an asterisk are from either Australia or New Zealand, while those without an asterisk are all from the United States.

Four products from pork are presented in figure 2.2, and it can be seen that these pork meats have a very low omega balance (less than 10 percent) compared with many other meats. Both the American and the Australian databases give the same low omega balance values for pork products (see appendix 1), and this likely reflects the high grain-feeding of pigs in both countries. The omega balance of the four lamb meats in figure 2.2 are similar (23–29 percent), with little difference between US and Australian lamb, likely reflecting the low degree of grain-feeding of sheep in both countries.

Apart from sheep, cattle, and pigs, many other mammals are consumed as "meat" throughout the world, and as can be seen in figure 2.2 the omega balance of meat from these other mammals is similar to other grass-eating livestock: one-quarter to half of the polyunsaturated fats are omega-3. Nowadays, what we call "meat" in the Western world is predominantly "skeletal muscle." But this has not always been the case, and it is also not currently the case in many parts of the planet. Other tissues ("offal") are also "meat," and many of them are good sources of omega-3 fats, with some being better sources than muscle. Brain has an exceptionally high omega-3 content and consequently a high omega balance. Although it varies, the omega balance of offal tissues generally reflects the omega balance of muscle from the particular species, and also shows the influence of grain-feeding versus grass-feeding. For example, although I have featured beef offal in figure 2.2, lamb is also an important source of offal. The USDA database provides two sets of information for beef offal. One set of data is from tissue analysis of US beef, while the other is for offal from New Zealand beef. The feed for US beef will be predominantly grain, while New Zealand beef will be grass-fed. While the omega balance of liver, heart, and kidney from US beef is

1–2 percent, the omega balance of the same tissues from New Zealand beef is 28–40 percent (appendix 1).

Dairy Foods and Animal Fats Are Sources of Both Omega-3 and Omega-6

The fats in milk and its fermented and non-fermented products are an important source of food for humans. Globally, in 2018, separate from the contribution from meats, the combined contribution from animal fats and dairy products provided 15g fat per person per day (about 17 percent of total fat) (see note 4). In the United States and Australia, the contribution of dairy and animal fats is greater than the global average, being 35–36g fat per person per day (20–23 percent of total fat supply).

The omega balance values of two animal-fats (lard and tallow), as well as of a variety of dairy products, are presented in figure 2.2. Lard is made from fat tissue of pigs and has an omega balance (9 percent) similar to pork-meat products. Tallow is made from the fat tissues of beef, and US tallow has an omega balance of 15 percent. In Australia, tallow is called "dripping" and has more omega-3 fats than US tallow, with an omega balance of 28 percent, indicative of the relative importance of grain and grass in cattle-feed of the two countries.

There is a consistent difference in the omega balance of dairy products calculated from the US and Australian databases. Milk (whole-fat and reduced-fat), butter, cream, and cheeses from the United States have omega balance values in the 10–15 percent range, while the same dairy foods from Australia have omega balances in the 25–55 percent range (see figure 2.2 and appendix 1). Although different types of cheeses vary in their omega balance, they have values similar to many other dairy foods and also show large differences between the United States and Australia.

Poultry and Poultry Products Are Low in Omega-3 Fats

Poultry meat and eggs together were calculated to provide 7g fat per person per day to the total fat in the global food supply in 2018. This was 8 percent of the total fat in the food supply. In both the United States and Australia, poultry meat provided about 3–4 times more fat per person than the global average (see note 4).

Chicken meat and eggs contribute predominantly omega-6 fats and relatively little omega-3 to the food chain, having omega balance values generally less than 10 percent. This is not restricted to chicken: similar omega balance values are calculated for several other poultry products (turkey, quail, ducks, and emus) as illustrated in figure 2.2. There are essentially no differences in the omega balance values calculated from the US and Australian databases for poultry and poultry products.

Seafood Is High in Omega-3 and Low in Omega-6 Fats

Finally, we consider seafood. According to the FAOSTAT database, seafood contributes very little fat to the world's food supply. Globally, in 2018, its contribution was approximately 1 percent of total fat, with the same contribution for the United States and Australia (see note 4). Nowadays, when you mention "omega-3" to someone, the most likely association that immediately comes to their mind is either "fish" or "fish oil." This association is justified but also oversimplified. As pointed out in chapter 1, like other animals, fish cannot synthesize omega-3 (nor omega-6) and must obtain them pre-formed in their food. Fish in general have a high omega balance, and are thus good sources of omega-3 fats. The fish illustrated in figure 2.2 include both marine and freshwater species, as well as oily and non-oily fish, and all have more omega-3 than omega-6. Wild-caught individuals of these species have omega balance values of 63–83 percent compared to values of 13–67 percent for "farmed" individuals of the same species (appendix 1). However, not all fish have a large predominance of omega-3 fats. For example, tilapia have an omega balance of 47 percent and while wild-caught catfish have an omega balance of 63 percent, farmed catfish have an omega balance of only 13 percent. The difference between wild-caught and farmed fishes is likely due to the composition of the food provided in the farmed situation.

Seafood other than fish, also has high omega balance values and is a good source of omega-3. For example, lobsters, scallops, oysters, and calamari (squid) have values ranging from 71 to 96 percent. This is because, like fish, they don't make omega-3 fats but must obtain them from the marine food chain. Algae—the plants at the base of marine food chains—can be considered "leaves" and do not produce "seeds." Consequently, the predominant polyunsaturated fats they contain are omega-3. For example, edible seaweeds and algae have omega balance values of 60–70 percent.[10] The preponderance of omega-3 in the marine food chain is superbly illustrated by measurement of the fatty acid composition of fat from a marine mammal, the bowhead whale. The blubber of this whale has an omega balance of 99.5 percent.[11] Measurement of Inuit traditional foods gives similar values, with blubber from seals and whales having omega balances of 81–92 percent, and the flesh of seals, whales, and walrus having values of 66–86 percent.[12]

Some fish products are also included in figure 2.2 and appendix 1. For example, caviar (fish eggs) has an omega balance of 92 percent, while smoked salmon (lox) has an omega balance of 53 percent compared to 83 percent for wild salmon.

Fish is also available as canned food, and I have included two examples, tuna and sardines. The specific fish can be canned "in oil," "in water," or "in tomato sauce." However, the oil that is used for canned fish is vegetable oil rather than fish oil. The supermarket decision to purchase either the fish canned in water or that canned in oil will have very different consequences. For tuna canned in water the omega balance is 90 percent, while for tuna canned in oil the value is 16 percent. Similarly, sardines canned in tomato sauce have an omega balance of 80 percent compared with 31 percent for sardines in oil.

Key Influence of "Seeds" and "Leaves" on Omega Balance of Animal Foods

To stress again, because animals are unable to synthesize either type of polyunsaturated fat, their diet is the source of both omega-3 and omega-6 fats found in their body. Consequently, the type of plant food at the base of their specific food chain has a fundamental influence on their omega balance. As emphasized in the previous section, because the algae and plants at the base of marine food chains can be loosely considered as "leaves," the omega balance of marine animal-based food favors omega-3 fats over omega-6 fats.

Because the poultry we eat are primarily domestic fowl, which are generally fed a grain-based diet, both poultry-meat and eggs have a low omega balance. The fact that this is fundamentally due to their diet can be illustrated if we compare their omega balance with those of the other birds from the wild. For example, one study that analyzed tissues from two birds (partridges and geese) hunted by Canadian Inuit, shows their meats to have average omega balance values of 13 and 29 percent, with eggs of the geese having an omega balance of 30 percent.[13] This is higher than the values of poultry and eggs in figure 2.2. which are below 10 percent (see appendix 1). Similarly, breast muscle from 18 non-domestic bird species feeding in aquatic and terrestrial ecosystems had an average omega balance of 41 percent.[14]

It's understandable that the livestock that our ancestors first domesticated and farmed included mammals that were able to survive on food that often provided little nutrition apart from energy. As described in chapter 1, many of these animals essentially "made" their own nutrients from this low-nutrient feed by maintaining and growing large microbial populations in their gut. Over time, our ancestors started to keep these animals indoors during winter, providing them with fodder stored from the summer growth period. Gradually, the food provided changed. In the United States grain-feeding started in the late 1930s and has now become the conventional method of raising cattle whereby they are maintained in intensive feed-lots and food is brought to them. Because of its energy density, grain was increasingly added to the cattle feed over time to produce what came to be called "concentrate." In the United States, corn (maize) has become the most common grain used in such concentrate. This method of raising livestock increased dramatically in the 1960s, and nowadays it is increasingly being introduced both to other species and to other parts of the world. It was not appreciated when it started that grains contained predominantly omega-6 and relatively little omega-3 compared to grass. It is the reason why I obtained lower omega balance values for beef and dairy products when I used the US food composition database compared with using the Australian database.

There is considerable literature examining the influence of feed type on composition of various livestock and their products. A comparison of the influence of grain-feeding and grass-feeding on the omega balance of a variety of animal-based foods is shown in figure 2.3. For beef,[15] for cow's milk,[16] and for lamb,[17] the comparison is between animals provided with the grain-based concentrate feed used in the conventional feed-lot method and animals that are solely grass-fed. For the other animals—goats,[18] pork,[19] and rabbits,[20]—the comparisons are less rigid, and these examples compare animals with access only to grain-based pellets ("grain-fed") with animals that have access to both pasture and pellets (labeled as "grass-fed"). For example, the data for pork compares meat from free-range pigs, allowed access to pasture grass and acorns as well as a grain diet, which had an omega balance of 10 percent compared with 3 percent for meat from pigs enclosed in a shed and fed solely the grain diet. Similarly, meat from wild boars has an omega balance of 17 percent compared with 7 percent for domestic pork.[21] Although not illustrated in figure 2.3, a separate study shows that milk from goats fed hay has an omega balance of 31 percent compared with 9 percent for milk from goats given corn-based feed.[22]

All of these comparisons show the same effect—namely, increasing the "seed" component of livestock-feed at the expense of the "leaf" component results in a lowering of the omega balance of

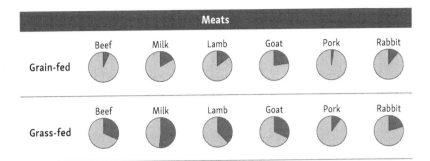

Figure 2.3 Comparison of omega balance of beef, milk, lamb, goat, pork, and rabbit—either grain-fed or grass-fed. In each pie chart, the dark sector represents omega-3 PUFA, while the light sector represents omega-6 PUFA. See text for details and sources.

the food derived from that livestock. The use of grain-feeding in the finishing of cattle is perceived as beneficial because it results in a different meat quality. Grain-fed meat is more "marbled" than grass-fed meat, and this marbling is because the meat has more intramuscular fat, which gives it a different flavor and tenderness. If the fat is not within the muscle tissue it is called separable fat. In comparison, "leaf-eating" game animals provide relatively lean meat with very little fat. Ever since we domesticated cattle and sheep, in our desire to maximize weight gain from feed provided, over time we have slowly selected for livestock that have substantial amounts of body fat. We have effectively selected and produced "obese" animals, especially compared with their game cousins. The recent shift to grain-feeding is a further extension of this process, and the consequent increase in intramuscular fat in such livestock has interesting and fascinating parallels to the increased intramuscular fat in humans with obesity and diabetes. Human obesity and the potential role of dietary omega balance will be considered in chapter 6.

The Importance of Meals Rather than Individual Foods

Our diet consists of everything we put in our mouth and swallow. We generally consume food items in combinations, as part of a meal. As opposed to the usual "minimum requirements" approach used in nutrition advice, the key concept of this book—that of "balance" of two essential nutrients—emphasizes the importance of the whole diet for proper nutrition. In a way, it stresses the need to consider the omega balance of meals over individual foods.

In the publication in which I and colleagues first proposed the use of the omega balance concept (we called it *PUFA balance*),[23] we also analyzed the composition of 23 whole meals. Some of the meals were purchased as "fast food," some came from restaurants or cafes, some were bought at supermarkets as frozen meals, and some were home-cooked. The omega balance values for these whole meals are presented in appendix 1, while the complete composition details can be found in the original publication. The importance of considering meals rather individual foods is illustrated by comparing the three "fish" meals included in the study. The "salmon & salad" meal had the highest omega balance, with a value of 80 percent. The "Filet-o-Fish & fries" meal had an omega balance of 13 percent and the "fish & chips" meal had an omega balance of only 4 percent. All three meals are described as 'fish' meals, and thus popularly considered as being healthy meals (as they all contain omega-3 fats), however, they will have different consequences after being eaten. Only the "salmon & salad" meal will increase the omega balance of an individual following its consumption, and the "fish & chips" meal is likely to decrease the individual's omega balance. The potential health consequences of such a difference are covered in the second half of this book.

The "fish & chips" example above illustrates another important consideration. The low omega balance of the fish & chips meal is due to vegetable oil taken up by both the fish and chips during the cooking process. Most of the omega balance values I have listed in appendix

1 are for the raw rather than cooked versions of the particular food. If a food is cooked in a way that does *not* involve added fat, then the omega balance of the cooked version of the food is essentially the same as that of the raw version. In appendix 1, I have included a few examples of cooked and raw versions of the same food to illustrate this point. However, if the food is cooked with added fat, as is the case for the fish & chips meal, then this needs to be taken into account when considering the omega balance of the total meal.

Some General Principles

I hope this chapter has already led you to some generalizations about the omega balance of foods. Knowing these generalizations, you don't have to learn a long list of omega balance values for different foods but rather, by knowing where a particular food comes from, you can make a reasonable assessment of its balance between omega-3 and omega-6 fats.

I am not concerned with total fat, saturated fats, or monounsaturated fats, but only the polyunsaturated fats in food. While "total fat" is often relatively obvious in food, the polyunsaturated fats are not so. As an example, spinach is rarely spoken about as providing "fat," yet all whole foods (foods that contain plant or animal cells) contain fat, because all cells have membranes and all membranes contain "fat." Membrane fats will feature in the rest of this book, and they are the important location of polyunsaturated fats. They are the "invisible" fats in our food.

The total PUFA content varies between foods. For many foods, the total PUFA content is less than 1g PUFA/100g food, but for some foods it is much greater. Food items that have a low water content will often have a high total PUFA content. Vegetable oils (which are 100 percent fat) can also vary in their PUFA content. For some oils, PUFA constitute more than half their total fatty acids (safflower oil, soybean oil, sunflower-seed oil, cottonseed oil, and corn oil), but in others less than one-tenth are PUFA (palm oil, coconut oil, and palm kernel oil), while others are intermediate in PUFA content (canola oil, peanut oil, rice-bran oil, and olive oil).

The most important principles can be described by the following generalizations:

- Seeds and their products generally contain little omega-3 and have omega-6 as their predominant polyunsaturated fat. The exceptions include some beans. Some seeds provide *no* omega-3 and only omega-6.
- Leaves and their products contain predominantly omega-3 fats and have very small amounts of omega-6 in their polyunsaturated fat.
- Meats and animal products provide both omega-3 and omega-6 fats but these vary in their relative proportions between different types of animal-products depending on their diet. Animal-products (dairy and eggs) have essentially the same omega balance as the animal itself. The omega balance of meat and dairy is lower from grain-fed animals than from grass-fed animals. Seafood, both fish and non-fish, are high in omega-3 compared to omega-6.

Having sketched a general idea about the relative abundances of the two types of polyunsaturated fats in different foods, the next two chapters will examine what we know about the diet of our ancestors and the changes over the last half-century.

CHAPTER 3

EARLIER DIETS

From Paleo Times to the Mid-Twentieth Century

Insights from Our Anatomy and Physiology

The first insights into humankind's early diet must surely come from the anatomy and physiology of our digestive system. Comparison of the human digestive system with that of dogs and sheep (mammals with different diets but similar in size to humans) shows that the human digestive system is similar to the dog's but quite different from the sheep's (table 3.1).[1] Plants' cell walls are made of cellulose, but mammals cannot make an enzyme to digest cellulose and consequently are unable to break down the walls surrounding plant cells. In contrast, many bacteria, fungi, and protozoa have this enzyme and thus can access the nutritious contents of plant cells. Herbivorous mammals, such as sheep, overcome their inability to produce this enzyme by maintaining large microbial populations in their gut and providing them with a regular supply of plant material. The herbivores themselves use the microbial waste products as a source of energy and then also digest the microbes to obtain essential nutrients.

The fundamental requirement for this symbiotic relationship is an expanded space in the gut. While some herbivores (sheep, goats, cattle, deer, kangaroos) provide this space early in the digestive tract, in an expanded fore-gut, other herbivores (horses, rabbits, rodents) provide the space in an expanded hind-gut, either an expanded cecum or colon, or both. Herbivorous mammals display other adaptive features. Their teeth and jaws are organized to mechanically

grind and break down plant food and facilitate the enzymatic breakdown by the gut microbes. The expanded fore-gut does not secrete
acid; it is only the very last chamber of the stomach that secretes
acid in such herbivores. This last, strongly acidic, chamber is where
the process of digesting and consuming gut microbes begins. The
human digestive system displays none of the adaptations to a plant
diet manifest in sheep.

Our closest living primate cousins are the great apes (gorillas,
orangutans, and chimpanzees), and comparison with their digestive systems provides additional insight. These apes are mainly plant
eaters, typically consuming ripe fruit and young leaves, although

Table 3.1 Human, Dog, and Sheep Digestive Systems

	Human	Dog	Sheep
Feeding	intermittent	intermittent	continuous
Teeth			
incisors	both jaws	both jaws	lower jaw only
canines	small	large	absent
molars	ridged	ridged	flat
Jaw movement	tearing-crushing	tearing-crushing	grinding
Stomach			
capacity (liters)	1–2	1–2	30–50
emptying time	about 4 hours	about 4 hours	never
acidity	strong	strong	limited
microbes present	no	no	plentiful-vital
cellulose digestion	no	no	considerable
Small intestine length*	3	3	22
Cecum length*	0.03	0.11	0.32
Colon length*	0.6	0.4	4.5

Source: Data are from mixed sources (see text note 1).

*Expressed relative to total body length

some chimpanzees kill and eat vertebrates.[2] In all three species, as might be expected of plant-eaters, the colon (together with the cecum) is the most voluminous part of their gut, comprising more than half of the total gastrointestinal tract. In contrast, the colon of humans is relatively small, and our small intestine constitutes more than half the total gastrointestinal tract (table 3.2).

The human digestive tract and its physiology are relatively simple and show little evidence of specific adaptation to a dominantly plant-based diet. It exhibits adaptations suggestive of a more carnivorous diet than our close cousins. As with the dog, such a system does not exclude the consumption of plant food, and we can be considered omnivores. It should also be noted that we have evolved many food-preparation practices (including the use of fire for cooking) that allow the preliminary breakdown of food outside of the human body. This shifted the selective pressure for obtaining energy and nutrients from our digestive anatomy and physiology to cultural practices.

So, apart from the evidence that our digestive system suggests about our early diet, what is the direct evidence of what our ancestors ate?

Table 3.2 Relative Sizes of Parts of Gorilla, Orangutan, Chimpanzee, and Human Gastrointestinal Tracts (as percent of total gastrointestinal volume)

	Gorilla	Orangutan	Chimpanzee	Human
Stomach	17	25	20	24
Small intestine	27	14	23	56
Colon + Cecum	56	61	57	20

Source: Data are from Milton K (2003). The critical role played by animal source foods in human (*Homo*) evolution. *J. Nutr.* 133:3886S–3892S, fig. 1, https://doi.org/10.1093/jn/133.11.3886S.

The Use of Isotopes to Determine Past Diets

Once is pretty good, but twice is nice. To be responsible for one signif-icant scientific discovery is a great pleasure, but to be responsible for two significant findings is a blessing. George Burr not only discovered that certain fats were essential nutrients for animals; he also was the first to discover that there were at least two types of photosynthesis in plants.[3] After the Second World War, he tried to repeat the exper-iments on sugar cane that others had done on green algae. The pre-vious scientists had found that during photosynthesis, the carbon atoms of carbon dioxide end up in a 3-carbon molecule. Burr found that in sugar cane they end up in a 4-carbon molecule. We now know that there are at least two types of plants, called either C3 plants or C4 plants. Both types eventually make the same carbohydrates but by slightly different pathways. There are other types of photosynthesis in plants, but they need not concern us here.

Most plants are C3 plants, including green algae, most trees, and some agricultural crops. The C4 plants perform better than C3 plants under certain conditions and include sugar cane, maize, sorghum, and millet. About half of C4 plants worldwide are "grasses." The reason we are interested in these two types of plants here is that they handle carbon atoms slightly differently.

For most atoms, there is more than one type that differ in what they weigh (called isotopes). Some isotopes are stable, and the others are unstable. The vast majority of the carbon atoms in the natural environment weigh 12 units (written as ^{12}C) while some others weigh 13 units (written as ^{13}C). When C4 plants convert carbon dioxide into carbohydrates during photosynthesis they favor those carbon dioxide molecules made of ^{12}C atoms over those in which the carbon atoms are ^{13}C. The result is that the abundance of ^{13}C relative to ^{12}C in the molecules that eventually make up the plant is less than that in the environment. The difference is called the delta ^{13}C (written $\delta^{13}C$) and applies to all C atoms in the plant. It has a negative value because ^{13}C relative to ^{12}C is less in the plant than in the environment. The C3 plants show even greater favoritism, and consequently the $\delta^{13}C$ value for C3 plants is even more negative than for C4 plants. The animals that consume these plants retain their $\delta^{13}C$, and the $\delta^{13}C$ of an animal's proteins can tell you whether it ate C4 or C3 plants, or a mixture of the two types of plants.

Proteins contain nitrogen atoms, and there are also two forms of nitrogen atoms. The majority of nitrogen atoms in nature weigh 14 units (^{14}N), while some weigh 15 units (^{15}N). When an animal metabolizes protein from a plant, it favors the ^{15}N atoms over the ^{14}N atoms. Consequently, the proteins of herbivorous animals have a higher ratio ($\delta^{15}N$) than that found in the plants they eat. If a predator eats that animal, it will have an even higher $\delta^{15}N$ value than its prey.[4] In this way, it is possible by measurement of $\delta^{15}N$ to differentiate between plant-eaters (herbivores) and meat-eaters (carnivores) and even to estimate whether the mammal is a top predator. It is also possible to estimate the relative proportions of meat and plant food.

By extracting the distinctive proteins of either bone (collagen) or hair (keratin) and measuring their $\delta^{15}N$ and $\delta^{13}C$ values, it has been possible to estimate the diet of past humans.[5] Many archaeological investigations often include the bones of other animals whose modern diet is well known. This comparison of isotopes allows us to determine the types of food eaten by humans (and other animals) from past times by analysis of their bones or hair.

Paleolithic Diets: Neanderthals and Early Modern Humans

Food is not the only reason to hunt and kill large mammals. The skins of large mammals would have provided blankets and ready-made fur coats, just the right size for early naked apes in cold climates, as well as material for tentlike shelters. As long as 300,000 years ago, early humans (likely Neanderthals) left evidence of manufacturing spears and butchering horses.[6]

Measurement of bone collagen from Neanderthals suggests that these early humans were top-carnivores who derived their protein mainly from animal sources.[7] One study from France suggests that the main protein sources included antelopes, bison, deer, goats, and horses.[8] Bones from the original location in Germany suggest that Neanderthals derived most of their protein from terrestrial mammalian herbivores, such as deer, with neither fish nor terrestrial plants being significant sources.[9] An extensive study of Late Pleistocene fossils (approximately 40,000 years old) in Belgium compared bones from both Neanderthals and mammals that included herbivores (reindeer, horses, aurochs, woolly rhinoceros, and mammoths), omnivores (cave bears, brown bears), and carnivores (wolves, cave lions, spotted hyenas) and revealed that Neanderthals belonged to the carnivore group. Detailed analysis suggested they were the dominant predators of mammoths.[10]

Modern humans joined Neanderthal humans in Europe about 60,000 to 40,000 years ago, and measurements of their bone collagen suggests that their main source of dietary protein was of animal origin but was more varied than that of the Neanderthals and included aquatic animals. There is little evidence that Neanderthals ate small game such as birds or fish, but there is evidence that early modern humans ate such small game, both in Europe[11] and in China.[12] Bone collagen from three humans who lived in North Wales about 12,000 years ago suggests that about one-third of their dietary protein was most likely marine mammals.[13]

Measurements of bone collagen from Neanderthals and early modern humans suggest that animals provided 60–80 percent of their protein intake. Fatty acid composition of meat, fat, bone marrow, and brain of three herbivores (deer, antelope, and elk) that were likely part of the diet of these early humans[14] provides an omega balance that averaged 32 percent, suggesting a good dietary balance of omega-3 and omega-6 fats in these early humans.

The Diet of Recent Hunter-Gatherers: The Ethnographic Evidence

Ethnography can help to understand the diet of human groups that maintained a hunter-gatherer lifestyle into historical times. An ethnographic atlas comparing 1,267 of the world's societies and specifying the degree to which the economic subsistence of each society depended on (1) gathering of wild plants and small land fauna, (2) hunting, (3) fishing, (4) animal husbandry, and (5) agriculture, has been used for such insight.[15] Of these societies, 229 (or 18 percent) had zero subsistence from animal husbandry and agriculture, and they can therefore be regarded as hunter-gatherer societies.

Substantial variation existed among the diets of these modern hunter-gatherer societies. However, there was not a single hunter-gatherer society that depended solely on "gathered plant food" and in only 8 out of 229 did "gathered plant foods" constitute more than 65 percent of their subsistence.[16] The importance of animal food in these modern hunter-gatherer societies can be estimated by combining the "fished" and "hunted animal food" categories; after these are combined, the category of 86–100 percent subsistence from animal foods includes the greatest number of worldwide hunter-gatherer societies. Ethnographic analysis supports the conclusion that animal foods dominated in most hunter-gatherer societies. The broad analysis of the 229 modern "hunter-gatherer" societies was based on subjective estimates by ethnographers. However, more precise quantitative studies of thirteen modern "hunter-gatherer" societies come to the same conclusion, providing average values of 65 percent subsistence on animal food and 35 percent on plant food.[17]

Underlying these average values, there is a large amount of variation. For some groups their diet is primarily plant-based; for the Gwi of Africa, it is reported to be 74 percent plant food and 26 percent animal food. For the Nunamiut from Alaska, the breakdown is 99 percent animal and 1 percent plant food, while for the Inuit from Greenland, it is 96 percent animal food and 4 percent plant food. It should not be assumed that human groups living in environments such as the arctic, where there are negligible plants, are the only ones that have a completely animal-based diet. For example, the traditional food of the Maasai of Africa is milk, blood, and meat, which obviously is a diet of 100 percent animal origin. The Maasai, though, are not hunter-gatherers; they are nomadic pastoralists, having quite sophisticated animal husbandry practices.

Characteristics of a Contemporary Paleolithic Diet

A few years ago, Loren Cordain, an advocate of the Paleo Diet, made up a contemporary diet based on Paleolithic food groups but using modern ingredients and calculated its nutritional characteristics.[18] The diet consisted of vegetables (15 percent of total energy), fruits (15 percent), nuts/seeds (15 percent), seafood (27.5 percent), and lean meat (27.5 percent). One day's menu was cantaloupe with broiled or grilled salmon for breakfast, while lunch was broiled or grilled lean pork loin with vegetable salad and walnuts. Dinner consisted of roast lean beef sirloin tip with steamed broccoli and a vegetable avocado/almond salad with dessert being strawberries. Throughout the day, snacks consisted of an orange, as well as sticks of carrot and celery. The macronutrient content of the day's diet was protein as 38 percent of energy, carbohydrate as 23 percent of energy, and fat as 39 percent. Importantly for our purposes, the polyunsaturated fats in the diet had a good balance between omega-3 and omega-6 fats, with an omega balance of 40 percent.[19]

Neolithic and Later Diets: The Beginnings of Agriculture

The "Neolithic and later" started about 12,000 years ago and marks the beginning of agriculture and farming. The transition from hunting-and-gathering to farming is the first agricultural revolution and marks the beginning of increased human population growth. The domestication of plants and animals took place independently, in at least seven to eight separate places around the world and represents a form of co-evolution of humans with specific plants and animals. The native wild characteristics of the plant or animal change, and it becomes dependent on humans for its protection, growth, and reproduction. Of course, it is symbiotic, and humans also become dependent on the animal or plant.

Fig trees, wheat, and barley were domesticated in the Middle East; rice, millet, soybeans, and oranges in East Asia; corn, dry bean, and tomatoes in Central America; potatoes, peanuts, and strawberries in South America; sorghum in Africa; sugar-beet in Europe; sugar cane in New Guinea; apple, almond, and alfalfa in Eurasia.[20] Dogs were the first animals to be domesticated, likely when humans were still hunter-gatherers and before they were agriculturalists.[21] Sheep were domesticated in Anatolia; goats in Iran; pigs in the Near East and China; cattle in Western Asia and India; cats in Western Asia; chickens in India and Southeast Asia; guinea pigs in Peru; donkeys in Egypt; ducks in China; horses in Eurasia; and the process continues to this day.

The diversity of the human diet continued into the Neolithic. Bones from deposits near the Mediterranean coast of Spain show that approximately 7,500 years ago marine food was significant but not the dominant source of protein.[22] In some places there were dramatic changes. Isotopic measurement of human bones indicates that there was a sudden and near-complete change from a marine-based diet to a terrestrial-based diet among both coastal and inland dwellers in Britain about 5,000 years ago.[23] Britain has provided considerable diet information during this period because several cemetery populations have been analyzed. Items accompanying the burials (such as chariots, barrows, and other goods) have allowed things such as social status to also be determined. Bones from an Iron Age cemetery indicated that the human diet was high in animal protein but with no evidence of significant marine food and little diet variation associated with age, gender, or social status.[24]

Although there was little contribution from marine food sources on mainland Britain, this was not the situation on the Orkney Islands.

Bones from human burials, as well as animals, for the period AD 600 to AD 1500 showed that some individuals had a diet with 50 percent of their protein from marine sources (likely seals). Males had more marine protein than females, and there was an increased consumption of marine food in the tenth and eleventh centuries, coinciding with the Viking and medieval periods.[25]

A study of animal bones and human burials around the city of York in Britain dating from the late second to the early nineteenth century investigated 1,500 years of human diet in the region.[26] This study clearly showed the reintroduction of significant amounts of marine food in the eleventh century. It was suggested by the authors that this was a response of the populace to introduction of church rules that dictated "fasting" (abstinence from eating meat) for nearly half the year.

Human bone collagen from three burial sites in the same area of Britain (combined with animal bones) also suggests a mixed diet of terrestrial, freshwater, and marine food.[27] The human bones were from a hospital cemetery, an Augustinian friary, as well as a mass-grave of soldiers from the Battle of Towton in AD 1461. The results are presented in figure 3.1 and show that the three different human populations had very similar bone isotope values. They had $\delta^{15}N$ values similar to those of two carnivorous fish species, one fresh-water (eels) and the other marine (herrings) but considerably greater than the herbivorous mammals from the same sites.

Evidence from other parts of the world also suggests a mixed diet with significant amounts of animal protein, often including marine food. Just because a society was located on the coast does not necessarily mean that its diet was primarily marine food. For example, a Korean coast site that dates from about 2,500 to 1,900 years ago shows isotope values that suggest the diet was primarily terrestrial with only a very small marine component.[28]

Bone collagen measurements can also give insight into the domestication of plants. For example, millet agriculture began in northern China about 8,000 years ago, but measurement of human bone

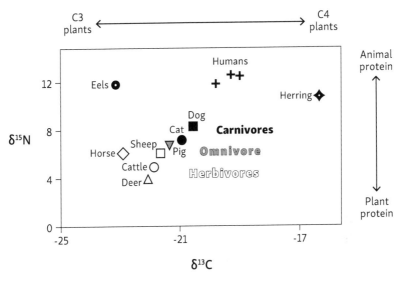

Figure 3.1 Comparison of $\delta^{15}N$ and $\delta^{13}C$ values of collagen from bones of humans and animals from three late medieval sites in northern England. Data from Muldner G, Richards MP (2008). Fast or feast: reconstructing diet in later medieval England by stable isotope analysis. *J. Archaeol. Sci.* 35:2960–2965, https://doi.org/10.1016/j .jas.2004.05.007.

collagen suggests millet (a C4 plant) contributed only one-quarter of dietary protein at that time, and it was not until approximately 1,000 years later that all dietary protein came from C4 plants (likely millet).[29]

In August 1999, three hunters found a naturally mummified body in Canada. This young male was named Kwaday Dan Ts'inchi (meaning "Long-Ago Person Found") and was approximately 20 years old when he died about 550 years ago. Although he was found more than 100 kilometers inland, bone collagen suggested that his diet was dominated by marine food, while a microscopic analysis of contents of his digestive tract revealed pollen of an intertidal salt-marsh plant and pieces of a marine crustacean.[30]

Isotopes in Hair Keratin:
Important Evidence of Early Diets

Hair keratin has the advantage over bone collagen in that it can be easily experimentally validated as a measure of previous diet. For example, isotope measurement of hair keratin from an individual eating a vegan diet after an omnivorous diet has shown the predicted changes, after allowing for the six-day period for hair to emerge from the skin.[31]

Because hair grows, measurement of isotope composition of different sections of hair can provide a time-course of dietary changes. For example, the Inca performed Capacocha rites that involved the sacrifice of children, and analysis of the hair from frozen child mummies, discovered between 1996 and 1999 in the high Andes, show that the preparation included a dramatic increase in meat consumption during the year before sacrifice.[32]

Otzi the Iceman, a well-preserved, naturally mummified human body who lived about 5,300 years ago, was found on a glacier in the European Alps in 1991. Hair analysis concluded he was omnivorous. His stomach contents, moreover, showed that his last meal included a high proportion of fat (approximately 46 percent), most likely from the ibex goat. This was supplemented with fresh or dried wild meat and a large amount of an early wheat (see note 31).

Pottery: What Was Stored or Cooked in It

Pottery was first used by hunter-gatherers and predates the invention of agriculture by about 10,000 years. The earliest pottery comes from China and is dated from approximately 20,000 years ago.[33] Pottery is very helpful for two reasons: first, it is plentiful, and second, potsherds are often the remnants of vessels used for storing or cooking food. Unglazed ceramic vessels absorb a substantial amount of the organic matter from the commodities stored or processed in them. Fats are the best preserved of these absorbed materials, and even if the fats themselves break down over time, the degradation products are distinctive for particular fatty acids, and powerful modern analytical techniques enable determination of what was stored or processed in these ceramic vessels.[34] For example, specific breakdown products from waxes in the leaves of plants have demonstrated that some of these ancient ceramic jars were used for cooking leafy vegetables, such as cabbage.

Analyses show that the incidence of degraded animal fats in ancient domestic pottery is very high. It is often possible to measure the particular "signature" of the degraded fat in the vessel and determine the particular species that the fat came from.[35] Some of the ceramic pieces come from lamps, and thus the presence of animal fat reflects its use as the source of oil for the production of either heat or light. This practice continues to this day with the use of yak-butter lamps in Tibetan Buddhist temples and monasteries. One collection of English potsherds from the Middle Ages includes both lamps and "dripping dishes," which were used to collect fat from carcasses during spit-roasting. The fats from the "dripping dishes" appeared to come from pigs, while that from lamps came from sheep and cattle. The specific signature of the fat clearly excluded vegetable oils as the source of fat in the ancient lamps (see note 35).

The Emergence of Milk and Dairy in the Adult Diet

Pottery remains have provided significant insights into the role of dairy food in the early human diet. Milk fats and carcass fats of mammals differ in their specific fatty acid composition, and modern sophisticated analytical techniques can determine whether a pottery vessel was used to store or process milk.[36]

This new technique has shown that milk and milk products were used very early in the history of animal domestication, as early as 8,500–9,000 years ago in Anatolia (present-day Turkey).[37] Analysis of the earliest Neolithic pottery show that the residues from milk fats were more common than residues from body fats. Furthermore, the evidence is that milk was processed at this time, being possibly made into cheese, butter, ghee, lighting oil, and so on. Such practice allows surplus milk to be used at a later date.[38]

An emerging picture is that dairy food was not a late product following the domestication of animals but rather was associated with beginnings of various domestications. Of course, you don't need to domesticate animals to eat them, but you certainly need to domesticate them to milk them. It is tempting to speculate that the use of milk and milk-products was a primary driving force for the domestication of several species of mammal.

All female mammals produce milk for their newborn, and several species have been domesticated for milk production. For example, communities of modern Kazakhstan use horses for both their meat and milk; recent evidence shows that as early as 5,500 years ago horses were a source of milk and milk products in this area.[39]

The mammary gland commences milk-production prior to the birth of the young and it continues as long as there is a suckling stimulus. The composition of mammalian milks, the relative proportions of fat, protein, and sugar varies between species.[40] Lactose, a specific sugar synthesized solely by the mammary gland, is a distinctive feature of milk, and requires a specific intestinal enzyme (lactase) in the suckling young before it can be absorbed. This lactose-lactase connection is essential for the mammalian milk-feeding system, and in human young, lactase activity peaks at birth. Congenital lactase deficiency is lethal (if not recognized very early).[41] In most mammals, lactase activity declines dramatically at weaning, with the consequence that the adult is unable to digest lactose. This condition can produce the symptoms of "lactose intolerance" in some humans, which include diarrhea, bloating, abdominal pain, gas, nausea, and borborygmi (pronounced: bawr-buh-rig-mahy; these are the rumbling or gurgling noises made by the movement of gases and fluids in the intestines; I often wondered what these noises were called). The threshold for lactose intolerance depends on the amount of lactose consumed, gut-transit time, the microbial population in the gut, other dietary components, as well as the residual lactase activity (see note 41).

In some human populations, genetic changes have essentially abolished the decline in lactase activity after weaning, and "lactase persistence" into adulthood has become common. These populations are descendants from the humans that first introduced dairy into the adult diet. Lactase persistence is high in northern European humans (about 90 percent) and very low in Asia (about 1 percent in China). In Africa, lactase persistence is variable, being very high in some pastoralist populations but low in other populations.[42] This increased gene frequency of lactase persistence in adult humans is calculated by some to be the strongest selection pressure for any gene in the human genome yet observed.[43]

One of the advantages of lactase persistence in adults is an increase in acquisition of energy from dairy food. One liter of cow's milk provides energy equivalent to about 40 percent of the daily energy requirements of a resting adult if fully metabolized, but the liter provides 12 percent less energy if the lactose is not digested. Human milk has one of the highest lactose concentrations and one of the lowest protein concentrations of mammalian milks. For example, cow's milk has less lactose, more protein, and about the same fat content as human milk (see note 40). Because milk from domesticated livestock has a lower lactose content than human milk, the consumption of cow's milk in the adult human diet resulted in approximately 30 percent less lactose consumption compared to the same amount of human milk.

Another way to reduce lactose intake is to consume processed milk-products rather than milk itself. When milk coagulates, it separates into curds and whey. The curds contain the milk fats and milk proteins, while the whey contains the water-soluble lactose. The removal (by straining) of the whey (and thus lactose) from the curds is an early step in making cheese. Consequently, production of cheese from milk has the dual advantages of allowing the storage of dairy food for consumption at a later time as well as reducing lactose consumption. It is of interest that some pottery from early Neolithic sites in Europe are pierced with many small holes. Recent measurements of such pottery pieces show the presence of abundant milk fat residues[44] and suggests these vessels were cheese strainers. This is evidence that herders were producing cheese between 6,800 and 7,400 years ago.

Pastoralism, the herding and use of livestock, is common throughout the world, and some pastoralist communities are nomadic (especially in less fertile areas), moving their livestock to available pasture. In Africa, nomadic pastoralist populations are found among the Maasai, the Fulani, the Berbers, the Somalis, the Tuaregs, and the Turkana. In Asia, they are found among the Tibetans, the Mongols and Turkic peoples, while in Europe, among the Sami people, and in the Middle East among the Bedouin. In almost all pastoralist societies, milk and dairy is an important part of the diet. Depending on the society, milk is obtained from cattle, goats, sheep, yak, buffalo, horses, camels and reindeer, and the processing of milk into dairy products is prominent in those populations where milk is seasonally available. Yoghurt, butter, ghee, and cheese are manufactured from the milk of cattle, yak, buffalo, sheep and goats. Camel milk is used to produce yoghurt and cheese, while fermented milk is produced from horse and reindeer milk. Some nomadic pastoralist societies produce a wide variety of dairy products. In view of the fact that the livestock of pastoralists are eating "leaves" to produce their milk, all dairy food from these sources will provide a good balance of omega-3 and omega-6 fats.

Using the Maasai of East Africa as an example, a 1982–1983 survey showed average food availability was 1.9 liters of milk and 216 grams of meat per person per day.[45] Such availability would provide about 7,500 kJ energy (more than the daily energy requirements of a resting adult), and the milk would provide three times the energy and approximately 50 percent more polyunsaturated fats than the meat. Whole milk is the preferred form of milk used by Maasai, and it is either consumed directly or in the cooking of tea or porridge. Butter is made regularly, but sour milk is only made when milk is plentiful. Maasai do not consume meat and milk at the same meal. They consider it bad practice to have both dead (meat) and live (milk) animal products in the same place. They want a long and productive life for their animals, and while sheep and goats are slaughtered for their fat and meat, cattle are rarely slaughtered for nonceremonial purposes.[46]

In conclusion, the evidence concerning our earlier diet is that we are omnivores and that our food varied significantly between different groups and populations. While many populations consumed substantial amounts of animal-based foods as well as plant foods, some human populations had a diet almost completely composed of animal or animal-based products (including dairy). Because these animals consumed pasture, it is a reasonable estimation that the omega balance of our earlier diets was approximately 30 percent.

Before we examine, in the next chapter, the significant changes in the modern human diet that have occurred over the last half-century, I will take advantage of a unique dataset from the US Department of Agriculture, to examine changes in the US food supply over the first half of the last century.

Case Study 1: PUFA in the US Food Supply, 1910 to 1960

The US Department of Agriculture (USDA) has estimated annual US food supply and has calculated the provision of energy, macronutrients, and micronutrients. Among the macronutrients, they estimated polyunsaturated fats in the food supply and have calculated this data on a per-person basis for each year. They have also calculated the relative contribution from different food groups. This information is publicly available for the years 1909 to 2010.[47] To my knowledge, it is the most complete dataset provided by any nation, and before we examine, in the next chapter, changes over the last half-century, I will use this dataset to examine changes in the US food supply between 1910 and 1960.

In 1910 the US population was 92 million, and the US food supply provided 12g total polyunsaturated fats (per person per day). By 1960, the US population had increased to 228 million, and the daily supply of polyunsaturated fats had increased to 20g per person. This increase over the fifty years can be completely accounted for by an increase in polyunsaturated fats from plant sources, specifically vegetable oils (716 percent increase) and margarine (685 percent increase). These two sources went from representing 9 percent of total PUFA in 1910 to representing 45 percent of total PUFA in 1960.

There was essentially no change in the supply of PUFA from animal-based foods between 1910 and 1960, although there were small changes in the contribution from various *types* of animal-based foods. Decreases of 0.6g from lard and beef tallow and 0.4g from butter were compensated by increases of 0.6g from meat, poultry, and fish and 0.3g from 'other dairy' (excluding butter).

As well as calculating the contribution of various food groups, the USDA Food and Nutrition Service has also calculated the total supply (grams per capita per day) of individual fatty acids (see note 47). When these individual values are combined and an omega balance calculated, the US food supply in 1910 had an omega balance of 40 percent compared to 18 percent in 1960. The decrease in omega balance of the global human food supply over the last half-century, which I will describe in more detail in the next chapter, was already underway in the United States by 1960.

CHAPTER 4

THE OMEGA STORY

Diet Changes over the Last Half-Century

It is not easy to obtain information about what people eat: it is an expensive exercise, since as individuals we are very diverse in what we eat day-to-day, there is substantial variation between individuals, and we often have poor memories about what we ate and how much. Some of us notoriously tell untruths about what and how much we have eaten, both to the questioner and to ourselves. Consequently, diet questionnaires need to take these factors into account. Before examining the evidence from diet questionnaires, let's examine what the global food supply statistics tell us.

The Provision of Fat in the World Food Supply, 1961–2018

Using the FAOSTAT database,[1] I have plotted the changes from 1961 to 2018 in provision of fat (g per person per day) from plant-based and animal-based sources in the world food supply, as well as for major world regions (figure 4.1).

Globally, from 1961 to 2018, on a per-person basis, there was an 81 percent increase in fat provision in the food supply. In 1961 the food supply (per person per day) provided 23g of animal-sourced fat and 25g of plant-sourced fat. In 2018 the respective values were 38g of animal-sourced fat and 48g of plant-sourced fat. The dominant changes were an increase in "vegetable oils" in the plant-sourced fats, and in "pork and poultry" in the animal-sourced fats. In 1961 "vegetable oils" constituted 56 percent of all plant-sourced fats compared to 69 percent in 2018. The contribution of "pork and poultry" to animal-sourced fats was 20 percent in 1961 and 41 percent in 2018. In both cases, these two categories were responsible for 80 percent of the increase in plant-sourced and animal-sourced fat. Between 1961 and 2018, there was a dramatic worldwide increase in the supply of fats from sources that have very low omega balances (see chapter 2). This indicates that worldwide there has been a substantial decrease in the omega balance of the human food chain over the last half-century.

Fat from "vegetable oils" varied substantially between the continents, with North America having the greatest "vegetable oil" contribution throughout the entire period. Australia and New Zealand had low "vegetable oil" contribution (7g/person/day) in 1961, but had the second highest value in 2018 (61g/person/day). The absolute increase over this period was the same (about 52g) in both Australia and North America, which showed the greatest change of all the continents. The continent that had the least change was Africa. Fat supply from "all other plant sources" was relatively similar in all continents and showed essentially no change over this period.

Fat from "pork and poultry" was greatest in North America for the entire 1961–2018 period, while for both Australia and South America, the contribution from "pork and poultry" was at the world average level in 1961 and showed the greatest absolute increases (about 16g) over this period to be similar to North America and Europe in 2018. There was negligible change in fat supply from "pork and poultry" in Africa over this period. It was fat supply from "all other animal sources" that showed the greatest variation among the continents over the 1961–2018 period. There was little difference between 1961 and 2018 for Africa or Europe, whereas the values for Asia and South America increased, and those for North America and Australia decreased over this period. The "all other animal sources" value for Australia shows the most dramatic decline of all regions, and this is mostly due to an 80 percent decrease (or 22g) in fat supply from lamb ("mutton and goat") and a 65 percent decline (or 16g) in fat supply from butter, between 1961 and 2018.

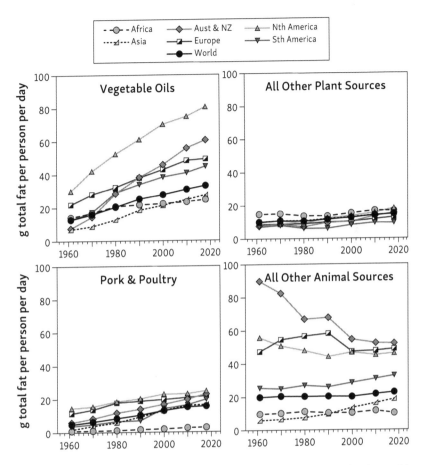

Figure 4.1 Provision of fat (g per person per day) in the food supply for the world and major continental areas, from 1961 to 2018. Plant-based fat provision is divided into contribution from "vegetable oils" and "all other plant sources." Animal-based fat provision is divided into "pork and poultry" and "all other animal sources." Data are from FAOSTAT online database.

Analysis of the world food supply data for the last half-century, provided by the FAO (see note 1), shows there has been a large increase in some food groups with a low omega balance. This is predominantly due to a dramatic increase in "vegetable oils," as well as an increase in "pork and poultry." These changes have varied between the different regions of the planet, but the variation has largely been one of degree.

It has been most pronounced in North America, followed by Australia, Europe, and South America. It is present, but less pronounced, in Asia and least manifest in Africa. These trends are likely related to the internationalization of the planet, especially the ultraprocessing and industrialization of food manufacture over the last half-century. There has been a significant shift in the omega balance, emphasizing omega-6 fats in the modern human food chain. The analysis in this section does not include the shift from grass-feeding to grain-feeding of cattle that has occurred in several countries over the same period; that particular shift has exacerbated the dominance of omega-6 and the diminution of omega-3 in the modern world's food supply.

The Global Commodity Boom in Vegetable Oils

The January 2013 issue of the World Bank's *Commodity Market Outlook* stated that "edible oils experienced the fastest consumption growth rates of all food groups during recent decades." The report continued: "as people become wealthier, they tend to eat more in professional establishments and also consume more pre-packaged food items, both of which are using more edible oil."[2] This text accompanied a graph covering the period 1964 to 2012 that is reproduced in figure 4.2.

The World Bank's "edible oils" are vegetable oils. There are two aspects we need to consider before fully appreciating the implications of this graph. First, the global population has also increased significantly over this period. Secondly, economic "consumption" is not the same as food "consumption." Vegetable oils are used for non-food purposes as well as for food. Oils and fats are used to make soap, cosmetics, paints, varnishes, floor coverings, and increasingly are also used to make bio-fuels.

In 1964 the global population was approximately 3 billion; by 2012 it had risen to approximately 7 billion. The dramatic increase in "global edible oil consumption" shown in figure 4.2, however, cannot be explained by global population growth. What about the "non-food" uses of vegetable oil? The FAOSTAT database also includes data for

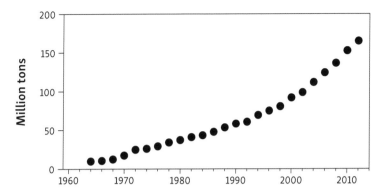

Figure 4.2 Global edible oil consumption from 1964 to 2012. Data are from World Bank's *Commodity Markets Outlook*, January 2013.

"other use" as well as for "food" (see note 1)· In 1964, 17 million metric tons of vegetable oils were used for "food," while 4.5 million were used for "non-food" purposes. In 2012, both "food" and "non-food" uses were approximately 80 million metric tons. There was a dramatic increase in "global edible oil consumption" for both types of use over this 48-year period.

The Dramatic Rise of Ultraprocessed Food

Much of the populace of the developed world nowadays obtains their food from large supermarkets or eating establishments. Just as the "growing of food" has become more industrialized so has the "production of food." Previously food was obtained as produce from markets or other sources, and meals were generally made at home. Nowadays, food is grown, harvested, separated into its various components, then modified and re-assembled into various "food-products" before it is sold, sometimes as individual food-products (breads, pastries, sauces, and so on) or already combined into pre-made meals. Just defrost and re-heat, or just add water and heat. While some foods were previously described as being "processed" foods, more recently many foods are described as "ultraprocessed" foods.

As large corporations have come to dominate many aspects of our society, especially over the last half-century, they have also been important in the industrialization of our food provision and especially in the manufacture of ultraprocessed food. Although this change has been happening for some time, it was not introduced as a concept until 2009, when the Brazilian nutritionist Carlos Monteiro initiated the NOVA classification system.[3]

The classification of "ultraprocessed" food refers to the transformation of substances derived from foods by processes such as baking, frying, extruding, molding, hydrogenation, and hydrolysis, followed by their reconstitution and mixing to provide durable, convenient, and palatable ready-to-eat or ready-to-heat food products to substitute for freshly prepared meals or to be consumed as snacks. A key aspect is shelf-life and low-cost ingredients They generally also include many additives such as preservatives, emulsifiers, sweeteners, colorants, and flavors, but little whole food.[4] Vegetable oils have featured prominently in this process, and the increase in vegetable oils over the last half-century, especially in high-income parts of the modern world (see figure 4.1) is connected with the dramatic rise of ultraprocessed foods.

Because of the high omega-6 content of vegetable oils, their increased use has been a dominant influence on the decrease in the diet omega balance in many countries. The often inferred omega-3 deficiency of modern populations is actually largely due to an overconsumption of omega-6, which, because it is the *balance* between omega-3 and omega-6 fats that is biologically important, can appear to many as an omega-3 deficiency. Ultraprocessed foods bear a significant responsibility for this situation.

Four examples will suffice to explain the increased intake of omega-6 at the expense of omega-3 fats in the consumption of ultraprocessed foods. These are; (1) the use of shortenings in baked goods, (2) the use of emulsifiers, (3) the consumption of snacks such as potato chips, and (4) the replacement of dairy food with non-dairy ingredients.

Shortening is used in the baking of pastries, pie crust, tarts, cakes, and modern breads to make them tender and flaky. Shortenings do this by preventing the cohesion of wheat gluten strands, and they are also used to add flavor and richness to some breads, in manufacture of icing and fillings, as well as for deep-frying. The original shortenings were made from animal fats, but in the late 1800s, vegetable oils started to be added to the animal fats and later became the dominant ingredients such that nowadays "shortening" refers to semi-solid vegetable oils. Initially, the main vegetable oil used to make shortening in the United States was cottonseed oil. Crisco (crystalized cottonseed oil) is a well-known shortening and frying fat. Later soybean oil was used, as well as palm oil. These are the dominant oils in most modern shortenings.[5] The use of shortening increased dramatically after the Second World War.

Many ultraprocessed foods, such as baked goods (breads, cakes, biscuits), confectionary (chocolate), as well as pre-mixed sauces and salad dressings contain emulsifiers that allow normally un-mixable ingredients to form stable mixtures. Pre-made sauces in which the fat and water components separated in the jar would likely not leave the supermarket shelf. Emulsifiers increase the "smoothness" of food and its "pourability." The original food emulsifier was egg yolk, which contained lecithin (derived from the Greek for "egg yolk"). Lecithin is a type of membrane fat and is present in egg yolk to make the cell membranes of the future chick. Nowadays, lecithin and several other emulsifiers (such as diglycerides and monoglycerides) are derived from vegetable oils. Soy lecithin, a common emulsifier, has the same polyunsaturated fatty acid composition and thus omega balance as other soybean products (see chapter 2). Emulsifiers are also made from other vegetable oils and as such will have a low omega balance.

Potato chips are a common snack food, and although potatoes themselves have a very little fat, the chips are fried in vegetable oils and thus constitute a significant source of omega-6 fatty acids. For example, the USDA FoodData Central database records a *"reduced fat* potato chip snack" having 12 percent of the chip as omega-6 fat and virtually no omega-3, giving it an omega balance of 1 percent (see appendix 1). In many ways, such potato chips epitomize ultraprocessed foods. One brand available in Australia, but made overseas contains dehydrated potato, vegetable oils, wheat starch, rice flour, emulsifier, maltodextrin, salt, and food acid. The most obvious manifestation of being produced by industrial processes is that the chips have the same size and shape, so much so that they can be very efficiently packed in cylinders. Because of their high vegetable oil content, chips provide significant amounts of omega-6 fats but negligible omega-3 fats.

A common practice in the manufacture of ultraprocessed foods is to replace dairy products with non-dairy substitutes. Vegetable oils are increasingly used in this role. For example, "coffee creamers" are made from hydrogenated vegetable oils, and increasingly vegetable oils are being added to ice creams. The rise of plant-based "milks" (soy milk, almond milk, hazelnut milk, oat milk) in place of normal milk (cow's milk, goat's milk) is also a significant contributor to the increased consumption of omega-6 fats and decreased consumption of omega-3 fats.

The intimate connection between "vegetable oils" and ultraprocessed food is illustrated by the fact that in a recent analysis of the 2006–2019 trends in ultraprocessed foods, the authors included "vegetable oils" as a separate category in the analysis.[6] This analysis showed substantial variation in the 2019 per capita sales of ultraprocessed foods between different regions of the world, ranging from 134kg in North America and Australia, 113kg in Western Europe, to 12kg in Africa, and 9kg in Southeast Asia. An alarming trend in this analysis was the projected growth in vegetable oil sales in Southeast Asia.

Case Study 2: PUFA in the US Food Supply, 1960–2010

I ended the previous chapter examining the changes in polyunsaturated fats in the US food supply from 1910 to 1960. The database I used also provides data up to 2010.[7] An account of the provision of PUFA in the US food supply from 1960 to 2010 is presented in figure 4.3.

There has been no change in total animal-sourced PUFA in the US food supply for a century. Between 1960 and 2010, the PUFA from animal sources in the US food supply remained unchanged at 7g per person per day. However, as can be seen from figure 4.3, the relative contributions from different animal food sources over the half-century have changed. The PUFA contribution from poultry increased by 264 percent (to become the largest contributor in 2010), while the contributions from meat, eggs, dairy, and animal fats, respectively, decreased by 27 percent, 24 percent, 28 percent, and 63 percent. The contribution from fish remained unchanged but, at 0.2g PUFA per person per day, it is a relatively insignificant contributor to total PUFA in the US food supply.

Plant-sourced PUFA, unlike that from animal sources, has increased dramatically over the last half-century. In 1960, plants contributed 13g PUFA per person per day, and this increased almost threefold over the next fifty years to 37g in 2010. Between 1910 and 1960 the increase in plant-sourced PUFA was 8g PUFA, while the increase between 1960 and 2010 was 24g PUFA per person per day. Almost all of the recent increase in the US food supply was due to a 23g increase in vegetable oils.

As can be seen from figure 4.3, there were changes in the relative contributions from other plant sources, but these appear trivial in comparison to the change in the contribution from "vegetable oil." There were small increases in the contribution from "grains" and from "legumes, nuts, soy," both of which were less than 1g PUFA person per day. "Margarine" and "shortening" are both made from vegetable oils. There was a decrease of about 2g PUFA in the contribution from margarine over the half-century that is almost solely due to a decline since the early 1990s. Shortening had an increase of about 1g PUFA per person per day from 1960 to 2010, and this is associated with a larger increase up until the early 2000s, followed by a decline since that time.

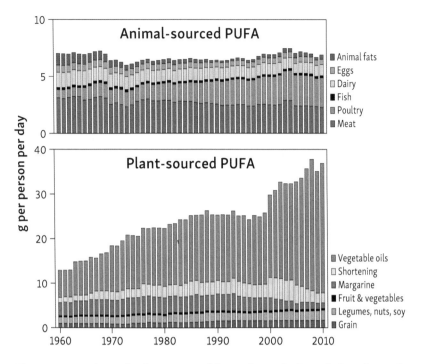

Figure 4.3 Provision of polyunsaturated fats in the US food supply from "animal-sources" and "plant-sources" between 1960 and 2010. Data are from US Department of Agriculture Food and Nutrition Service, Nutrient Content of the US Food Supply Reports. https://www.fns.usda.gov/resource/nutrient-content-us-food-supply-reports. Note different scales for "animal-sourced" and "plant-sourced" graphs.

Using the data-sheet for the supply calculated for individual fatty acids, in 2010 the US food supply provided 4.2g omega-3 fats and 39.5g omega-6 fats per person per day. This corresponds to an omega balance of 9–10 percent in 2010 compared to 18 percent in 1960.

The changes in the modern food chain have, so far, been determined from the analysis of the *supply* of food. Another analysis, that may confirm or contradict the perceived changes in supply, is to examine changes in the *consumption* of food. This is easier said than done.

Dietary Surveys of Different Populations

There are two common techniques to determine the dietary intake by individuals. The first is the "dietary recall" method, while the second is the "dietary record" technique. "Dietary recall" involves (1) the reporting of all food consumed by an individual over the previous period (normally twenty-four hours); (2) estimation of "portion size" of each food; and (3) calculation of daily intake of energy and/or nutrients from an appropriate composition database. It is retrospective of what was eaten and is often considered the "weakest link" in nutritional epidemiology. It has been described as "memories of perceptions of dietary intake," and its overuse in quantitative analyses has been strongly criticized.[8] "Dietary record" is a prospective technique that can be regarded as more accurate than "dietary recall." It involves recording both type and amount of food eaten—portion size can be either estimated or weighed—and then a composition database is used to calculate dietary intake.

In recent years, many countries have initiated national dietary surveys of large numbers of people, often using "dietary recall" to assess nutrition of the population. Many diet surveys have solely reported food types and have not calculated intakes of specific nutrients. Most diet surveys reporting intakes of types of fats have limited the breakdown to "saturated," "monounsaturated," and "polyunsaturated" fatty acids. None of these are satisfactory for my purposes. It is only relatively recently that some investigators have differentiated between omega-3 and omega-6 fats or reported intake of individual fatty acids.

The thrust of this book is that intakes of omega-3 fats and omega-6 fats need to be considered in relation to each other. The reason for this focus will become apparent in later chapters, but it is important to realize that this is not currently a common perspective. In order to calculate the dietary omega balance of various populations I have used either the "average" values or "median" values of both the omega-3 and omega-6 intakes.

Do dietary surveys support the conclusion from the food supply data? That is, do dietary surveys indicate that during the last half-century there has been a decrease in diet omega balance (an increase in omega-6 intake relative to omega-3 intake)?

The "Seven Countries Study," a multiyear study examining links between lifestyle, diet, and cardiovascular disease across seven countries, was begun in 1956. It involved extensive nutrition surveys of large population groups in seven countries in the 1960s, but did not differentiate omega-3 and omega-6 intakes. However, in 1987, duplicates of diets reported in the early 1960s were prepared and analyzed for their fatty acid composition. This was done for four of the seven countries; namely the United States, the Netherlands, Finland, and Japan.[9]

The diet of the US participants in the Seven Countries Study had an omega balance of 11 percent in the 1960s (although it should be noted that the actual foodstuffs measured were obtained in the late 1980s). Earlier in this chapter, the value estimated from the US food supply data for 1960 was 18 percent. In 1987-88, the USDA Nationwide Food Consumption Survey showed the US diet to have an omega balance of 10 percent.[10] Similar surveys gave a value of 9 percent in 1999-2000[11] and 10 percent in 2017-18.[12] In the United States, a decline in the omega balance of the diet was already underway by the 1960s (see chapter 3), and several dietary surveys have shown it to be approximately 10 percent in recent years. This value is the same as that determined, in the previous section, from the food supply data for 2018.

In the early 1960s, the Dutch diet had an omega balance of 17 percent (see note 9). The Dutch National Food Consumption Survey 2007-2010 reported the fatty acid intakes for adults, which provided an omega balance of 10-11 percent.[13] In the early 1960s, the diet of Finland had an omega balance value of 25 percent (see note 9). In 2007, a representative survey from five regions of Finland found the omega balance to be 21 percent.[14] In Japan, the 1960s diet had an omega balance of 25 percent (see note 9). A 2003 diet survey in Japan had an omega balance of 22 percent[15] while another survey in 2006 determined a value of 17 percent.[16] Thus, since the 1960s, dietary surveys report declines in the omega balance of the Dutch diet, nearly the same as that observed in the US diet, and smaller declines in the Finnish and Japanese diets.

The earliest Australian nutrition survey I can find that differentiates omega-6 and omega-3 intake is the 1995 National Nutrition Survey,[17] and the omega balance calculated from this survey is 11 percent. Almost certainly, the Australian diet in the 1960s would have had a much higher value. For example, the 1961 food supply data for Australia (see note 1) shows three-quarters of the fat supply was from lamb, beef, and dairy, which were all grass-fed. In my opinion, the omega balance of the Australian diet in the 1960s was likely approximately 20 percent. The omega balance calculated from the 2011–12 National Nutrition and Physical Activity Survey was 15 percent.[18]

Other examples of omega balance values calculated for other countries are: 17 percent from the 2008–9 National Diet and Nutrition Survey of the United Kingdom,[19] 14 percent from the Korea National Health and Nutrition Examination Survey of 2013,[20] and 6 percent from the 2006 National Nutrition Survey in Mexico.[21]

From both the food supply data in the previous section and the dietary survey data in this section I have calculated omega balance values for whole populations from the average intakes of omega-6 and omega-3. However, a disadvantage of this technique is that it is not possible to determine the variation in omega balance among individuals in a population. This is only possible if omega balance is calculated for each individual in a population.[22] In order to assess the degree of individual variation in diet omega balance in a population, I will use a study that reported the omega-6/omega-3 ratios calculated for individual diets of children and old adults combined for three U.S. studies between 2010–15.[23] This study reported that 7- to 12-year-olds had an average ratio of 9.2 (with a standard deviation of 2.8) while the average ratio for 65- to 79-year-old adults was 7.8 (with a standard deviation of 2.6). Using certain assumptions,[24] we can calculate that, while for children the average omega balance was 10 percent, approximately 68 percent of the children had values between 8 and 14 percent and approximately 96 percent of the children had diet omega balance between 6 and 22 percent. For the elderly adults, the average omega balance was 11 percent, and approximately 68 percent of the adult values ranged between 9 and 16 percent, while approximately 96 percent of the adult values were in the 7 to 21 percent range. Expression of average values can hide significant variation in diet omega balance of individuals.

Another advantage of diet surveys compared to analysis of food supply data is that one can compare groups with different eating behaviors. For example, measurement of fatty acid intakes of omnivores, vegetarians, and vegans found omega balance for diets for high meat-eating omnivores was 10 percent, for moderate meat-eating omnivores was 9 percent, for vegetarians it was 7 percent, while for vegans it was 5 percent.[25]

Changes in Traditional Diets: Maasai and Inuit as Examples

Some of the most dramatic changes of recent times have been to the traditional diets of indigenous peoples. I will consider two; the Maasai of eastern Africa and the Inuit of North America.

Nowadays, the Maasai are seminomadic pastoralists of Kenya and Tanzania who herd cattle, sheep, and goats. Their traditional diet was predominantly milk and associated dairy products, supplemented by blood and occasional meat from their livestock. They also collected some wild plant food, honey, and medicinal herbs, but these appear to have been relatively minor contributors to their energy and protein intakes. Over the twentieth century, land restrictions and reduced livestock numbers have resulted in a more sedentary and a more market-oriented lifestyle. This change has been associated with an increased plant contribution to their diet, mainly from maize-meal. The traditional milk, blood, and meat diet would have likely had an omega balance of about 30 percent (see figure 2.2). A comparison of the diet of Maasai groups between 1989 and 2007 shows an increase in food energy intake that was mainly associated with a more than twofold increase in consumption of maize.[26] The increase in maize constituted more than 70 percent of the increase in energy intake. Measurement of omega-3 and omega-6 intake in 2007 showed the Maasai to have a diet omega balance of 11 percent (see note 26)— essentially the same as the United States and Australia. An indication of the changes that had occurred is that previously "ghee" (a home-made butter fat) was traditionally used to prepare food, but by 2007 a substantial amount of the "ghee" previously used in food preparation had been replaced by "Kimbo" (a purchased commercial palm-oil based shortening). A cooking fat devoid of omega-3 had replaced almost half of the previous cooking fat, ghee, in which a third of the PUFA were omega-3 fats.

The Inuit are inhabitants of the Arctic whose traditional diet included fish and marine mammals (such as seals, whales, walruses) and land mammals (such as caribou, arctic hares, polar bears). Measurements of the fat composition of these animals show their omega balance to be high in the marine animals (85 percent in fish, 66–92 percent in marine mammals) and moderate in the land mammals (66 percent in polar bears, 15 percent in arctic hares).[27] Measurements of the diets of Inuit populations in northern Greenland in 2004 and in southern Greenland in 2006 have been compared with earlier studies of their diet in 1976.[28] Over this thirty-year period, intake of omega-3 fats had decreased by 80 percent, while omega-6 intake had increased by 64 percent. The Inuit diet in 1976 had an omega balance of 72 percent compared to 45 percent and 24 percent, respectively, in 2004 and 2006. The change was due to an increasingly "westernized" diet.

These two examples show the decrease in omega-3 fats relative to an increase in omega-6 fats in the human diet over the last half-century is not limited to western countries. The change in the types of polyunsaturated fats in the human food chain over the last half-century is due to a number of distinct trends in types of foods consumed.

I have concentrated on the influence of vegetable oils in this section, but there are four identifiable food trends responsible for a reduced omega balance in the modern diet. These trends have occurred in many parts of the world to varying degrees, but are most advanced in the developed world and have significant consequences concerning the health and happiness of the respective countries.

Trend I: The Shift from Animal Fats to Vegetable Oils

The shift from animal fats to vegetable oils in the food chain is worldwide and began over a century ago, when vegetable oils replaced animal fats in the first margarines and shortenings. The problem of vegetable oils being more "liquid" than animal fats was overcome by the introduction of "hydrogenation" which has been associated with the production of "trans fats" into the food chain (this topic will be covered later).

Although the shift began over a century ago, the pace of this transition has increased dramatically over the last half-century and is related to the dramatic rise of ultraprocessed foods. Globally, in 1961, the per capita supply of fat from vegetable oils exceeded that from animal fats by 60 percent in 1961 and by 360 percent in 2018. In the United States, vegetable oils exceeded animal fats by 40 percent in 1961 and by 624 percent in 2018. The shift was even more dramatic in Australia, with fat from vegetable oils being 73 percent *less* than from animal fats in 1961, but being 393 percent *more* in 2018. This shift was observed in many countries but was most pronounced in high-income countries. Not all vegetable oils contributed equally to this trend. The two largest contributors were soybean oil and palm oil.

The reason for the shift was likely primarily economic: vegetable oils are cheap to produce. At the time there were no expected health consequences, although the mistaken concern about saturated fat in the diet and the ignorance about the difference between the omega-3 and omega-6 fats, might have suggested to some that the shift was actually beneficial. Whatever the fundamental reason, the consequence was a *less* balanced supply of polyunsaturated fats in the food chain; a decrease in omega-3 coupled with an increase in omega-6 fats.

Trend II: The Grain Feeding of Livestock

Another influence on the imbalance between omega-3 and omega-6 fats in food chain is the practice of feeding grain, instead of grass, to livestock. Normally associated with industrial or feed-lot farming, the rationale is that it increases the energy density of the diet; it is more prevalent in some countries than others. In the United States, grain-feeding started in the 1930s and has now become the "conventional" method of raising livestock. A perceived advantage is that it results in an increased growth relative to feed consumption and also produces meat that has greater intramuscular fat: the meat is "marbled." It is arguable that it produces a more obese animal and, as will be considered later, the increased marbling of meat is remarkedly similar to the increased intramuscular fat associated with insulin-resistance in humans.

Change in feeding practices over the last half-century is not restricted to livestock such as cattle. As pointed out earlier, fish, like mammals, cannot make omega-3 fats and require them pre-formed in their diet (see chapter 1). Indeed, the manufacture of food for the farming of fish is one of the main users of industrially produced fish oils. As aquaculture has expanded, other sources have increasingly replaced the fish oil used to make fish food. These sources include various vegetable oils, as well as rendered poultry or animal fat, with the consequence that the omega balance of farmed fish has decreased in recent times. One Australian study measured the fatty acid composition of two farmed fish species over time. The omega balance of farmed Atlantic salmon decreased from 89 percent in 2002 to 45 percent in 2013, while the omega balance of farmed barramundi was 75 percent in 2002 and 64 percent in 2010.[29] It is quite possible that "fish oils ain't the oils they used to be" in that many fish-oil capsules made from farmed fish may have less omega-3 than indicated on the label.

Trend III: The Decline of Full-Fat Dairy

We obtain our omega-3 fats from "leaves" or from the meat or products of animals that eat "leaves." Dairy foods have been a significant source of high-omega balance food as long as the animal producing the milk is feeding on pasture or on forage made from "leaves." This is less so, if the milk-provider is grain-fed.

Moreover, there has been a shift in several countries from normal full-fat dairy to reduced-fat dairy. The prime reason for this has been the misguided belief that saturated fat is unhealthy and its intake should be minimized. Full-fat milk can be processed by a centrifugal treatment to reduce the fat content of milk. Such reduced-fat milk and other reduced-fat dairy products have increasingly replaced consumption of full-fat dairy. My own experience of visiting supermarkets over the years, shows shelf space for dairy is increasingly devoted to reduced-fat dairy. In 1960, the supply of full-fat milk in the United States was nearly nine-times that of low-fat milk, however by 2010 the situation had reversed, with the supply of full-fat milk being 38 percent of low-fat milk.[30]

The substitution of non-dairy "milks" (almond milk, soy milk, and so on) for dairy milks will have an even more dramatic effect, as many are devoid of, or have little, omega-3 fat. From an evolutionary perspective, I could never understand why a mother cow would feed its young calf with milk that had an unhealthy amount of fat. I've always thought that the fat content of normal milk was most likely near optimal. Human and cow's milk have approximately the same fat content.

Trend IV: The Rise of Pork and Poultry

The imbalance between omega-3 and omega-6 fats in the food chain has been exacerbated by changes among the "meats" consumed. The meats that have shown the greatest increases in provision of fat over the last half-century are the meats that have the lowest omega balances, namely pork and poultry (see chapter 2).

Globally, poultry meat showed the greatest relative change while pork had the largest absolute increase between 1961 and 2018. Over this period, the per-capita supply of poultry increased by 468 percent, while an extra 7.3g fat per person per day was contributed by pork (a 179 percent increase) (see note 1). There was essentially no change in the contribution of fat from beef, sheep, goats, and other meats over the same period.

In the United States and Australia, poultry was responsible for both the greatest absolute change and for the greatest percentage change. In the United States, poultry increased by 252 percent, or 10.8g fat per person per day, between 1961 and 2018. Perhaps the most dramatic changes occurred in Australia. In Australia, the respective changes were 931 percent and 12.5g fat per person per day. In 1961 Australians ate more lamb and beef than pork and chicken. In 2018 this had reversed. The rise in consumption of pork and chicken compared with other meats is a little appreciated factor in the increased imbalance between omega-3 and omega-6 fats in the modern human diet.

In conclusion, over the last half-century, for a variety of reasons there has been a decrease in omega-3 content and an increase in omega-6 content of the foods we eat. Because of individual variation it will be minimal (maybe even nonexistent) in some individuals and extreme in other individuals. In the second half of this book, I will posit that this change, relatively unknown by the public, is responsible for significant ill-health in modern societies and largely responsible for the increased prevalence of many chronic diseases grouped together as modern epidemics.

However, in order for you to fully understand this situation I need to first explain; (1) the different types of fats, (2) why polyunsaturated fats exist, (3) the role and importance of cell membranes in the function of cells and organisms, (4) the different effects of omega-3 and omega-6 fats on cell function, and (5) the influence of diet omega balance on membrane composition and thus cell function.

So, now for some biology.

CHAPTER 5

THE IMPORTANCE OF CELL MEMBRANES AND THE LINK WITH DIET

Visible and Invisible Fats

Fat has an image problem. In the age of DNA, it is perceived by many biologists as boring. This likely stems from our first experience of fat, which for most of us, is when it is pointed out as the highly "visible" cream-colored part of the meat on our dinner plate. This adipose tissue consists of specialized cells that store energy in the form of fat molecules. In evolutionary terms, fat is an ideal molecule to store energy for two reasons. The first is that fat molecules are overwhelmingly made of carbon and hydrogen (they are hydrocarbons) and consequently, on a weight basis, these molecules contain more than twice the amount of energy as carbohydrate or protein molecules. The second is that when energy is stored as fat, it contains very little associated water. When animals store energy as carbohydrate (or protein), they have to also store water with it—just over four times the mass of the carbohydrate. When both factors are taken into account, storing energy as carbohydrate requires nearly ten times the body mass as storing the same amount of energy as fat.[1]

The more interesting fat on our dinner plate is "invisible." It is found in all whole-foods because it is the fat that makes up cell membranes. This "invisible fat" is the fat in the spinach on our dinner plate (see chapter 2). All bacteria, fungi, plants, and animals are made of cells, and all cells have a "skin," a membrane, in which fats provide the underlying fundamental structure. Visible fats are "storage fats," while "membrane fats" are the invisible fats. These two differ-ent types of fat differ in their structure. Molecules of "storage fats" have three fatty acid chains (sometimes called triglycerides), while "membrane fats" contain only two fatty acid chains per molecule. Although there are many different types of lipids that make up mem-branes, for the sake of simplicity, I will group them all together as "membrane fats."[2]

The general structure of a "membrane fat" is that two fatty acids are attached to a head group (figure 5.1). While the two fatty acids are hy-drocarbon chains (generally 16–22 carbons long) and are consequently "water-fearing" parts of the molecule, the head group is a "water-loving" part of the molecule. This characteristic—that one end of the molecule is "water-fearing" while the other end is "water-loving"—is a distinctive and essential feature of all "membrane fat" molecules. Molecules with such a property are called "amphipathic."

The dominance of "storage fats" in both the initial awareness of fat and in the teaching of fat biochemistry is, in my opinion, unde-served as "storage fats" are the recent arrivals compared to more an-cestral "membrane fats." Most of our biochemistry was evolved by bacteria,[3] yet while synthesis of storage fats (triglycerides) is wide-spread among plants and animals, bacteria do not make storage fats.[4] The appearance of "membrane fats" likely preceded the appearance of "storage fats" by some 2 billion years. Furthermore, the biochem-ical processes that make triglycerides in animals essentially convert a "membrane fat" to a "storage fat" by replacing the "water-loving" head group of the membrane fat with a "water-fearing" fatty acid chain, thus turning an "amphipathic" molecule into a fully "lipo-philic" molecule.[5] This completely lipophilic nature of triglyceride molecules allows them to aggregate as globules, while the amphipa-thic nature of membrane fat molecules is fundamental in determin-ing how they relate to each other and also to how they self-organize to form the distinctive structure of membranes. The specific fatty acids in "storage fats" have essentially only a trivial influence on their func-tion as a source of energy. However, although we obtain our dietary omega-3 and omega-6 from both the "storage fats" and the "membrane fats" in our food, it is through their role in "membrane fats" that the omega-3 and omega-6 influence cell and body function and consequently health.

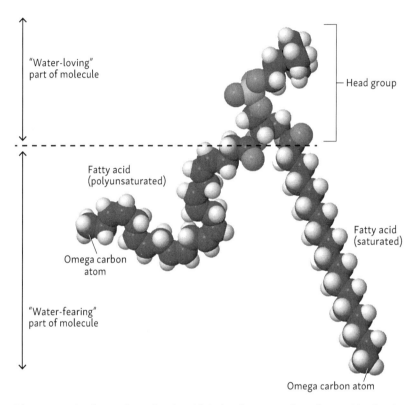

Figure 5.1 Membrane fat molecule with its head group and two fatty acid tails. The head group is "water-loving," while the two fatty acid tails are "water-fearing" (or "fat-loving"). The right-hand fatty acid is saturated (18:0), and the left-hand fatty acid is polyunsaturated (22:6ω-3). The "omega" carbon atoms of each fatty acid are the last carbon atoms in the fatty acid chain.

Membrane Composition: Membrane Fats and Membrane Proteins

Membranes are universal to life. All life consists of cells, and all cells are surrounded by a membrane "skin." Membranes also surround the internal compartments of animal and plant cells. All these biological membranes are a mosaic of "membrane fats" and "membrane proteins" (figure 5.2). It is the "membrane fats" that are fundamental to biological membranes, and I will spend a little time explaining this structure.

Membranes are unusual structures, in that the molecules that make up membranes are not covalently bonded to each other. Membrane fats like to "hang out" with each other because of their mutual "fear" of water, and when they "hang out" together, they do it in a special way. Membranes are thin; they are approximately 10 nanometers wide (one millionth of a centimeter) and are very organized in a bilayer structure.[6] Of course, molecules don't "like" or "love" or "fear" or "prefer." I have used the words for human emotions as an analogy to explain how these molecules respond to certain physical forces. You don't need to understand the physical forces, only their consequences, with respect to how the molecules will orient in certain environments. Later, I will describe the different "behaviors" of the different types of fats.

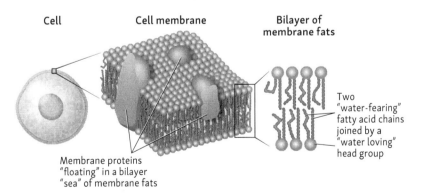

Cell   Cell membrane   Bilayer of membrane fats

Two "water-fearing" fatty acid chains joined by a "water loving" head group

Membrane proteins "floating" in a bilayer "sea" of membrane fats

Figure 5.2 Fluid mosaic structure of a cell membrane illustrating how membrane fat molecules form a fluid bilayer in which membrane proteins are located.

Imagine we added some "membrane fat" molecules to a bowl of water. We would find that all the "membrane fat" would float on the top of the water; if we could look at individual molecules, we would see that for every single membrane fat molecule, the "water-loving" part of the molecule in the water and the "water-fearing" fatty acid chains would be in the air above the water. Further, all the fatty acid chains would be closely grouped together because they all dislike being near water and consequently prefer being together: they are "fat-loving." This structure is very organized although the molecules are not bonded with each other. It is called a "monolayer." Monolayers of membrane fats exist in nature, often surrounding globules of storage fat, with the "fat-loving" fatty acids adjacent to the storage fat and the "water-loving" head-groups on the outside of the globule. In this manner, they allow fat globules to remain suspended in water solutions, to form emulsions. This is the case for milk-fat globules in milk. It is also the case for certain fat globules in blood, the lipoprotein particles measured in blood tests.[7]

Now imagine we can peel this "monolayer of membrane fats" off the surface of the water. In fact, imagine we have two monolayers that we have peeled off the surface of two bowls of water. We have these two monolayer sheets, one side of each sheet is "water-loving," the other side is "fat-loving," so if we could place these two monolayers such that the two "fat-loving" sides came into contact, they would rapidly come together and stay together. We would now have a "bilayer" in which the two outside surfaces are "water-loving" and the internal center consists of the "water-fearing," "fat-loving" fatty acid chains. Such a bilayer structure describes the basis of cell membranes. Because they are not chemically bonded to each other, membrane fats can undergo high-speed lateral movement in the membrane bilayer such that an average membrane fat molecule can circumnavigate a red blood cell in seconds.[8]

As well as membrane fats, cell membranes also contain membrane proteins, and different cells have different sorts of membrane proteins. The membrane proteins are embedded in the bilayer of membrane fats. In effect they can be thought of as floating in a sea of membrane fats. Some membrane proteins cross the entire membrane bilayer, while others are attached only to one side of the bilayer. Although the atoms that make up the membrane fat molecules are associated tightly with each other and the membrane proteins, there are no tight chemical bonds between the individual "membrane fats" nor are there tight chemical bonds between the "membrane fats" and the "membrane proteins." While many membrane proteins can also move laterally in the membrane, others cannot because they are anchored to a "skeleton" inside the cell. The membrane proteins are less mobile than the membrane fats. The presence of omega-3 and omega-6 fatty acids in membrane fats can influence the movement of membrane fats within the bilayer and consequently also the activity and movement of important membrane proteins.

Living systems require movement of molecules, so they may collide, vibrate, and interact. Life requires a "goldilocks" level of movement, not too much and not too little.[9] While movement of molecules in the water compartment of cells has been evident under the microscope for a long-time, it was not until 1970 that lateral movement of molecules in membrane bilayers was observed, as the rapid intermixing of different membrane proteins following the fusion of mouse and human cells.[10] Two years later, the "fluid mosaic" model of membranes was proposed,[11] and this is now the widely accepted understanding of the structure of biological membranes. That polyunsaturated fatty acids speed up such movement in membranes is the fundamental reason why they have come to exist. To understand this aspect, we first need to understand the structural difference between saturated, monounsaturated, and polyunsaturated fatty acids, as well as the difference between omega-3 and omega-6 fatty acids. We are going to enter the world of molecules, so fasten your seat belt and imagine yourself a hundred-million times smaller than you actually are.

Saturated, Monounsaturated, and Polyunsaturated Fatty Acids: The Differences

To be functional, biological membranes likely have to be of a minimum width. The most common fatty acid chains of bacterial membranes are 16 carbon atoms long, and thus a bilayer of such fatty acids is 32 carbon atoms wide. Bacteria, plants, and animals are all capable of making fatty acid molecules by a process called *lipogenesis*—the creation of fat—which in many ways is best thought of as fundamental to making membranes. It uses an enzyme complex called *fatty acid synthase* to make a 16-carbon saturated fatty acid called *palmitic acid.* While the fatty acid synthase of bacteria (and many plants) consists of seven separate enzymes (that is, seven separate proteins), the fatty acid synthase of vertebrate animals consists of one enzyme (one protein) with seven active sites that operate sequentially.[12] Such a change emphasizes the evolutionary importance of fatty acid synthesis for making membranes of cells. Seven genes had merged to become one gene. Seven separate "workshops" were reorganized to become an "assembly line of seven different stations." Evolution had preempted Henry Ford's invention of the assembly line by millions of years!

The product of fatty acid synthase, palmitic acid, is a 16-carbon saturated fatty acid and is the source from which the other fatty acids found in membranes are made. To make it easy to understand fatty acids, throughout this book I will refer to fatty acids by a numbering system (figure 5.3). This number will allow you to immediately recognize the type of fatty acid. (For names, see appendix 2.)

Palmitic acid is described as 16:0, and its structure is illustrated in figure 5.4, as are those of six other common fatty acids. Because the basic building block to make both palmitic acid and the other fatty acids is a 2-carbon unit, fatty acids generally consist of chains of an even number of carbon atoms.

A carbon atom is capable of sharing four electrons and can thus chemically bond with up to four other atoms. As can be seen from figure 5.4, the carbon atom in the 16:0 chain each has a chemical bond

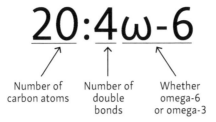

Figure 5.3 The numbering system used to identify individual fatty acids. The specific fatty acid identified is "arachidonic acid," an omega-6 polyunsaturated fatty acid. See text for full explanation.

with the carbon atoms before and after it in the chain, as well as with two hydrogen atoms each. Thus, each carbon atom has four bonds and could not share electrons with any more hydrogen atoms. It is "saturated" with hydrogen atoms and is thus called a *saturated* fatty acid. It is not the only saturated fatty acid, and 16:0 can be elongated (by an enzyme called an "elongase") to make 18:0, a longer saturated fatty acid known as stearic acid. The carbon atoms in fatty acid chains are numbered according to chemical conventions, with the first carbon atom in the chain known as the *alpha* carbon and the last carbon atom in the chain is known as the *omega* carbon. These carbon atoms are identified in figure 5.4.

The third fatty acid illustrated in figure 5.4 is also 18 carbons long but differs from 18:0, in that both "carbon 9" and "carbon 10" each have bonds with only one hydrogen atom; this hydrocarbon chain is thus not saturated with hydrogen atoms. To compensate, these carbon atoms share an extra electron with each other. They are consequently connected by a "double-bond" rather than a single-bond, as are the other carbon atoms in the chain. There is one double-bond in the hydrocarbon chain and this fatty acid is therefore a *monounsaturated* fatty acid, and is identified as 18:1 (it is named *oleic acid* after the Latin for *oil*).

The next fatty acid illustrated in figure 5.4 is also 18 carbons long, and as well as carbons 9 and 10, carbons 12 and 13 are also unsaturated with hydrogen, and they are also connected to each other by a

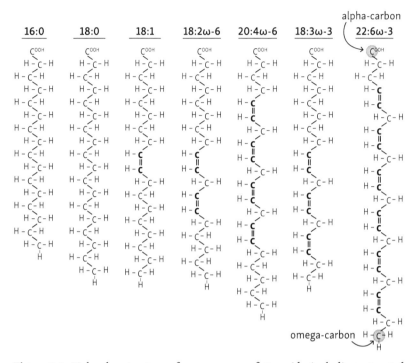

Figure 5.4 Molecular structure of some common fatty acids, including saturated fatty acids (16:0, 18:0), a monounsaturated fatty acid (18:1), omega-6 polyunsaturated fatty acids (18:2ω-6, 20:4ω-6) and omega-3 polyunsaturated fatty acids (18:3ω-3, 22:6ω-3).

"double-bond." Thus, this fatty acid has more than one double-bond, it is *polyunsaturated*. Furthermore, the second "double-bond" is six carbons from the omega-carbon of the chain, it is an *omega–6 polyunsaturated* fatty acid, and is identified as 18:2ω–6. You will notice it is not called an "omega 6 fatty acid" but rather an "omega–6 fatty acid." The "–" is a minus sign, not a hyphen, and is thus significant because it has a meaning.

The next fatty acid in figure 5.4 has been elongated to become 20 carbons long and also has four double-bonds. There are two important considerations: The first is that when a fatty acid is elongated, the 2-carbon building block is added to the *alpha-carbon* and consequently there is no change in the position of the double-bonds relative to the *omega-carbon*. This elongated product remains an omega-6 fatty acid. The second consideration is that when more double bonds are inserted into the hydrocarbon chain (by desaturase enzymes) they are also inserted on the *alpha-carbon* side of the initial double-bonds present in the chain, and thus also do not change its "omega-6" status. This particular fatty acid is identified as 20:4ω-6 (called arachidonic acid) and is a very important membrane fatty acid that we will later return to many times.

The last two fatty acids illustrated in figure 5.4 are both omega-3 polyunsaturated fatty acids. The first is 18:3ω-3, and it can be seen that the most terminal double-bond is three carbons from the *omega-carbon*. The second omega-3 fatty acid illustrated in figure 5.4 is 22:6ω-3 and is one of the longest and most polyunsaturated fatty acids found in membrane bilayers.[13]

Saturated fatty acids are the initial fatty acids synthesized from which the others are made. Monounsaturated fats are made by modifying saturated fats, and omega-6 fats are made from monounsaturated fats, while omega-3 fats are in turn made from omega-6 fats. Plants and some simple animals have all the necessary enzymes, but higher animals have "lost" the desaturase enzyme responsible for converting monounsaturated fats to omega-6, as well as the desaturase enzyme for converting an omega-6 into an omega-3 fat. This is the reason why both omega-6 and omega-3 fats are separate essential requirements in our diet.

It may have seemed to be a certain overkill to have gone into the detail of where the double-bonds are in certain fatty acids, but as we will see shortly, there is a big difference in the influence of single-bonds and double-bonds on the "movement" of a membrane fatty acid, and this has very important influences on membrane function and consequently body function.

The Importance of Membranes for Being "Alive"

We know that a warm corpse is not "alive," yet it has essentially all the molecules required for life. Similarly, our ancestors have known for a long time that depriving an individual of the ability to breathe air by suffocation will stop the process of living. Respiration and circulation are essential for being "alive" because they support cellular "energy metabolism," and membranes are central to energy metabolism.

In 1777, the French aristocrat and scientist Antoine Lavoisier named an important gas, both necessary for life and also constituting about one-fifth of the atmosphere, as "oxygen." He and his wife, Marie-Anne Paulze Lavoisier, showed that animal respiration was the process whereby oxygen from the air was combined with carbon and hydrogen from the body to produce heat, water, and "fixed air" (carbon dioxide). This process was similar to the burning of a candle, and furthermore the amount of heat produced from a certain amount of fuel was the same whether the process was combustion or animal respiration. Lavoisier thought that this process took place in the lungs and that the function of blood flow was to distribute the heat produced in the lungs throughout the body. Later it was shown that oxygen consumption took place in all the tissues throughout the body.[14] Nowadays, we name this process "energy metabolism" and the rate of oxygen consumption as the "metabolic rate." If an organism exhibits "energy metabolism," it is "alive."

In 1849, two Frenchmen, Henri Victor Regnault and Jules Reiset, reported that when they kept rabbits and dogs in an atmosphere that had two to three times normal oxygen levels, the rabbits and dogs had exactly the same metabolic rates as those measured in normal atmospheric oxygen. In other words, metabolic rate was an intrinsic characteristic of the species and was not normally limited by the supply of oxygen. In this way it differed from a burning candle.[15]

The basal metabolic rate (BMR) is used to compare the metabolic rate of different species.[16] It is analogous to measuring the fuel consumption rate of a car, when idling. The BMR of an adult human (weighing approximately 65kg) is approximately 14 liters of oxygen consumed per hour; when expressed in energy terms, it is equivalent to about 80 watts. It is still amazing to me, even after years of scientific investigation into energy metabolism, that it costs the same amount of energy to keep an adult human body alive as the energy consumed by an 80-watt incandescent light globe. Interestingly, a "standard candle" also consumes energy at the rate of approximately 80 watts.[17]

The existence of a lipid bilayer membrane allows the environment inside the cell to be different from the outside environment, and this ability is fundamental to energy metabolism. In bacterial cells, most oxygen is consumed by the last member of a series of membrane proteins that, as a group pump "protons" from inside the bacterial cell to outside, and consequently produce a transmembrane "proton" gradient. In animal cells, the same process takes place in "mitochondria" (sometimes called the "powerhouses" of the cell). Nowadays, mitochondria are thought to be evolutionary descendants of a symbiotic bacterial community that evolved to become animal cells.[18] Similarly, in plant cells, the capture of the energy in light is used to pump "protons" across the chloroplast membrane and thus create a transmembrane proton gradient.

A proton is a hydrogen atom that lacks its electron and consequently has a "positive" charge. It is written as H^+ and is the smallest ion (an atom or molecule with an electric charge due to loss or gain of electrons). The proton gradient across the mitochondrial membrane is equivalent to nearly 200 millivolts. This electrochemical gradient is used to make a high-energy molecule known as ATP, which in turn is used to carry out many energy-requiring processes in other parts of cells.[19] ATP is called a universal "energy coin" of life. In animal cells, ATP is used to pump sodium ions (Na^+) out of the cell, across the cell membrane, and consequently creates a transmembrane Na^+ gradient. Transmembrane ion gradients are a form of electrochemical energy that are continually being dissipated by "leaks"; we will see that their maintenance is a significant part of the basal metabolic rate of an animal. Together membrane pumps and leaks constitute about half the "cost of living." [20]

Membranes and the Cost of Living: Insights from Different Species

The "cost of living" is not constant among species but varies with body size. The basal metabolic rate (BMR) of a 65kg human is approximately 80 watts, which corresponds to 1.2 watts per kg. The BMR of a mouse is approximately 9 watts per kg, and for an elephant it is approximately 0.4 watts per kg. Metabolic rate of animals varies with body mass in a very systematic manner (see note 15). Why is the BMR (on a per-g body mass basis) of a mouse 7.4 times that of a human? Part of the explanation lies in the relative size of internal organs, but a significant part is also explained by the fact that on a per gram basis, the tissues from small mammals have greater metabolic rates than those from large mammals.[21] Similarly, small mammals spend relatively more energy on pumping Na^+ ions across membranes than large mammals, as with many other cellular activities.

Heart rate is a manifestation of these differences in metabolic intensity. In humans the resting heart rate is about 70 beats per minute, while for mice it is about 580 beats per minute.[22] In the late 1970s, an Icelandic biochemist, Sigmundur Gudbjarnason, reported a fascinating observation for which he had no ready explanation. He reported that the 22:6ω-3 content in membrane fats from the hearts of whales, humans, rabbits, rats, and mice increased in a systematic manner and was strongly correlated with the resting heart rate of these species.[23] I was intrigued by this observation and together with a colleague, Patrice Couture, decided to further investigate. We confirmed Gudbjarnason's finding for the heart and extended it to other tissues. Just as the metabolic activity of tissues (heart, liver, kidney, and muscle) increases in a systematic manner in smaller compared with larger mammal species, so does the 22:6ω-3 content of membrane fats. Higher metabolic activity was associated with higher 22:6ω-3 content.[24] The only exception was the brain, in which 22:6ω-3 content remained high, irrespective of the size of the mammal. In humans, 22:6ω-3 is higher in the brain than in other tissues, and it is consequently sometimes suggested that this highly polyunsaturated fatty acid has a special brain-centric function. However, this tissue difference in humans is related to the fact that we are a relatively large species of mammal. For example, mice have more 22:6ω-3 in the membrane fats from their heart and muscle than in those from their brain. The 22:6ω-3 content of membrane fats seems to be associated with fast membrane processes in general rather than with brain-specific activities. An interesting observation from this comparison of different sized mammals was that percent of total polyunsaturated fats in membranes of different-sized mammals was relatively constant with body size. The polyunsaturated fatty acids in membranes of highly active tissues of small mammals had a greater *degree* of "polyunsaturation" than those from larger mammals. Similar membrane fatty acid relationships have also been shown to exist in birds of different sizes.[25]

It is a consequence of geometry that metabolic intensity needs to decrease as species get larger. Let's compare mice with men. What would be the consequence if a human suddenly had the metabolic intensity of a mouse? If BMR of a human increased 7.4-fold? With no change in insulation, a 7.4-fold increase in BMR would require a 7.4-fold increase in the temperature gradient to lose the heat from this increased BMR. In other words, if environmental temperature was 27°C, then body temperature would need to be about 100°C, an obviously lethal body temperature. If mammals, regardless of size, are to maintain a body temperature around 37°C, then it is essential that they decrease their metabolic intensity the larger they become.

Another manifestation of large differences between species in metabolic rate is the difference between "warm-blooded" (or endothermic) animals, such as mammals and birds, and "cold-blooded" (ectothermic) animals, such as reptiles, amphibians, and fish. This difference is several-fold and despite the name is not related to their body temperature. About forty years ago, a colleague, Paul Else, and I set out to understand this difference by investigating matched "endotherm-ectotherm" species. The first was a comparison of mice with an Australian desert lizard of the same size (about 30g) and body temperature (about 37°C) as the mouse. Later we changed the comparison to rats and a different lizard species, similarly with the same mass (about 300g) and temperature (about 37°C). Still later, we changed the comparison to that of the laboratory rat with the "cane-toad," a Central American amphibian that has become a feral pest in Australia. All three comparisons gave essentially the same results and for the sake of brevity I will treat them as a single "endotherm-ectotherm" comparison.

When measured at the same body temperature, the BMR of the endotherm is about five times that of the ectotherm. As with the body size comparison, this is due to both relatively larger organs and a greater metabolic rate per g of tissue.[26] About 40 percent of cellular metabolic rate was devoted to providing energy for the sodium pump in both endotherm and ectotherm.[27] This was because endotherm cells are several-fold leakier to Na^+ ions than ectotherm cells; later measurements extended this generalization to other vertebrates. Rat and pigeon cells are much leakier to Na^+ ions than cells from lizards, toads, and trout.[28] Further investigation revealed that endotherm and ectotherm tissues did *not* differ in the number of sodium pumps but instead differed in their activity. A sodium pump from endotherm cells operated between 6,000 and 12,000 cycles per minute, while those from ectotherm cells operated at much slower rates: between 1,500 and 2,500 cycles per minute.[29] As well as having faster sodium pumps, membranes from the endotherm cells contained about twice the content of both 22:6ω-3 and 20:4ω-6 than did the cell membranes from the ectotherm.[30]

Sodium pumps operate only when they are in membranes, and we designed some experiments to examine whether the difference in membrane fat composition was responsible for the large difference in pump activity. When rat sodium pumps were surrounded by toad membrane, they exhibited toad activity and vice versa.[31] In a series of additional species "cross-over" studies (involving cattle and crocodiles) it was confirmed that it was the surrounding membrane that determined the activity of the sodium pump (a membrane protein).[32] Further, it was shown that the physical membrane properties of the membrane fats (such as lateral pressure) were significantly correlated with the activity of the sodium pumps.[33]

Similar to cell membranes from rats being much leakier to Na^+ than cell membranes from reptiles, we found that mitochondrial membranes from the mammal were both much leakier to H^+ and contained significantly more 22:6ω-3 compared to those from the reptile.[34] Furthermore, when we measured the activity of a foreign membrane protein (valinomycin, an antibiotic from fungi) we observed that it operated at three times the rate in the more polyunsaturated membranes from the mammal than it did when in the reptilian membrane.[35]

The consistent insight from these studies investigating the metabolic activity of different species was that membrane-associated processes are significant components of metabolic activity, and that faster membrane-associated processes are associated with membrane fats containing highly polyunsaturated fatty acids, especially 22:6ω-3. We found that the connection was physical rather than chemical, and was likely due to the "movement" of polyunsaturated fatty acid chains in the membrane bilayer.

The Behavior of Membrane Fats: Fluidity and Membrane Remodeling

Drawings of what a molecule looks like are only partly true, because even if we ignore the fact that drawings are two-dimensional while molecules are three-dimensional, the drawing is static while the molecule is vibrant. "Temperature" is a measure of molecular movement in a system, and the higher the temperature the greater the movement. This movement means that molecules in a system collide with each other, and these collisions will cause small changes in the shape of the molecule. In a way, at temperatures consistent with life, molecules can be thought to vibrate. So it is with fatty acids. More importantly, the type of bonds connecting the carbon atoms in a fatty acid chain will strongly influence this movement. Without going into the physics, "double-bonds" strongly influence the movement of fatty acid chains.[36]

Although the structures of the various fatty acids shown in figure 5.4 shows them all as "straight chains," this is a very false depiction of their individual shapes. These straight chains are an artifact to easily illustrate the differences in how the carbons atoms are attached to each other. A more real representation is presented in the picture of a typical membrane lipid in figure 5.1 (in which the two fatty acids are 22:6ω-3 and 18:0), but even this representation is not completely true. Although we draw a polyunsaturated fatty acid such as 22:6ω-3 with a particular shape, it doesn't have a *single* shape. At normal temperatures, there are hundreds of equally probable shapes. It is a molecule in vibrant motion. The greater the number of double-bonds in the chain, the more vibrant will be the movement of the whole chain. If we could see the relative movement of these two fatty acid chains in this membrane lipid (figure 5.1), we would see that the highly polyunsaturated 22:6ω-3 chain has much more violent movement compared to the more sedately moving saturated fatty acid chain.[37] This is the reason why, at room temperatures, unsaturated fats are liquid while saturated fats are generally solid. Shortly, we will see this violent movement of 22:6ω-3 is very important for its function in cell membranes.

This difference in movement of fatty acids is manifest in their different melting temperatures. The more "double-bonds," the lower the temperature at which they solidify. Melting temperature of 18:0 is 69°C, for 18:1 it is 13°C, while for 18:2ω-6 it is –5°C, for 18:3ω-3 it is –11°C, and for 22:6ω-3 it is –44°C.[38] These differences have significant biological implications. Bacteria that had membrane fats with only saturated fatty acid chains would have only been able to survive in hot springs and similar environments. This is because at temperatures below about 50°C, their cell membrane bilayers would no longer be "fluid," and instead would "solidify."[39] However, by replacing one of the saturated fatty acid chains in their membrane fats with an unsaturated fatty acid, they would be able to maintain "fluid" membranes and thus survive in lower-temperature environments. This is what they do, and they do it *very* rapidly. The membrane fats of the common intestinal bacteria, *E. coli*, contain mixed pairs of 16:0, 18:0, 14:0, 16:1, 18:1, and 14:1 and when subjected to lower temperatures, they actively replace some of the 16:0 chains in their membrane fats with 18:1. This change is very fast, being evident within 30 seconds of the temperature change.[40] This rapid alteration of membrane fatty acid composition enables the bacterium to maintain a constant membrane fluidity.[41] The response is now known to occur in plants and animals as well as bacteria. It has been especially studied in fish, and is the reason why cold-water fish are generally a richer source of highly polyunsaturated omega-3 fats than are warm-water fish. It also provides additional evidence of the effect of membrane fats on the activity of membrane proteins. For example, membrane lipids extracted from cold-acclimated fish cause greater reactivation of de-lipidated membrane enzymes than do those from warm-acclimated fish,[42] and the activity of sodium pumps is increased in cold-acclimated fish but is not due to a change in the number of sodium pumps.[43] There are two pathways for a fatty acid to appear in a membrane fat; the first is through de novo synthesis of a membrane fat molecule, while the second is via "remodeling" of an already existing membrane fat molecule. A study of liver cells found sixteen different fatty acid pair combinations make up about 90 percent of all membrane fat molecules. Of the sixteen pair combinations, only four are the product of *de novo* manufacture, which together constitute about 30 percent of total membrane fats, while the remaining 70 percent are products of the *remodeling* process.[44] The *remodeling* process is carried out by a range of membrane enzymes.[45] We are still learning much about membrane remodeling, but it is ideally situated to regulate membrane composition because the responsible membrane proteins can be both "sensors" and "effectors" of the membrane bilayer in which they are located. Some are responsive to the fatty acid composition of the membrane surrounding them.[46]

Membrane remodeling process can be extremely rapid. For example, one study has shown that polyunsaturated fatty acids in membrane fats that have been damaged (by oxidative stress) can be removed and replaced with undamaged polyunsaturated fats as fast as they are damaged, thus maintaining a constant membrane fatty acid composition.[47] An especially important finding by William Lands, is that although an acyltransferase enzyme (one of the remodeling enzymes) can be highly selective for polyunsaturated fatty acids, it does not discriminate between omega-6 and omega-3 fatty acids.[48]

Diet Fat and Membrane Composition:
An Experiment with Rats

For obvious ethical reasons, there are limits to using humans to understand human biology. This is especially true for biochemistry. In human diet experiments it is common for plasma or red blood cells to be analyzed. However, red blood cells are not "typical" cells (they lack a nucleus). Most of our knowledge comes from experiments on other species, and the laboratory rat (*Rattus norvegicus*) is often used. All indications are that the results achieved and conclusions reached in such experiments apply to *Homo sapiens*.

Following an invitation to write a review about "Dietary fats and membrane function: implications for metabolism and disease,"[49] I and my colleagues searched the scientific literature and found that relatively little was known of the relationship between diet and membrane composition for most tissues under normal situations.

We were interested in the "normal" situation and decided to use the "conformer/regulator" paradigm to examine the influence of diet composition on membrane composition. We chose outbred adult rats (because of genetic diversity) and fed them one of twelve diets, which were complete in all respects except they differed in their fatty acid composition. To emulate the average human diet,[50] all were "moderate-fat" (25 percent energy) with a wide range of fatty acid compositions. Saturated fat content ranged from 8 percent to 88 percent, monounsaturated fat from 6 percent to 65 percent, total polyunsaturated fat from 4 percent to 81 percent. The dominant fats were 18-carbon fatty acids, the "normal" situation for both rats and humans.[51] The omega balance of the twelve diets ranged from 1 percent to 86 percent. Rats were fed the diets for eight weeks (equivalent to approximately one year in humans on a metabolic rate comparison) following which they were euthanized and tissues (brain, heart, liver, kidney, adipose tissue, red blood cells, and plasma) removed, with the fatty acid composition of both membrane fats and storage fats measured.

This extensive study showed that although "storage fats" reflected the fatty acid composition of the diet, for "membrane fats" this was not the case. In all tissues, the saturated, monounsaturated, and total polyunsaturated fatty acid composition was constant irrespective of wide variation in diet fatty acid composition. With respect to these three classes of fatty acids, membrane composition was *not* influenced by changes in their relative abundance in the diet; it was homeostatically regulated.

Although content of total polyunsaturated fatty acids was relatively constant irrespective of diet content, both membrane omega-3 and membrane omega-6 were more responsive to the diet. In all tissues, membrane fatty acid composition was responsive to the omega balance of the diet. Membrane omega balance was especially responsive to diet when diets had an omega balance less than 15 percent. Diets with higher omega balances had small but significant influence on membrane omega balance, while for diets with an omega balance less than 15 percent, the membrane fats were essentially "diet-conformers."[52] The average omega balance of the modern US diet, and that of Australia as well as several other developed countries is about 10 percent.

In presenting this information at scientific talks, a common comment was "but this is only in rats." Convinced that the relationship was likely important and that it was also a general finding applicable to humans, I decided to experiment on myself.

Diet Omega Balance: An Experiment on Myself

I had just over a month free from other commitments and set upon the following schedule; 11 days on high omega-6 diet, then 13 days on high omega-3 diet, followed by 12 days on the original high omega-6 diet. On waking each morning, I thoroughly rinsed my mouth and strongly wiped a sterile gauze swab on the inside of my cheek to collect cheek mucosa cells, which I immediately froze for later analysis. I wanted my diets to be reasonably "normal" and as similar as possible, except for their fatty acid composition. I decided to change only the evening meal and keep everything else the same for the 36 days of the total experiment. The evening meal for the high omega-6 diet consisted of grilled chicken, vegetable oil–coated potatoes, and microwaved frozen vegetable mix. For the high omega-3 diet, my evening meal was grilled salmon, microwaved baby potatoes (non-coated) and microwaved spinach. Both diets provided about 9,850 kJ energy and 79g fat per day. My weight remained constant throughout the experiment.

The high omega-6 diet had an omega balance of 8 percent compared with 49 percent for the high omega-3 diet. The omega balance of membrane fats extracted from my cheek cells during the experiment is shown in figure 5.5. There was no influence of diet on the total polyunsaturated fat content of my cheek cells (about 30 percent of total fatty acids) throughout the entire experiment. However, my cheek cells responded relatively rapidly to the change in the omega balance of my diet. My cheek cell omega balance was relatively constant during the first omega-6 diet period but rose upon the change to the omega-3 diet. On return to the omega-6 diet, this situation reversed. I was surprised by the speed of the response to diet change.

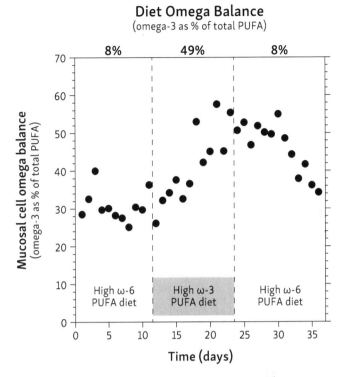

Figure 5.5 Changes in the omega balance of my cheek mucosal cells during my 36-day diet experiment. See text for details.

Susan Allport, the author of *The Queen of Fats*,[53] is passionate about omega-3 fats and has also experimented on herself. She changed her diet to a high omega-6 diet for a month and had daily blood samples analyzed for their fatty acid composition.[54] At the beginning of her experiment, her blood omega balance was 34 percent; by two weeks, it had decreased to 15 percent; and at the end of the experiment, it was 13 percent. The rapid decrease in the first two weeks is a similar time course to the changes in my own cheek cells. Both of our experiments show that membrane composition is very responsive to diet omega balance. In both of our experiments, the rapid change in the omega balance was not associated with any change in total PUFA content.[55]

Although changes in diet omega balance have rapid effects on the omega-3 and omega-6 content of membrane fats, does it matter? Do omega-3 and omega-6 have different effects on membrane processes?

Omega-3 and Omega-6: Different Effects on Membrane Processes

Although the experiments I have described earlier suggest a connection between membrane fats and the activity of membrane proteins, they do not necessarily indicate a difference between the effects of omega-3 and omega-6 fatty acids. Normally, biological membranes have a large number of different membrane fat molecules, and it is difficult to allocate particular effects to specific fatty acids. However, there is a series of experiments that are relatively little known but, in my opinion, have *very* significant implications for understanding the difference between omega-3 and omega-6 fatty acid chains. They were carried out by Drake Mitchell and colleagues at the US National Institutes of Health (NIH) and involve the membrane processes that occur in retina of the eye.[56]

Retinal cells, responsible for detecting light energy, are densely packed with membranes. The concentration of 22:6ω-3 is especially high in these membranes, which also contain four types of membrane proteins, that operate in a "cascade" to convert the presence of photons (light) into neuronal information. The first protein, rhodopsin, carries the visual pigment and after it is "activated" by a photon, it then collides with and activates another membrane protein, a G-protein. The "activated" G-protein in turn collides with and activates a third membrane protein (an enzyme), which causes the fourth membrane protein (a Na^+ channel) to close, resulting in neuronal impulses in the optic nerves.[57] Although I've just described a one-on-one sequence, it is more than that. An activated rhodopsin molecule can collide with and activate several hundred membrane-bound G-proteins, and once the enzyme (the third protein) has been activated, it can also act on several hundred molecules. Consequently, this G-protein cascade can greatly amplify a signal. It has been calculated that *one* photon can result in the conversion of thousands of molecules by the third protein in the series.[58]

The NIH researchers made artificial membrane vesicles containing the first three proteins of this G-protein cascade, and then measured the enzyme activity after stimulation with light (at the level normal to retinal cells). Control vesicles were made of membrane fats with 18:0–22:6ω-3 fatty acid pairs (which is the dominant membrane fat in retinal membranes). When they substituted 22:5ω-3 for 22:6ω-3 to make their vesicles, there was no change in enzyme activity per photon. However, when they substituted 22:5ω-6 for the 22:6ω-3, enzyme activity per photon was *halved*. In this experiment, it was the position of double-bonds and not the number of double-bonds in the membrane fatty acids that determined the amplification of the G-protein cascade. When the membrane was made with omega-3 fatty acid chains, it had twice the amplification compared to being made with equivalent omega-6 fatty acid chains (see note 56). The only difference between the two systems was that when carbons 19 and 20 in the fatty acid chain were connected by a "double-bond," the amplification of this G-protein cascade was twice the amplification when they were connected by a "single-bond." The interactions involved in the G-protein cascade don't all occur in the membrane; they take place between G-proteins (attached to the membrane) in the water compartment inside the cell.[59] Thus, this experiment also shows that changes deep in the middle of a membrane bilayer can significantly influence events occurring on the surface of the membrane.

The reason why this finding is so important is that over the years, "G-protein cascades" have been found to be very common in biology. They have two important features: (1) they amplify a signal from a "receptor" to an "effector," and (2) they can involve a wide variety of "receptors" and "effectors." The receptors are called "G-protein-coupled receptors" (GPCRs) and include receptors for a large number of signaling molecules including hormones, neurotransmitters, inflammatory mediators, and for the senses of taste, smell, touch, as well as sight. An indication of both their widespread occurrence and importance in biology is that, since 1947, nine Nobel Prizes have been awarded for various aspects of GPCR and G-protein signaling.[60]

I suggest the different effects of omega-3 and omega-6 described by this experiment are not restricted to the visual system and are likely widespread. For example, when rats are maintained on an omega-3 deficient (but omega-6 adequate) diet, they display not only visual deficiencies, but also loss of cognitive skills, as well as deficits in odor and spatial discrimination.[61] Such observations imply more widespread effects of omega balance on other G-protein cascades in other types of cells.

In the rat diet experiment, 22:6ω-3 was the most abundant of all omega-3 in membrane fats of all tissues, especially in the brain, where 22:6ω-3 on average constituted 97 percent of all brain omega-3. The high concentration of 22:6ω-3 in brain membranes likely maximizes the speed of other G-protein cascades such as those involved in neurotransmission at synapses.

An Important Membrane Fatty Acid: Arachidonic Acid, 20:4ω-6

Polyunsaturated fatty acids consumed in the diet are predominantly 18-carbon fatty acid molecules, while the PUFA in membranes include significant amounts of 20-carbon and 22-carbon fatty acid molecules. This diet-membrane difference applies to both omega-6 and omega-3 fats, but it is most pronounced for the omega-3, and it applies to both humans and rats. For example, in the US dietary survey of 1999–2000, more than 99 percent of omega-6 consumption was 18:2ω-6 and about 95 percent of the omega-3 consumed was 18:3ω-3 (see note 51). In the total blood lipids (both storage fats and membrane fats) of US citizens in 2003–2004, long-chain (20- and 22-carbon) fatty acids constituted more than one-fifth of omega-6 and more than three-quarters of omega-3 fatty acids.[62]

The processes involved in the elongation and desaturation of the 18-carbon PUFA to the longer-chain PUFA appear to take place predominantly (but not solely) in the liver, and this is the tissue where the enzymes involved in the transformation are most abundant.[63] The most common long-chain omega-3 in membranes is 22:6ω-3, while the most common long-chain omega-6 in membranes is 20:4ω-6, known as arachidonic acid. Once 20- and 22-carbon PUFA have been made from 18-carbon PUFA, they can become part of membrane fat molecules either via the de novo synthesis or the remodeling pathway. Investigations using rat liver cells suggest 22:6ω-3 enters membrane fat molecules predominantly via the de novo pathway, while 20:4ω-6 enters via the remodeling pathway (see note 44).

These two PUFA molecules seem to differ significantly in their role in membranes. For example, the human brain has about 5 grams of 22:6ω-3 and about 4 grams of 20:4ω-6. Although there is approximately same amount of these long-chain PUFA in the brain, they differ greatly in their turnover. The half-life of 22:6ω-3 molecules is 773 days compared to 147 days for 20:4ω-6 molecules. This difference corresponds to about 5mg per day for 22:6ω-3 compared to about 18mg per day for 20:4ω-6.[64]

The importance of 20:4ω-6 in membranes is illustrated by a couple of findings in rats. When 20:4ω-6 is available in the diet of rats, very little is metabolized for energy, compared with other fatty acids, and it is preferentially and strongly directed to incorporation into membrane fats, compared with other dietary fatty acids.[65] In the twelve-diet experiment with rats described previously (see note 57), an unexpected finding was that 20:4ω-6 was the fatty acid that showed the greatest variation in membrane composition of all fatty acids, although it was not available in the diet. In liver, the 20:4ω-6 content of membrane fats ranged from 13 percent to 31 percent between diet groups, in muscle the range was 7 percent to 21 percent, in heart it was 14 percent to 25 percent, in red blood cells it was 14 percent to 28 percent, while in plasma it was 8 percent to 28 percent. In all these tissues, it was by far the fatty acid that showed the greatest variation between the twelve diet groups. In all these tissues, 20:4ω-6 was more abundant in membrane fats than was 22:6ω-3. In brain, the tissue that showed the lowest variation with respect to diet (brain is the most homeostatically regulated of all tissues) 20:4ω-6 ranged from 9 percent to 11 percent, while 22:6ω-3 ranged from 12 percent to 14 percent of membrane fatty acids.

Neither of these long-chain polyunsaturated fatty acids was provided in the diet, which contained only 18-carbon PUFA. Another surprise in this study was the relationship between 20:4ω-6 content of membrane fats and diet content. Although all 20:4ω-6 in membrane fats has been made from 18:2ω-6 in the diet, for all tissues dietary omega-6 content (18:2ω-6 content) was a relatively *poor* predictor of membrane 20:4ω-6. The *best* predictor was diet omega balance. This result was consistent for all tissues. Whereas variation in diet omega-6 could explain, on average, about 38 percent of the variation in membrane 20:4ω-6 content, diet omega balance could explain about 90 percent of variation in membrane 20:4ω-6 content.[66] Two previously mentioned observations come to mind: (1) 20:4ω-6 enters membranes via membrane remodeling, and (2) the enzyme fundamentally responsible for such membrane remodeling (acyl-transferase) is specific for polyunsaturated fatty acids but is *poor* at differentiating between omega-6 and omega-3. This likely explains the strong predictive capacity of diet omega balance for ascertaining membrane 20:4ω-6 content.

All the diets in the twelve-diet rat experiment were moderate-fat (25 percent energy) diets. Does the strong influence of diet omega balance on membrane 20:4ω-6 content also occur at other levels of dietary fat? In his earlier experiments, Ralph Holman fed rats a fat-free diet and gave them mixtures of very small quantities of 18:2ω-6 and 18:3ω-3 directly into their mouth by use of a micro-syringe.[67] The total amount of fat provided averaged 0.9 percent of dietary energy, and when I compared the 20:4ω-6 content of brain, heart, and liver membrane fats relative to both 18:2ω-6 content and omega balance of the eighteen different mixtures in the diet, the same relationship is observed as for the medium-fat diets. Namely, even in very low-fat diets, the content of 20:4ω-6 in membranes is better predicted by diet omega balance than it is by diet omega-6 content.

During the remodeling of a membrane fat, whether an omega-3 or omega-6 is added to the membrane fat will depend upon the relative abundance of omega-3 and omega-6 in the environs of the enzyme. While the most abundant omega-3 and omega-6 fats in the diet are 18:3ω-3 and 18:2ω-6, quantitatively the most abundant omega-3 and omega-6 fats in membranes are 22:6ω-3 and 20:4ω-6. As we will see in the second part of this book, membrane 20:4ω-6 content is the source of several important signaling molecules that include, for example, mediators for inflammation, appetite, and fat cell development. Because the balance between omega-3 and omega-6 fats in the diet strongly influences the amount of 20:4ω-6 in membranes, it will also affect the production of these various signaling molecules which, in turn, will have health consequences.

The Omega-Story So Far

Before we start the Consequences and Solutions part of this book, let me summarize the omega-story so far (figure 5.6). In the twentieth century, it became obvious that neither omega-6 and omega-3 fats can be made by humans and both are thus separate essential requirements in our diet (chapter 1). Both are made by plants at the base of the food chain, and as a generalization, the "leaves" of plants are the original sources of omega-3 while the "seeds" of plants are the source of omega-6 fats. The balance between omega-3 and omega-6 in animal-based foods (meats and dairy) depends on the relative balance between "leaves" and "seeds" in the food of the particular animal (chapter 2). All evidence suggests our ancestors were omnivorous, and had a good balance between omega-3 and omega-6 fats in their diet (chapter 3). Changes over the last half-century have resulted in a dramatic increase in omega-6 fats at the expense of omega-3 fats in much of the developed world (chapter 4). In order to understand the effects that changes in the relative abundance of omega-6 and omega-3 fats in the modern diet may have, it is necessary to understand the structure and function of the bilayer membranes of cells and how diet omega balance affects the structure and function of cell membranes. The dominant omega-3 in membranes is 22:6ω-3, while the dominant omega-6 in membranes is 20:4ω-6. As a generalization, these two different polyunsaturated fats exert their main influence on biological systems by different pathways, with changes in membrane 22:6ω-3 affecting "movement" in biological membranes and 20:4ω-6 affecting a variety of signaling systems. (chapter 5). In the following chapters, the evidence concerning a range of chronic disease epidemics will be examined with the view to see whether there are any connections linking the relatively recent change in the omega balance of the modern food chain and the increased prevalence of ill-health.

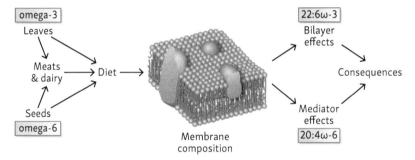

Figure 5.6 The omega story, so far. The presence of the labels "omega-3" and "omega-6" as well as "22:6ω-3" and "20:4ω-6" in their respective locations signify generalized and not absolute differences.

PART II

CONSEQUENCES
and
SOLUTIONS

CHAPTER 6

OBESITY AND DIABETES

The Obesity Epidemic Is Not a Morality Tale

The "obesity epidemic" is sometimes presented as a morality tale: too much gluttony, too much sloth. The response of many is "just control yourself, eat less, and exercise more." Yet it is not this simple.

Body Mass Index (BMI), often used to classify whether an individual is obese, is calculated as body mass (kg) divided by the square of the individual's height (m) with BMI = kg/m². Values above 30 are conventionally regarded as "obese." While the BMI has the advantage that it is an easily determined diagnostic, it is not a perfect indicator, as it has the disadvantage that it is influenced by body build. Such a disadvantage, however, does not apply for comparisons over time of populations with the same body build. Many studies show that there has been a dramatic increase in the prevalence of obesity over the last half-century. It is often referred to as an "obesity epidemic."[1]

Although there is no agreed explanation for this epidemic, the most common explanations are "excessive food intake" and "inadequate exercise," but these explanations are essentially superficial truisms about weight change. Individuals maintaining their weight constant, whether lean or obese, are by definition in "energy balance." The question really is: Why do some individuals regulate around a high body fat content and others regulate around a low body fat content?

We are more complicated systems than the simple "energy in–energy out" concept implies. First, we don't eat energy; we eat food, and not all energy in food is equally available. For example, both sugar and fiber are carbohydrates, but they differ in their provision of energy. Similarly, the "energy-out" pathway is not restricted to exercise, and non-exercise activities such as basal metabolism, the processing of food (especially protein) are significant components of energy expenditure.

Although we metabolize the protein, carbohydrate, and fat in our food to obtain energy, when we store energy, it is primarily as fat. We do not "store" protein, but during starvation, we consume body protein to make glucose molecules for energy.[2] In the normal situation carbohydrate and protein excess to our energy needs is converted to "storage fat." This storage of energy as fat is not simply leftover unused energy but involves complicated biochemical and physiological processes.

Food intake is governed by appetite (the desire to eat) and satiety (cessation of this desire), regulated by neural and hormonal signals involving the brain, the digestive tract, and adipose tissue. Nerve cells of the hypothalamus, one of the main regulatory centers, are influenced by hormones from both the digestive system and adipose tissue to modulate food-seeking behavior. Ghrelin, secreted by the stomach, stimulates food-seeking behavior, while leptin, secreted by adipose tissue, inhibits food-seeking behavior. Obesity was important in the discovery of these appetite and satiety regulatory pathways. In 1949, the sudden appearance of obese individuals in a breeding colony of normal-sized mice signaled the appearance of a mutation in the gene later identified as being the gene for "leptin." In the 1960s, the unexpected appearance of obese mice in a normal-sized colony signified a mutation in the gene for the brain "receptor" for leptin. Leptin would no longer bind to this "altered" receptor, and thus food intake was not inhibited.[3]

Obesity is a multi-factorial disease, and not all cases of obesity will have the same cause. For some individuals, there will be a genetic or hormonal basis to their obesity. However, the increased prevalence of obesity over recent times suggests that it is not due to genetic changes or hormonal imbalances; rather, environmental change has driven this epidemic. Is it sloth, gluttony, or something else?

Low Energy Expenditure, High Food Intake,
or Something Else?

The assumption that obesity is associated with a low energy expenditure is likely incorrect. For example, one study compared energy expenditure in lean individuals (BMI = 23) with three groups of progressively obese individuals (BMIs = 32, 38, 46).[4] Comparing the "most obese" and the "lean" groups, the investigators found that total daily energy expenditure averaged 14 megajoules in "most obese" but only 10 megajoules in "lean" individuals. Resting metabolic rate constituted 58 percent of total energy expenditure in the "most obese" and 55 percent in "lean" individuals. Obesity was associated with less voluntary physical activity with, for example, the "most obese" averaging about 6,600 steps per day compared to about 10,000 steps per day in lean individuals. However, because of the greater body mass that needs to be moved, the calculated daily energy expenditure associated with activity was greater in the "most obese" group (about 4.4 megajoules) compared to "lean" individuals (about 3.5 megajoules).

Another study also measured total energy expenditure in lean and obese subjects and compared it to "self-reported" food intake.[5] Total energy expenditure was 11 megajoules in lean adults compared to 12 megajoules in obese adults. Self-reported daily food intake averaged 9 megajoules for lean adults and 7 megajoules for the obese adults, and is obviously thus not a reliable indicator of energy expenditure. Intriguingly, although obese individuals self-reported a *lower* daily food energy intake than the lean humans, their actual measured energy expenditure was *greater* than the non-obese individuals.

Reality television has not ignored the obesity epidemic, and following its inception in 2004, the program *The Biggest Loser* has been franchised around the world. The program subjected very obese individuals to a period of vigorous exercise and a reduced food intake in order to lose weight in a competitive format. For the fourteen original contestants (BMI = 50), the average weight loss after 30 weeks was 58kg, of which 47kg was body fat and 11kg was lean body mass.

At the beginning, their daily total energy expenditure averaged 16 megajoules; after 30 weeks, it was 13 megajoules.[6] Although it was "exercise" that featured on television, the reduced food intake is estimated to be responsible for about 55 percent of weight loss, with the increase in vigorous exercise responsible for about 45 percent.[7]

Although physical activity is beneficial for good health in general, and increased physical activity is used in many weight-loss programs, the role of physical activity in obesity is not as simple as the naïve observer may think. Others have made a case that reduction in physical activity does not influence the risk of obesity in individuals.[8] A common experience after weight loss is that despite conscious effort to avoid it, the lost weight is regained over time. For example, when the fourteen *Biggest Loser* contestants were reexamined six years after their initial weight loss success, they had regained 41kg (about 70 percent of their initial loss) (see note 6). This suggests that although a new body weight was achieved at the end of the TV program, the "set-point" for body mass was relatively unchanged, resulting in a return to the obese state during the following years.

I am not convinced that reduced physical activity is the cause of the "obesity epidemic," and, for a number of reasons, I suggest the decreased omega balance of the modern food chain is at least partly responsible. There are at least three possible mechanisms that can connect a low diet omega balance to obesity; I will consider these in more detail shortly. The increase in obesity has also been associated with other chronic diseases, with obesity often described as a "risk factor" for these diseases. Obesity is not the cause of the other "epidemics," and such associations should be more properly simply described as "correlations." For me, there are a number of diseases that have increased in recent times (sometimes described as "epidemics") that can all plausibly be explained by changes in the omega balance of the human food chain.

The link between diet omega balance and the other disease epidemics will be covered in later chapters. This chapter considers obesity and will also consider the "epidemic" often closely associated with obesity—namely, diabetes. But before these considerations, I want to examine another commonly believed cause of obesity: that there is *too much* fat in the modern diet.

High-Fat Diets?

"Eating lots of fat will make you fat" is a common belief. The general public has been told for a long time there is a problem with "fat" in the diet. For example, the amount of shelf-space devoted to "low-fat" or "reduced-fat" dairy products in today's supermarkets exceeds that devoted to normal "full-fat" dairy. Similarly, the advertising that a product is "99 percent fat-free" rather than being described as having "1 percent fat" is another illustration.

Initially, it was not "obesity" but "heart disease" that was associated with a high-fat diet. In 1952, Ancel Keys published a graph of deaths from heart disease for six countries against fat as a percentage of the national diet. This famous graph showed a dramatic upward curve that was understandably alarming. Keys proposed the "diet-heart" hypothesis, which for various reasons, dominated the following years, and although he was most concerned with the influence of high-fat diets on heart disease, he also thought they would make humans fat. Keys featured on the cover of the magazine *Time* in 1961, and in the same year the American Heart Association recommended a "low-fat diet" for heart health reasons. This report suggested that "animal fats" should be replaced with "vegetable oils" because they contained less saturated fat. Low-fat diets contained less energy per gram and were also thought to be beneficial for losing weight. In 1977, the US Senate Select Committee on Nutrition and Human Needs published *Dietary Goals for the United States,* which proposed that too much fat is "directly linked to heart disease, cancer, obesity and stroke." For the first time, the government suggested the US population eat fewer high-fat foods and suggested they substitute nonfat milk for whole milk. A further important influence came in 1983, when an article based on extensive study of heart disease cited obesity as a risk factor. Dietary fat was increasingly blamed for obesity as well as heart disease.[9]

Although, at the time, this demonization of "fat" was challenged by some (for example, by John Yudkin),[10] it became what could be reasonably described as dogma in the 1980s and beyond. In recent times, this dogma has been increasingly challenged. Two science journalists have produced works of merit in this challenge; Gary Taubes with his *Good Calories, Bad Calories*[11] and Nina Teicholz with *The Big Fat Surprise*.[12]

While the quantity of fat in the human diet is not as important for ill-health as previously thought, diets described as being "high-fat" are still used as a common experimental treatment to produce obesity in laboratory rodents. Unfortunately, this description is misleading, not in describing the diet as being "high-fat" but in paying no attention to the type of fat in the diet, and specifically to its omega balance. It has encouraged the continuation of the simplistic "eating fat will make you fat" belief.

High-fat diets were first used in the 1940s and have become the standard method of inducing obesity in laboratory rodents. Almost 10,000 scientific papers were published in the decade 2004 to 2014 that featured the feeding of "high-fat" diets to laboratory animals.[13] Unfortunately, almost all use "vegetable oils" as the source of dietary fat. Commercial providers of food for laboratory rodents offer a number of "high-fat" diets; for example, I calculated the average omega balance of seven "Teklad Custom Research Diets for diet induced obesity" (available in 2018) to be 6 percent.[14] As part of her PhD project, one of my former students calculated the omega balance of high-fat diets used by scientific researchers in 2008. She found the average omega balance was 7 percent, and the median omega balance was just 4 percent.[15]

There are challenges in translating the "high-fat-fed" rodent model to human obesity. One is that few investigators pay attention to the type of fat in the diet. Another is that not all strains of laboratory rodents become obese on a high-fat diet.[16] In one study comparing seven different high-fat (60 percent energy) diets fed to mice, the diets varied only in the source of the fat. [17] The mice fed high-fat diets with a high omega balance both gained the least weight and had the least body fat. Mice fed the high-fat diet using fish oil, had a weight gain *lower* than that of control mice fed a low-fat diet (11 percent energy) even though they ate the most food. This demonstrates it is not the *amount* of fat but rather the *type* of fat in the diet that determines whether obesity results in these rodents.

Diet Omega Balance and Human Obesity

There have been many experiments on laboratory rodents but fewer on humans. The only study I know of that has examined effects of changing diet omega balance in non-obese humans is one from the mid-1990s in which healthy non-obese adults (BMI = 22) were fed a control diet, ad libitum for three weeks and their food intake, metabolic rate, and body fat were measured. Ten to 12 weeks later, they were fed the same diet for three weeks except that daily 6g of the visible fat was replaced with 6g of fish oil. They lost more body fat during the "fish oil" period than during the "control" period, without any change in food intake nor metabolic rate. [18]

Studies examining the effect of diet omega balance on obese subjects outnumber those on non-obese subjects. In one study, obese women (BMI = 30) were provided with either 3g per day fish-oil capsules or placebo capsules for two months. At the end of this period, blood plasma omega balance was 15 percent in the fish-oil group and 9 percent in the placebo group. Although there was no change in food intake, the fish-oil group lost more body fat and had smaller fat cells than the placebo group. [19]

In 2004–2005, a multinational study (Iceland, Spain, and Ireland) prescribed a 30 percent energy-restricted diet for obese adults (BMI = 30) which were randomly divided into four groups; (1) the control group had sunflower oil capsules but no fish, (2) one experimental group had fish-oil capsules but no fish, (3) another experimental group had lean fish (cod), and (4) the other experimental group consumed oily fish (salmon). After eight weeks, the three groups that consumed either fish oil or fish had a significantly greater weight loss (about 1kg greater) than the non-fish control group. The red blood cell omega balance differences were relatively small but were 25 percent in the control group compared to 27 percent for the lean-fish group and 30 percent for the fish oil and oily-fish groups.[20] A smaller Australian study confirms that fish oil supplementation can significantly enhance weight loss when obese subjects go on an energy-restricted diet.[21]

Use of fish or fish oil in the diet is not the only omega-3 treatment facilitating weight loss in humans. Flaxseed (also known as linseed) has an omega balance of 79 percent, with all of the omega-3 being 18:3ω-3. A meta-analysis of randomized controlled trials concluded that diet supplementation with whole flaxseed results in a significant decrease in BMI, as well as a decrease in waist circumference and body weight.[22] Evidence from experiments that directly increase the omega balance of the diet shows that such interventions can decrease obesity.

Membrane Omega Balance and Human Obesity

Descriptive evidence of a mechanistic link between omega balance and obesity would be provided if obese individuals differed in membrane fat composition compared to non-obese individuals.

When an Australian group of researchers combined data for individuals from three populations for which they had both membrane fatty acid composition of skeletal muscle and BMI, they found a strong inverse correlation between membrane omega balance and BMI. They found that a muscle omega balance of 19 percent is associated with a BMI = 24 (non-obese), while an omega balance of 2 percent is associated with a BMI = 40 (obese).[23]

In 2005, I was awarded a Fulbright Senior Scholar award and traveled to City College, New York to jointly investigate, with Rochelle

Buffenstein, the membrane fat composition of the naked mole-rat (*Heterocephalus glaber*), the longest-living rodent. Being a zoologist, my research has involved a wide variety of different animal species, and although I was developing a burgeoning interest in topics such as human obesity, until 2005 my research had never involved human subjects. While in New York, the possibility arose to obtain tissue samples from humans undergoing obesity surgery. After the various ethics approvals, and payment of the appropriate costs and fees, I obtained tissue samples and measured the fatty acid composition of "membrane fats" and "storage fats" from skeletal muscle (from the surgical incision), adipose tissue, and blood plasma from eighteen obesity-surgery patients (average BMI = 45).[24] For every tissue, these obese subjects had *lower* omega balance value than that reported in the literature for non-obese individuals. For membrane fats from muscle, the omega balance of obese subjects was 3 percent compared to 9 percent for non-obese controls; for adipose tissue the comparison was 5 percent versus 8 percent, and for plasma it was 9 percent versus 14 percent. For storage fats, the comparisons were: 4 percent versus 12 percent for muscle, 5 percent versus 10 percent for adipose tissue, and 5 percent versus 10 percent for plasma.

Other investigators have also reported that tissues from obese individuals differ in membrane fatty acid composition compared to those from non-obese humans. The omega balance is reduced in the membrane fats of liver,[25] red blood cells,[26] and plasma or serum[27] from obese subjects compared to non-obese controls.

Why should a low omega balance of membrane fats be associated with obesity? When presented with a correlation, for me scientific curiosity requires a feasible mechanism to explain the correlation. There are at least three possible ways that a low diet omega balance might result in obesity: (1) omega-6 enhanced adipogenesis, (2) omega-6 enhanced production of endocannabinoids, and (3) omega-6 enhanced conversion of diet carbohydrate to storage fats.

Omega-6 Fats and the Development of Fat Cells

The amount of adipose tissue in a human body is determined by the number of fat cells (adipocytes) and the average size of these fat cells. Adipocytes specialize in storing energy as storage fats (triglycerides) and are made from pre-adipocytes that lack the capacity to make storage fat. The process of cell differentiation is called "adipogenesis" and is one of the most intensely investigated processes of cell differentiation and proliferation. Gerard Ailhaud and colleagues have drawn attention to the fact that products made from $20:4\omega\text{-}6$ are important factors in stimulating adipogenesis. He has suggested that the recent shift in the human food chain emphasizing omega-6 fats at the expense of the omega-3 fats is an important contributor to the obesity epidemic through the effects of such omega-6 metabolites on the development and proliferation of adipose tissue.[28]

In humans, the number of adipocytes increases during childhood and adolescence, but after the age of about 20 remains relatively constant for the remainder of adulthood. The number of adipocytes varies between obese and non-obese individuals, with obese adults estimated to have 75 billion adipocytes compared to 45 billion in non-obese adults.[29] Most obese adults have been obese since childhood, with over three-quarters of obese children becoming obese adults, while less than 10 percent of normal-weight children go on to develop adult obesity.[30] Growth in adipocyte number begins earlier in obese children (at the age of 2 compared with 6 in non-obese children) and also ends earlier (about 17 compared with 19). During this period of growth, the relative increase in adipocyte number in obese children is about twice that in the non-obese children (see note 29).

Although the number of adipocytes during adult life is relatively constant, there is a continual turnover of them in both obese and non-obese individuals. This was revealed by using the nearly two-fold increase in radioactive ^{14}C in the atmosphere from 1955 to 1963, due to above-ground testing of nuclear weapons. This ^{14}C entered the food chain and consequently human DNA, and after a cell has gone through its last cell division, its DNA is stable and the relative abundance of ^{14}C in its DNA can thus be used to date the time of birth of the cell. Measurement of the ^{14}C in DNA of adipocytes from humans born both before and after the nuclear tests revealed that fat cells are continually dying and being replaced during adult life. There was no difference in the turnover of adipocytes between obese and non-obese adults, with about 8 percent of adipocytes dying and being replaced every year. In both obese and lean humans, the average age of an individual fat cell was nearly 10 years. The production rate of adipocytes is estimated to be about 8 billion cells per year in obese compared to about 3 billion cells per year in lean humans (see note 29).

When humans lose weight, it is largely due to a reduction in the size rather than the number of adipocytes. Following bariatric surgery (reduction of the stomach to facilitate reduced food energy intake) subjects exhibited loss of body weight and a change in fat cell volume but no change in the total number of fat cells in their body (see note 29). It is this constancy of fat cell number that is probably the reason why the common response following major weight loss is a slow return to original body weight. Dieting can shrink fat cells but not eliminate them.

The metabolites of 20:4ω-6 involved in the stimulation of adipogenesis are called prostacyclins, and they stimulate the conversion of pre-adipocytes to adipocytes through cell membrane receptors as well as receptors in the cell nucleus that control the genes involved in the production of mature fat cells.[31] While several studies using rats and mice show that diet omega balance influences adipose tissue development, the experimental evidence is more limited for human adipocytes. For example, addition of 18:3ω-3 to the diet of rats prevents the growth of adipose tissue.[32]

Additional evidence of a connection between omega balance and human obesity includes a study of mother-young pairs from midpregnancy to three years after birth. Obesity of the children (at age 3) was significantly associated with the relative abundance of omega-6 and omega-3 in umbilical cord blood collected at the time of their birth. The lower the omega balance of cord blood lipids, the greater the degree of obesity in the 3-year-old child.[33] A study of 10- to 12-year-old children from Cyprus and Crete showed that the 20:4ω-6 content of adipose tissue fats was significantly correlated with their BMI.[34] Another study that examined the newborn of mothers who had elected not to breast-feed also found a relationship between 20:4ω-6 content of blood plasma fats and body weight at 120 days of age. The newborn babies were fed different milk formulas that varied in omega balance from 2 percent to 17 percent, and at 120 days of age there was both significantly lower 20:4ω-6 in the plasma, as well as a lower body weight (by about 1kg) of the babies fed the high omega balance milk formula.[35]

A 1966 study involved elderly males living in an institution, with a control group that ate the normal institution diet (40 percent energy as fat), while the experimental group had the same diet but with vegetable oil replacing the saturated fat in the control diet. The experimental group gained weight over the following year, and the elderly men with the greatest increases in 18:2ω-6 content showed the largest gains in body weight.[36]

Experimental data on laboratory animals and some more limited data on humans supports Ailhaud's proposal that the obesity epidemic can be partly explained by increased adipogenesis associated with increased omega-6 (that is, a lower omega balance) in the food chain. One of the most worrying aspects of this link is that it suggests that if the diet of children has a low omega balance, the consequence is that more adipocytes are produced during childhood and adolescence, and likely destines the individual to a continual and difficult battle to control body weight throughout their adult life.

"Munchies" and the Endocannabinoids

Cannabis has a record in China as a plant cultivated since Neolithic times, about 6,000 years ago, for textile, food, and medicinal purposes.[37] Reports that cannabis use stimulates appetite, the "munchies" of modern times, date from AD 300,[38] but it was only in 1964 that the active ingredient of cannabis was isolated and identified as tetra-hydrocannabinol (THC).[39] The search for how THC might exert its effects led to the discovery in 1988 of a specific cannabinoid receptor (CB1) in the rat brain,[40] and this was followed by the discovery of a second receptor (CB2) in 1993.[41] The discovery of these receptors raised a question. THC is a plant product and not made by animals; thus obviously the receptors were unlikely evolved for use by THC. What were the normal molecules in an animal's body for these cannabinoid receptors? There must be an *endocannabinoid* that can bind to these membrane-located receptors. One, identified in 1992 was called "anandamide" (AEA),[42] and another, identified in 1995, was called "2-arachidonoylglycerol" (2-AG).[43]

A very significant fact is that both endocannabinoids are made from membrane fats that contain 20:4ω-6. Together, the endocannabinoids, their receptors, and the separate enzyme systems responsible for their synthesis and degradation make up the "endocannabinoid system." This system has been much researched over recent decades, and it has become apparent that the system is more widespread than originally thought. As well as being part of appetite- and satiation-control systems, it is intimately involved with lots of physiological systems having neurological, immunological, cardiovascular, and psychiatric effects as well as influencing food intake.[44]

A seminal example of the endocannabinoid system regulating food intake is manifest in the observation that blocking the CB1 receptors in newborn mice abolishes the suckling reflex and consequent ingestion of milk.[45] Endocannabinoids have been measured in the milk of many species, including humans, and it has been suggested they are important factors in maintaining food intake by suckling young.[46]

The endocannabinoids can modulate taste and smell sensations and act via different brain regions to stimulate food intake. Injection of endocannabinoids into the hypothalamic and mesolimbic regions of the rat brain stimulate food intake. The hypothalamus is the brain region for maintaining "homeostasis," while the mesolimbic system is the brain region for "reward." Although both endocannabinoids are made from 20:4ω-6, and both stimulate food intake, they have separate identities to some extent. There are two types of "appetite"; one is driven by energy shortage and has been called "homeostatic" appetite, while the other is driven by pleasure and is called "hedonic" appetite because it is reward-driven. While AEA seems to be associated with "homeostatic" feeding, 2-AG is more associated with hedonic feeding.[47]

Research shows that the endocannabinoid system and obesity are strongly connected, and although I have concentrated on food intake here, the endocannabinoids have other relevant effects including stimulation of fat accumulation by adipose tissue. Although measurement of circulating endocannabinoids is a common method of assessing the activity of the endocannabinoid system activity because they are rapidly synthesized and degraded in many tissues, it is not clear that blood levels of endocannabinoids are useful biomarkers of their concentration in tissues such as the brain.[48] Nevertheless, in recent times several studies have compared blood endocannabinoid levels in lean and obese humans. Some report significantly greater levels of both AEA and 2-AG in obese individuals,[49] some report significant increases only in AEA,[50] while others report significant increases only in 2-AG.[51] None report lower levels of endocannabinoids in obesity.

Is the association of higher levels of circulating endocannabinoids with obesity cause or effect? Does abundant adipose tissue result in greater synthesis of endocannabinoids? Or, does a high level of circulating endocannabinoids result in more adipose tissue? The observation that mice without the CB1 receptor do not develop diet-induced obesity[52] suggests that obesity is the result of elevated circulating endocannabinoids and not the reverse. Similarly, mice with their CB1 receptors blocked by the inhibitor Rimonabant also do not develop diet-induced obesity.[53]

The endocannabinoid receptor inhibitor Rimonabant was developed in 1994, only six years after the discovery of the CB1 receptor, and was proposed as one of the first anti-obesity drugs. Following

Phase 3 trials it was approved by the European Union in 2006 as an anti-obesity drug. In 2007, the US Food and Drug Administration rejected it because of concerns about adverse psychiatric side-effects (increased anxiety). The European authority removed their approval in 2008, and many pharmaceutical companies suspended their research into CB1 receptor inhibitors as potential anti-obesity drugs.[54] The pharmaceutical approach dominates our approach to medical conditions, often at the expense of diet modification. Because the endocannabinoids are manufactured from membrane 20:4ω-6, which is elevated by a low diet omega balance (see chapter 5), understanding the influence of dietary omega-6 and omega-3 on many of the other endocannabinoid effects, especially those connected with mental health, is in my opinion, an exciting future frontier. But back to obesity and the endocannabinoids.

Several investigators have shown that low omega balance diets (more omega-6 relative to omega-3) are associated with higher endocannabinoid levels in a number of tissues.[55] One study deserves particular mention because it concluded that it is the amount of 18:2ω-6 (and *not* the total amount of fat) in the diet that elevates endocannabinoid levels and induces obesity.[56] It also demonstrated that diet omega balance influences endocannabinoid levels when only 18-carbon polyunsaturated fats make up the diet.

Human experiments show the same influence of diet omega balance on endocannabinoid levels as those with laboratory rodents. Feeding of krill oil to obese humans for four weeks reduced plasma 2-AG levels with a significant relationship between omega balance of plasma fats and 2-AG concentrations.[57] Similarly, krill powder fed to mildly-obese men for 24 weeks dramatically reduced plasma AEA concentrations.[58]

I find one human study especially enjoyable because the experimental treatment involved changes at the base of the food chain. It involved comparing consumption of normal sheep cheese (Pecorino cheese) with consuming the same type of cheese made from sheep fed a linseed-enriched diet. The respective omega balance of the two cheeses were 21 percent and 48 percent. The experiment had a crossover design, and when subjects included 90g per day of the enriched cheese in their normal diet for three weeks, they had a reduced plasma AEA (about 40 percent lower) than when their diet included the same amount of nonenriched cheese.[59] Because other fatty acids in the cheeses also changed, it is not possible to definitively ascertain that the higher omega balance was responsible for the reduced endocannabinoid concentration.

In conclusion, there is a strong connection between diet omega balance, the endocannabinoid system, and obesity. An increased diet omega-6 relative to omega-3 results in elevated endocannabinoid activity and greater obesity. Part of the explanation for the obesity epidemic is likely a diet-induced "munchies" due to a reduced omega balance of the modern diet.

Role of PUFA in Making Fat from Excess Dietary Carbohydrates

This is the third potential mechanism whereby diet omega balance will influence the development of obesity. A diet low in omega-3 but high in omega-6 will enhance the production of "storage fats" from dietary carbohydrate.

The process of making "new" fat molecules is called *lipogenesis* (the creation of fat). There are three important enzymes involved, called ACC, FAS, and SCD.[60] All cells have the metabolic machinery for lipogenesis, but it is especially emphasized in two tissues: liver and adipose tissue. The three enzymes—ACC, FAS, and SCD—are essential to convert excess carbohydrate into fat, and when this process is required, more of these enzymes are produced in liver and adipose tissue. Because of the difficulty of measuring the process of lipogenesis in adipose tissue, most of our knowledge is limited to lipogenesis in the liver. The new storage fat molecules made by lipogenesis leave the liver as part of the VLDL (very low-density lipoprotein) particles and are then generally transferred to adipose tissue for longer-term energy storage.

In humans, lipogenesis is a minor pathway under normal dietary conditions. For example, it is estimated to produce only 1–2g fat per day compared to 50–150g fat per day in the diet.[61] Carbohydrate intake is first used to (1) increase glycogen (the storage form of glucose) in liver and muscle and (2) to produce energy. It is only when carbohydrate intake exceeds total energy requirements that its conversion to storage fat (through lipogenesis) becomes significant. Comparison of lipogenesis in non-obese and obese humans eating a normal diet showed the process produced about 2g per day in non-obese individuals and about 6g per day in obese subjects.[62] Although lipogenesis normally appears to be a relatively minor contributor, there is an indication that the balance between omega-3 and omega-6 fats in the diet influences this pathway. A low omega balance diet (one emphasizing omega-6 fat at the expense of omega-3) will boost the conversion of carbohydrate to storage fat. I don't know of an experiment that has investigated this proposal in humans but want to share with you the results from an experiment on mice.

In this experiment, mice were fed one of three diets which all had identical protein content.[63] One diet was a high-carbohydrate, low-fat diet, while the other two diets were high-fat, low-carbohydrate diets that differed in the type of fat (high omega-6 safflower oil versus high omega-3 fish oil). In this experiment, the two high-fat diets had *opposite* effects. The high omega-6 diet resulted in increased body fat, while the high omega-3 diet resulted in reduced body fat. Compared to the high-carbohydrate fed mice, those mice fed the high-fat omega-6 diet had *increased* levels of storage fat in their liver (48 percent increase), plasma (40 percent increase), and adipose tissue (250 percent increase). The mice fed the high-fat omega-3 diet had a *decreased* level of storage fat in liver (43 percent less), plasma (10 percent less), and adipose tissue (one-third less) compared to the high-carbohydrate fed mice.

This dramatic difference between the two high-fat diets was manifest in changes in the enzymes responsible for lipogenesis. Understandably, the mice fed the high-carbohydrate diet had the highest message levels for the three lipogenic enzymes. While the message levels to produce these enzymes were reduced in both low-carbohydrate, high-fat diets, the level of reduction was much greater in the high omega-3 diet compared to the high omega-6 diet.[64] This difference indicates a reduced capacity to convert excess dietary carbohydrate to body fat stores on an omega-3 diet compared to an omega-6 diet.

In conclusion, there are at least three possible means by which a low diet omega balance will favor the development of obesity; (1) increased production of fat cells, (2) enhanced appetite and food intake, and (3) enhanced ability to convert excess diet carbohydrate to body fat. The evidence suggests all three mechanisms are involved. Of course, there also may be others.

The Diabetes Epidemic: Emergence of Syndrome X

Diabetes is one of the earliest described diseases, being first recognized as the passing of very large amounts of urine. It was noticed that for some people with diabetes, their urine attracted ants because it was sweet. These individuals were diagnosed to have *Diabetes mellitus* (*mellitus* = honey). Although diabetes has been recognized for a long time, the understanding of its causes, and the ability to treat it date from only the last century. Initially, it was discovered that groups of cells ("islets") in the pancreas produced a substance that remedied the symptoms and the lethality of diabetes in dogs. This substance was called *insulin* after the Latin word for *island*.

There are two types of *Diabetes mellitus*. Type 1 was initially described as "juvenile-onset diabetes" as it usually appeared in young patients of normal or less-than-normal body weight, who had little or no insulin in their blood. Type 2 was initially described as "mature-onset diabetes" because it usually appeared in middle age or later in patients who were often obese and had significant (sometimes very large) amounts of insulin in their plasma. In 1936, Harold Himsworth showed the two types differed fundamentally in that Type 1 diabetics are "insulin-sensitive," while Type 2 are "insulin-resistant."[65] Type 2 diabetes is the more common form (more than 90 percent) and is no longer described as "mature-onset" because it is increasingly being diagnosed in young individuals and is associated with obesity.

Insulin-resistance is the basis of Type 2 diabetes, and after many years investigating this and other conditions, Gerald Reaven was invited to give the 1988 Banting Lecture. In this lecture, Reaven drew together a number of conditions: (1) resistance to insulin-stimulated glucose uptake, (2) glucose intolerance, (3) hyperinsulinemia, (4) increased blood VLDL (very low-density lipoprotein) triglyceride, (5) decreased blood HDL (high-density lipoprotein) cholesterol, (6) high blood pressure, and together labeled them "Syndrome X."[66] He proposed that resistance to insulin-stimulated glucose uptake was the cause of three related diseases: Type 2 diabetes, hypertension, and coronary artery disease. Although his initial proposal did not include "obesity," because Type 2 diabetes was already associated with obesity, it rapidly also became part of the syndrome. For a variety of reasons, "Syndrome X" was later renamed the "Metabolic Syndrome."

Metabolic Syndrome, Insulin Resistance, and Membranes

In some ways, this is where this book begins. In the late 1980s, I met Len Storlien, and he introduced me to "Syndrome X." Up until this time, I had paid little attention to medical research. Storlien had researched insulin-resistance in rats and had used the standard high-fat (59 percent energy) feeding paradigm to produce obesity and insulin-resistance in his rats.[67] To make his diets, he had used safflower oil (because of its easy availability), which is the same vegetable oil used to intravenously feed Shawna Strobel, highlighted at the beginning of this book. Safflower oil contains only omega-6 and no omega-3 fats. Storlien had come across a 1971 paper about the blood lipids of Greenland Inuit and was struck by the comment that diabetes mellitus was extremely rare in Greenlanders. This inspired him to examine the influence of the high omega-3 fish oils on insulin-resistance in his rats. When he replaced some of the safflower oil in the rat diet with fish oil, his rats no longer became insulin-resistant.[68] This was remarkable: the development of insulin resistance was dependent not on the *amount* of fat but on the *type* of fat in the diet. If the diet omega balance was 0 percent, then the rats became insulin-resistant, but if the diet omega balance was 20 percent (my calculations), then no insulin-resistance developed.

Later Storlien and colleagues compared six different diets to explore which type of dietary fat might be particularly important.[69] The concept of omega balance was not used at the time (1991), so I have calculated the omega balance of the diets they used. Three of the diets had minimal omega-3 (omega balances of 0, 1, and 7 percent), and all three diets resulted in insulin-resistant rats. Of the remaining diets, one repeated the earlier fish-oil diet (omega balance of about 20 percent) and, as previously, produced rats that were sensitive to insulin. The other two diets used 18:3ω-3 (from linseed oil) as the source of omega-3. In one, the linseed oil was mixed with safflower oil (high in omega-6) while in the other diet, it was mixed with tallow (high in saturated fat). The omega balances of these diets were, respectively, 15 percent and 68 percent. The rats on the linseed-safflower oil diet were insulin-resistant, while those that ate the linseed-tallow diet were sensitive to insulin. This detailed study demonstrated that in rats, normal insulin-sensitivity requires a diet omega balance of about 20 percent or greater. Storlien's research also showed that the different diets resulted in different amounts of 22-carbon omega-3 in muscle membranes, which in turn was strongly associated with the insulin-sensitivity of the muscle. This study also showed that the omega-3 in the diet did not need to come from fish oil but could be in the form of 18:3ω-3 (as long as there was little competing omega-6 in the diet). Other researchers have also shown that substituting 18:3ω-3 for 18:2ω-6 in the diet of rats improves insulin sensitivity.[70] Both of these rat studies emphasize that it is not the presence of omega-3 per se but that rather it is the *relative balance* between omega-3 and omega-6 in the diet that is important in determining whether tissues are responsive to insulin.

What about insulin-resistance in humans? Insulin is a protein hormone and thus not able to enter cells. It is secreted into the blood in response to elevated blood glucose and exerts its effects by binding to the *insulin receptor* on the cell membranes of responsive cells. The main tissues that respond to insulin are muscle cells, fat cells, and liver cells. The membrane surrounding each of these cell types contains insulin receptors that span the membrane bilayer. When insulin binds to the part of the insulin receptor outside the cell, the insulin receptor is changed, and the part of the insulin receptor inside the cell initiates certain actions. In muscle and fat cells, these actions allow glucose molecules to enter the cell and thus lower the blood glucose level. This is an important negative-feedback process responsible for blood glucose homeostasis. The "gold standard" way to measure insulin-resistance is to measure the entry of glucose into the cells of the body in response to the blood insulin level. If the muscle and fat cells are "insulin-resistant," blood glucose will rise, and, in response, the pancreas will secrete more insulin with the consequence that insulin-resistance is associated with elevated levels of blood insulin (*hyperinsulinemia*). The measurement of "fasting blood insulin" is sometimes used as an indicator of insulin-resistance. The higher the "fasting blood insulin" the more insulin-resistant the individual.

As noted by Storlien, the absence of *Diabetes mellitus* in Greenland Inuit suggested that a diet high in omega-3 was protective against insulin-resistance in humans. Changes in the fatty acid composition of the membrane bilayer surrounding the insulin receptor is a possible mechanism for insulin-resistance, and Storlien and colleagues measured the membrane fatty acid composition of muscle samples from three groups of humans that had varying levels of insulin-resistance. From the first group (healthy Australian adults undergoing elective surgery), they obtained an abdominal muscle sample as well as a blood sample following an overnight fast.[71] The second group (healthy normal Australian volunteers) provided a fasting blood sample and muscle biopsy sample and had their insulin-resistance measured by the "gold-standard" method described previously (see note 71). The third group consisted of volunteer Pima Indians participating in a longitudinal study of the development of Type 2 diabetes.[72] The Pima Indians of Arizona had the highest reported incidence of Type 2 diabetes in the world.[73] The Storlien group found several correlations between muscle fatty acid composition and insulin-resistance. Here, I will concentrate on one relationship observed when the results of all three groups were combined. They observed a statistically strong relationship between fasting blood insulin values and the omega-6:omega-3 ratio of muscle membrane fats.[74] Using fasting insulin as a measure of insulin resistance and converting the ratio values to omega balances, the relationship can be described thus: insulin resistance is low at omega balances of about 15 percent but gradually increases as muscle membrane omega balance decreases from 15 to 5 percent; muscle membrane omega balance values less than 5 percent are associated with substantial insulin-resistance. These human results are similar to the situation Storlien had previously observed in rats.

Storlien and colleagues were able to also obtain small samples of blood and muscle from 56 normally nourished infants undergoing elective surgery but otherwise healthy. They showed that for breast-fed infants, muscle membrane omega balance was 10 percent compared to 7 percent for muscle from formula-fed infants. Furthermore, there was an inverse correlation between muscle 22:6ω-3 content and blood glucose levels.[75]

An extensive epidemiological study over a 10-year period in England found an association between type of dietary fish intake and the risk of Type 2 diabetes. This was especially the case if the fish were "oily fish." However, there was no association if the fish intake were "fried fish."[76] This difference is interesting in that the fish were almost certainly fried in a vegetable oil and would consequently have a low omega balance (see "The Importance of Meals" section in chapter 2).

Mention "omega-3" to the average person, and most will immediately think "fish oil." This became very apparent to me in 2004

following an account of our research on an Australian television program. After the program, I received many enquiries from the general
public and the majority just wanted to know which "fish-oil capsules"
I recommended. I spent much time trying to convince these enquirers
that I was emphasizing a "whole-of-diet" approach, an "everything
you put in your mouth and swallow" approach, when considering
the balance between omega-3 and omega-6 in the diet. The dominant perspective of omega-3 fats as a supplement is a problem that
even permeates many scientific investigations. For me, it is the likely
explanation as to why the evidence connecting omega-3 intake and
Type 2 diabetes is regarded by some scientists as ambivalent. This is a
conclusion common to various "meta-analyses," because while some
studies report that fish oil reduces insulin resistance in humans,
others report no effect.

Let's consider two such studies. Both used 27 subjects diagnosed
with Type 2 diabetes (average BMI = 30 in both studies). Study 1
supplemented the normal diet for eight weeks with 3g/day of either
fish oils (= 1.8g omega-3) or a placebo (paraffin oil).[77] Study 2 supplemented the normal diet for nine weeks with 20ml/day of either
fish oils (= 5.9g omega-3) or a placebo (corn oil).[78] Study 1 found no
effect on insulin-resistance, while Study 2 found a significant reduction in insulin-resistance. The studies differed in that Study 1
was on females in France, while Study 2 was on males and females
in Norway, but the likely explanation of the different results is the
amount of fish oil used as the treatment. Both studies were for relatively short periods. An eight-week experiment in humans is equivalent to an approximately eight-day experiment in rats (on a metabolic
rate comparison). Although both demonstrated changes in plasma
fatty acid composition, they likely resulted in very small changes
in the membrane composition of body tissues. For example, fish-oil
treatment of Study 2 produced a change in plasma omega balance
from 21 to 41 percent, however the change in the omega balance of
adipose tissue was only from 10 to 11 percent. Because of their significant fat stores, obese subjects will be especially slow to change

membrane composition. The fact that it is the omega balance of the *entire* diet that is important, experiments designed to test the effects of omega-3 in humans have to both have treatments large enough to cause significant changes in omega balance and go on for a long enough time to change membrane composition of appropriate tissues. Use of relatively small supplements for a small time is unlikely to produce significant changes, especially if the background diet is high in omega-6 fats.

The influence of enhanced dietary omega-3 on Type 2 diabetes is not restricted to the 20–22-carbon PUFA found in fish oils. For example, a randomized crossover experiment demonstrated that flaxseed bread (high in 18:3ω-3 but low in omega-6) in the diet for 12 weeks reduced insulin-resistance in human subjects compared with consumption of a high omega-6 wheat bread.[79] A meta-analysis examining the influence of fruit and vegetable intake on Type 2 diabetes found a significant benefit of increased consumption of green-leaf vegetables but no influence of increased consumption of fruit, vegetables, or fruit and vegetables combined.[80]

Diet Omega Balance and Glucose Tolerance: My Own Experiment

My opinion expressed above—that many of the experiments examining the effects of omega-3 have a misguided "supplement" or "drug" approach—motivated me, during the preparation for this book, to do a small experiment on myself at home. I had previously shown that I could change my cheek cell membranes by changing the omega balance of my daily diet so I decided to repeat this experimental design and check whether I could also influence my response to an oral glucose test (a test of my insulin-resistance).

For two weeks I ate the same high omega-6 diet each day, then for two weeks I ate a high omega-3 diet each day, followed by two weeks eating the original high omega-6 diet each day. Both diets were precisely weighed and measured each day. Both diets provided essentially the same energy, protein, carbohydrate, and total fat per day. The differences were the following: (1) The high omega-6 diet included a slice of bacon for breakfast; ham and margarine were part of my lunchtime sandwich, and dinner was chicken, potatoes, and peas. (2) The high omega-3 diet omitted the bacon, substituted sardines for the ham and butter for the margarine for lunch, and dinner was salmon, spinach, and potatoes. The high omega-6 diet contained 50g of PUFA with an omega balance of 3 percent, while the high omega-3 diet contained 44g of PUFA with an omega balance of 70 percent. For the last two days of each fortnight, I would delay breakfast and carry out a glucose tolerance test, which involved drinking 75g of glucose in solution and then resting and measuring my blood glucose at 1, 2, and 3h after the ingestion. Excess blood was separated into plasma and red blood cells and frozen for later fatty acid measurement.

As with my earlier experiment analyzing my cheek cells, the two diets affected the omega balance of my plasma and red blood cells. After two weeks on the omega-6 diet, two weeks on the omega-3 diet followed by two weeks on the omega-6 diet, the omega balance values of my plasma were 4 percent, then 19 percent, then 5 percent, while the respective values for my red blood cells were 2 percent, then 6 percent, then 5 percent. More significantly, after ingestion of glucose, my blood glucose level peaked one hour later followed by a continual decrease at hour 2 and hour 3. The rate of decrease between hour 1 and hour 3 is an indication of the rate at which glucose leaves my plasma and enters my tissues, and was nearly twice as fast after the omega-3 diet than it was after both omega-6 diets (decrease in mM blood glucose per hour was 1.6 then 3.2 then 2.1). Assuming my pancreas secreted the same amount of insulin after each consumption of glucose, this is evidence that my cells are less insulin-resistant on the high omega-3 diet than on the high omega-6 diet.

This experiment deepened my conviction that diet omega balance is an important determinant of insulin-resistance. In changing from the high omega-6 to the high omega-3 diet, my daily intake of omega-3 PUFA had increased from 2g to 31g per day. Assuming the average fish-oil capsule contains about 0.5g of omega-3, I would have needed to consume 58 capsules per day to achieve this change! Actually consuming 58 fish-oil capsules per day while eating the omega-6 diet, my diet omega balance would have only changed from 3 percent to 39 percent. This is because the whole-of-diet change also involved a decrease in my daily intake of omega-6 fats (from 48g to 13g). If there had been no decrease in my omega-6 intake and I wanted to achieve a diet omega balance of 70 percent solely by consumption of fish-oil capsules, I would have needed to have taken 224 capsules per day! It is an important concept that omega-3 and omega-6 need to be considered in relation to each other, and further they need to be considered in a whole-of-diet perspective.

A Larger Syndrome?

A syndrome is a group of symptoms that consistently occur together; the implication is that they have a common cause. Although obesity was not included in Gerald Reaven's original description of Syndrome X, it has become central to the Metabolic Syndrome. So central in fact, that obesity is often implied as the cause of the other symptoms. Yet there is no fundamental mechanism whereby obesity might cause these other conditions of the Metabolic Syndrome. Reaven proposed that "resistance to insulin-stimulated glucose uptake" was primary and that the other symptoms were secondary consequences. However, he did not suggest a cause for the insulin-resistance. That obesity does *not* cause insulin-resistance is supported by a 1998 experiment by James Barnard and colleagues.[81] One group of rats was fed a low-fat complex-carbohydrate diet, while another group was fed a high-fat refined-carbohydrate diet (the "modern Western" diet), and the rats were then measured at various times later. The fat in the "modern Western" diet was lard and thus had a low omega balance. Resistance to insulin-stimulated glucose uptake and an increased plasma insulin were both manifest after two weeks on the "modern Western" diet and were its first significant effects. By eight weeks, there was an increased size of fat cells. Obesity (different body weights between the groups) was not manifest until 20 weeks and hypertension (blood pressure difference between the groups) not until 12 months on the "modern Western" diet. This experiment on rats demonstrated that insulin-resistance preceded obesity and thus obesity cannot "cause" insulin-resistance.

Despite much research, there is still no general agreement as to the "cause" of the Metabolic Syndrome. Indeed, the syndrome seems to be growing larger. Each year sees more symptoms associated with obesity, and many of these conditions are described as "epidemics" because their incidence has increased over recent times.

One example is fatty liver disease, which "is a burgeoning health problem that affects one-third of adults and an increasing number of children."[82] It is strongly associated with obesity and insulin-resistance, begins with an accumulation of storage fats in the liver, and if not stopped, can proceed to liver cirrhosis and liver cancer. It is strongly associated with inflammation. Although there is currently no generally agreed cause or treatment for the "epidemic" of fatty liver, I would suggest that it is another consequence of the relative imbalance between omega-3 and omega-6 in the modern human diet. In mice, omega-3 PUFA alleviate liver inflammation and reduce fat content in fat-enlarged livers.[83] It is sadly insightful that foie gras is a luxury food product made from the fatty liver of ducks or geese over-fed with corn, a "seed" with negligible omega-3.

Another tissue that accumulates storage fat is muscle, and the studies of Storlien and colleagues show that insulin resistance in humans is associated with elevated levels of intramuscular storage fats.[84] In many ways, this is not dissimilar to the increased marbling of meat when livestock are grain-fed as opposed to being grass-fed.

A 2017 review of the public health consequences of the rising prevalence of obesity included a table listing diseases associated with obesity.[85] They included

- Metabolic syndrome
- Diabetes mellitus

- Hypertension
- Non-alcoholic fatty liver disease
- Cardiovascular disease
- Stroke
- Atherosclerosis
- Gall bladder disease
- Polycystic ovary disease
- Osteoarthritis
- Back pain
- Gout
- Cancers (liver, breast, endometrial, colon, rectum, lung)
- Mental health disorders (including depression).

There are other conditions not included in this list that have also increased in recent times with no generally accepted explanation. They include "asthma" and "food allergies."

In the following chapters, I will consider the role of the imbalance of omega-3 and omega-6 in the food chain in the increased incidence of several of these disease conditions. I am not suggesting that the diet omega imbalance is necessarily the "cause" of each disease, but I will suggest that the imbalance is differentially affecting individuals predisposed to the various conditions. While this imbalance may not cause the disease, it can still be responsible for an increased "ill-health" associated with the particular disease.

CHAPTER 7

CARDIOVASCULAR DISEASE AND INFLAMMATION

Ancel Keys and the Emergence of the Diet-Heart Hypothesis

Cardiovascular disease includes coronary heart disease (CHD), myocardial infarction (MI, a "heart attack"), and stroke (disrupted brain blood flow). Much cardiovascular disease related to the heart is the result of atherosclerosis, which is the build-up of plaque between the endothelium cells lining the inside of the artery and the muscle in the wall of the artery. Plaque is a collection of mostly white blood cells (macrophages) that have taken up low-density lipoproteins (LDL) particles containing cholesterol. After macrophages accumulate large amounts of fatty material, they become "foam cells," which in turn produce signaling molecules that attract more macrophages. The plaque can grow to have a lipid core high in cholesterol, or it can harden and calcify. Sometimes the plaque ruptures releasing its contents which then initiates a clot of red blood cells that further interferes with blood-flow.

The initiation of atherosclerosis involves inflammation, and most adults will have some atherosclerotic plaques in their arteries when they die, with plaques having been noted even in Egyptian mummies. The fact that plaques have a high fat content (including cholesterol) has been known for a considerable time and has been a significant influence on our attempt to understand it.

Mortality rates from heart disease increase sharply with age, and heart disease is the single largest cause of deaths worldwide.

Although initially high, over the last quarter-century mortality has decreased in many high-income countries, largely due to medical intervention rather than changes in diet. There is a more than twenty-fold difference in mortality rates from heart disease between countries.[1] Mortality from cardiovascular disease in the United States increased during the twentieth century, such that by the 1940s cardiovascular disease was responsible for half of the deaths of Americans. This was perplexing to many as it was thought that affluence generally should be associated with reduced mortality from disease. Heart disease was described as a "disease of affluence." It was the first of the modern "epidemics" and was thought to be due to some aspect of the modern lifestyle.

In 1945, President Franklin D. Roosevelt died prematurely from hypertensive heart disease and stroke, and in 1947, the US Public Health Service started planning for a long-term epidemiological study of the development of heart disease in a "normal" US population. Framingham, Massachusetts, was chosen as the location, and in 1948, after the US Congress passed the National Heart Act, the Framingham study began and continues to this day. The Framingham study is responsible for renaming many "correlates" of disease as "risk-factors."[2] There was much scientific interest in possible causes of heart disease, and Ancel Keys was one of the interested scientists. Keys, who started his scientific career as a zoo-physiologist researching fish physiology, became interested in human physiology and was responsible for the development of the K-ration for the US Army. During the Second World War he also carried out a famous study on starvation using "conscientious objector" volunteers, with the results published in 1950 as a two-volume classic, *The Biology of Human Starvation*. His interest in cardiovascular disease was influenced by his travels and awareness of the difference in mortality from heart disease between countries. In 1953, he published a scientific paper titled "Atherosclerosis: A Problem in Newer Public Health,"[3] which included a graph that must surely be a contender for the "most societally influential scientific graph" (if there were such a prize). This graph plotted death from degenerative heart disease in middle-aged men from six countries against the amount of total fat in the diet for the same six countries. The "tightness" of the data and the upward nature of the relationship were understandably both dramatic and alarming. Ancel Keys had a powerful personality and substantial influence (being involved with United Nations Food and Agricultural Organization). Later, he reported that it was not "total fat" in the diet that was associated with heart disease but it was the "saturated fat" in the diet.[4] Keys created the "diet-heart" hypothesis, which proposed that saturated fat in the diet was the cause of heart disease through its effects on blood cholesterol.

Another important event in the "saturated-fat-is-bad" story was the release of the "Dietary Goals for the United States" in 1977 by a committee of the US Senate.[5] This report proposed a reduction in the consumption of fat, especially saturated fat. Significantly, it also recommended the *increased* intake of polyunsaturated fats, which at the time were regarded as a single category, with no differentiation between the types of polyunsaturated fats and no awareness that omega-6 and omega-3 had quite different effects.

This "saturated-fat-is-bad" perspective still dominates. It is found in the current "Dietary Guidelines for Americans, 2020–2025" from the US Department of Agriculture[6] which suggests a low saturated fat intake (replaced by increased polyunsaturated fats, but with no differentiation between omega-6 or omega-3). They also suggest fat-free or low-fat dairy replace normal full-fat dairy food, and recommend the consumption of "oils" (but with no differentiation between omega-3 and omega-6 oils). The most recent Australian dietary guidelines mimic those of the United States, also suggesting reduced saturated fat intake, substitution of low-fat dairy for the full-fat dairy, and making no differentiation between omega-3 or omega-6 fats.[7] The "saturated-fat-is-bad" guidelines have been challenged,[8] and heart disease has been the subject of much research over the last half-century. A meta-analysis in 2010 examining the evidence as to whether there is any association between dietary saturated fat and cardiovascular disease concluded that there was *no* significant evidence that dietary saturated fat was associated with heart disease.[9] In 2020 both a "state-of-the-art" review by the *Journal of the American College of Cardiology* and a report in the *British Medical Journal* found *no* evidence that saturated fat was associated with mortality from cardiovascular disease.[10] However, the early concern about dietary saturated fat and heart disease did have a beneficial side effect. It stimulated two Danish doctors to study the purported association.

A Trip to Greenland: The Inuit Paradox and Omega-3

Hans Olaf Bang, a Danish physician, had visited Greenland in the 1950s and was looking for an opportunity to return.[11] In May 1969, he read a Danish weekly for physicians that pointed out that Inuit died predominantly from tuberculosis and infection and not from the diseases of the arteries or heart. This was of interest because Inuit traditionally ate a diet extremely rich in saturated animal fat, living almost exclusively on meat, especially whale and seal blubber, and fish. This represented what I have called the "Inuit paradox," a highly saturated fat diet but low heart disease. Bang suggested to Jorn Dyerberg, that they should go to Greenland and measure the Inuit's blood lipids. They chose a location, Umanak, on the west coast of Greenland, where most of the residents were hunters and fishermen. On this first trip (they would make a total of four trips over the years), they took fasting blood samples, measured blood lipoproteins, and froze plasma samples to be transported back to Denmark for later measurement of fatty acid composition.

The results from the first trip showed the Greenland Inuit had lower blood cholesterol and triglyceride levels and also lower VLDL and LDL than Danes living in Denmark. This was not surprising in view of their low incidence of coronary heart disease but was surprising with respect to their diet, which was high in saturated fat and cholesterol. They also measured Inuit living in Denmark who ate a Danish diet, and found these Inuit had blood lipid profile that was different from that of the Greenland Inuit but similar to that of Danes eating a normal Danish diet. This demonstrated it was the Inuit diet, and not their genes, that was responsible.[12]

On a later trip, in 1974, they collected samples of the food eaten by Greenland Inuit for later diet analysis. Fat constituted 37 percent of diet energy and had an omega balance of 51 percent compared with 21 percent for the Danish diet.[13] When omega balance is calculated for plasma triglycerides and plasma phospholipids from Greenland Inuit, the values are, respectively, 45 and 53 percent compared with the respective values of 24 and 11 percent for Danes and 14 and 6 percent for Inuit living in Denmark.[14] The Greenland Inuit had blood lipids with both a higher omega-3 concentration and a lower omega-6 concentration than Danes and Inuit living in Denmark.

This "Inuit paradox" and the measurements by Bang and Dyerberg mark the beginning of the modern awareness of the health benefits of omega-3 fats, and their findings have stimulated many studies over the years that examine the influence of omega-3 and omega-6 on coronary heart disease. Most have concentrated on the effects of fish oils.

Diet Omega Balance and Cardiovascular Disease

In 1961 the American Heart Association recommended that saturated fat in the human diet be replaced with polyunsaturated fats, especially fats from vegetable oils.[15] To my knowledge, there had been no trial to test this proposal prior to the advice. In 1966 a randomized controlled dietary trial to test the recommendation, the *Sydney Diet Heart Study*, was begun and continued until 1973. Men (30–59 years old) who had attended hospitals for nonlethal heart attacks and had agreed to join the trial were randomly divided into a control group that received no dietary advice and a dietary intervention group that was instructed to reduce their saturated fat intake to less than 10 percent of food energy and increase their polyunsaturated fat intake to about 15 percent of energy. To achieve these targets, they were provided with both safflower oil and a safflower-oil based margarine.

This is a significant aspect of the study because 18:2ω-6 is the *only* polyunsaturated fat in safflower oil. Although we don't know the omega balance of the total diets of the groups, we can definitively conclude that the diet of the intervention group had a *lower* omega balance than that of the control group.

Following baseline measurements of blood cholesterol and triglycerides, subjects were regularly monitored over five years, including dietary surveys that confirmed the advised dietary fat intakes were achieved.[16] The results were the *opposite* of those expected. Survival was worse in the intervention group than the control group. In 1978, the investigators published a minimal report that noted overall survival was about 81 percent but was contrary to initial expectations. The conclusion was *not* that the "diet-heart" hypothesis was refuted but that the trial design was flawed. Recently, the data from this trial was recovered and reanalyzed. The 2013 reanalysis confirmed that the findings were the *opposite* of what was predicted from the "diet-heart" hypothesis. Although the substitution of omega-6 for saturated fat in the diet lowered blood cholesterol (and blood triglycerides) as expected, it did not provide the intended benefits; instead it "increased all-cause mortality, cardiovascular death, and death from coronary heart disease."[17] A larger randomized controlled diet experiment was commenced in 1968 in the United States to similarly test the "diet-heart" hypothesis. This trial was called the "Minnesota Coronary Experiment," and the principal investigators were Ancel Keys and a University of Minnesota colleague, Ivan Frantz Jr. It continued until 1973 and involved 9,570 patients (ranging from 20 to 97 years old) from one nursing home and six state mental hospitals in Minnesota. At each institution, subjects were randomly allocated to either a control group that received the normal institutional diet, or an intervention group that received the same institutional diet but with some saturated fat replaced by corn oil or corn oil–based foods (butter was replaced by corn-oil margarine). Corn oil contains predominantly omega-6, having an omega balance of 2 percent. Although the diets differed among the seven institutions, in all of them there was a significant replacement of saturated fat with omega-6. The average decrease in saturated fat was about 50 percent and the average increase in omega-6 was about 290 percent. All intervention diets had a *reduced* omega balance compared with the control diets.

As predicted, there was a significant decline in blood serum cholesterol, but contrary to the "diet-heart" hypothesis there was *no* effect on mortality. As with the Sydney Diet Heart Study, there was minimal reporting of the results of this large experiment, with a single paper appearing in 1989 (sixteen years after the end of the experiment) authored by Franz and colleagues (but not including Keys). It included the following sentence: "For the entire study population, no differences between the treatment and control groups were observed for cardiovascular events, cardiovascular deaths, or total mortality."[18]

Christopher Ramsden has been called the Indiana Jones of biology.[19] He was one of the researchers involved in reanalyzing the data from the Sydney Diet Heart Study and set about to reanalyze the Minnesota Coronary Experiment. Both principal investigators were by this time deceased (Ancel Keys died in 2004, and Ivan Frantz died in 2009), but Ramsden set about trying to find the data from the Minnesota Coronary Experiment. In 2011 he sought out one of Ivan Frantz's sons. Robert Franz, a physician at the Mayo Clinic, drove to the family home and eventually found several unlabeled boxes containing old yellowed documents and old magnetic computer tapes in a dusty corner of the basement. He sent an email headed "Eureka" to Ramsden. After recovering the data and fully analyzing it, Ramsden and colleagues (including Robert Frantz) published their results.[20] They confirmed that replacing saturated fat with corn oil lowered blood cholesterol (by about 14 percent) but found there was *no* decrease in mortality (either from coronary heart disease or all-cause mortality). Unexpectedly, they found the greater the decrease in serum cholesterol, the greater the risk of death.

The conclusion from both of these trials is that replacement of saturated fat with omega-6, a treatment that will lower the omega balance of membrane fats in the body, lowered blood cholesterol as expected but had *no* beneficial effect on death from cardiovascular disease. Indeed, in the Sydney Diet Heart Study replacing saturated fat in the diet with omega-6 *increased* mortality from cardiovascular disease.

What about the influence of an increased dietary omega balance? Following the findings of Bang and Dyerberg, there have been many studies examining the effect of fish oils on cardiovascular disease; one is the GISSI-Prevenzione Trial. It involved 11,324 patients who survived a recent heart attack and were randomly divided into four groups; one group took fish-oil supplements (about 1g omega-3 daily) for three and a half years; another group took vitamin E (300mg daily); the third group took both fish oil and vitamin E; while the control group took no supplements. The GISSI findings were that fish-oil supplements decreased cardiovascular-related mortality by about 30 percent (although there were no clinically important changes in blood cholesterol). Vitamin E had no effect.[21]

Other studies have also shown beneficial effects of omega-3 on cardiovascular health. For example, the greater the degree of fish consumption, the greater the survival free of congestive heart failure.[22] However, not all studies have shown beneficial effects of fish-oil supplements. A 2018 Cochrane meta-analysis combined the results of up to 39 previous random controlled trials and concluded there was little or no effect of increasing long-chain omega-3 on all-cause mortality, nor on cardiovascular mortality, nor on coronary heart disease mortality.[23] As I described in chapter 6, for me many omega-3 studies have the deficiency that they adopt a "diet-supplement" perspective when planning their experimental treatment rather than a "whole-of-diet" perspective. The vast majority of studies use a fish-oil supplement as the treatment, and often the amount of additional omega-3 fats consumed by subjects is relatively small. For example, in this 2018 meta-analysis, the experimental intervention in 85 percent of the studies was consumption of fish-oil capsules. Furthermore, the median treatment of studies that examine both overall-mortality and cardiovascular disease mortality was 1.3g of omega-3 per day (see note 23). If we assume a daily intake of 13.4g omega-6 and 1.2g omega-3, which is the median intake of US adults,[24] the treatments effectively only increased diet omega balance from 8 percent to 16 percent. This comes nowhere near the comparison that Bang and Dyerberg made between the Danish and Inuit diets, which had respective omega balances of 21 percent and 51 percent (see note 13). I'm not surprised the meta-analysis was equivocal about any omega-3 effect: the treatments are relatively trivial. Inuit do not take fish-oil capsules; rather, they have a "whole-diet" rich in omega-3 and low in omega-6. Many of the trials examining effects of omega-3 have ignored this "whole-of-diet" perspective for examining the influence of diet omega balance on cardiovascular disease.

When the "diet-heart" hypothesis was first proposed in the 1950s, only six countries were used in initial analysis. It was realized early on that not all countries showed an association between saturated fat consumption and heart disease. Two notable exceptions were France and Israel. France had a high saturated fat diet but a low incidence of heart disease, while Israel had a diet low in saturated fat without the predicted low mortality from heart disease. Like the Inuit paradox, both France and Israel were thus also paradoxes.

The French Paradox: Wine or Cheese?

The *French paradox* as a phrase was first used in the late 1980s to describe the observation that France did not conform to the "diet-heart" hypothesis. There have been a variety of explanations attempted for this paradox.[25]

One proposal—that it is a statistical illusion is—not true. The *European Cardiovascular Disease Statistics* gives heart disease mortality rates for European countries between 1972 and 2005.[26] As an example, in 1998 France had the *lowest* mortality from coronary heart disease for Europe, with values (per 100,00) of 22 for men and 4 for women, compared with respective values of 98 for men and 27 for women for Europe as a whole. In 1998, France also had the *highest* saturated fat consumption of all European countries, with 16 percent of food energy compared with an average value of 10 percent for the whole of Europe. The French Paradox is real. It is also not restricted to France, in that Switzerland in 1998, had the second highest saturated fat consumption and the second lowest coronary heart disease mortality rate for men and fourth lowest rate for women (see note 26).

What might explain the French Paradox? A well-known and widely publicized proposal by two French scientists[27] attributed it to the high red wine consumption in France (see note 25). While this proposal animates many dinner party conversations and has been well received by wine producers, it cannot explain this paradox. Various components of red wine have been suggested as important factors, but calculations of how much wine would need to be consumed rule out red wine as a realistic explanation. (Although I'm sure that will not stop the conversations at dinner parties during the consumption of red wine.)

The answer might lie in the dietary source of the high saturated fat intake. The French diet is especially rich in dairy fat. In 1998, dairy (milk, cream, and butter) provided 47g fat per person per day in France but only 26g per person per day in Europe as a whole. Of interest is that the value for Switzerland was 38g fat per person per day (see note 26). Consumption of dairy has been shown to be associated with better cardiovascular health. A large multinational study of 134,384 adults showed that dairy intake was associated with lower risk of mortality and major cardiovascular disease. Furthermore, the greater the consumption of dairy, the greater the benefit.[28] The French Paradox of a low mortality from heart disease is likely related to the high content of dairy fat, butter, cream, cheese, and milk in the traditional French diet.

Because normal full-fat dairy products contain saturated fats, they have been especially vilified in the dietary advice provided by many countries to their citizens. Yet when dairy comes from "pasture-fed" cattle, it has a good balance of omega-3 and omega-6 fats. For example, the omega balance of "pasture-fed" butter is 32 percent; for cream, it is 49 percent. The low incidence of death from cardiovascular disease in France is likely associated with the high incidence of dairy fat (and its good omega balance) in the French diet. The French Paradox is likely related more to the consumption of cheese (and butter and cream) than to the consumption of red wine.

The Israeli Paradox: Omega-6 and Heart Disease

The *Israeli Paradox* comes from the other side of the "diet-heart" hypothesis and was first used as a term in 1996.[29] It referred to the fact that although the Israeli diet was very low in saturated fat, this was not associated with a low incidence of (or mortality from) cardiovascular disease. For example, in 1981, the food supply of Israel provided 108g fat per person per day, which was close to the average 115g for Europe in general.[30] The difference was that for Europe two-thirds (73g) of the fat was from animal sources, compared with only one-third (38g) for Israel. Since most saturated fat intake comes from animal-sourced fats, this was indicative of a low saturated fat content of the Israeli diet. Vegetable oils contributed 60 percent (64g) of total fat in the Israeli food supply, compared with only 29 percent (33g) for Europe in general. Relative to the European food supply, the Israeli food supply was low in saturated fat but high in omega-6. According to both the diet-heart hypothesis and the 1961 advice from the American Heart Association, it should have also had a low mortality from cardiovascular disease. However, in 1981 the age-adjusted mortality rate (per 100,00) from heart disease was 59 for Israel and 60 for Europe in general.[31] In 1996, the medical scientists, who originated the term "Israeli Paradox," wrote "there is paradoxically a high prevalence of cardiovascular diseases ... and ... diseases associated with insulin resistance syndrome ... and ... increased cancer incidence and mortality." They warned of the possible dangers of a high omega-6 diet (see note 29). Although the Israeli diet has changed little with respect to the importance of vegetable oils in the food supply, there have been dramatic changes in cardiovascular disease mortality. Vegetable oils in the Israeli food supply had increased in absolute terms (to 76g per person per day) but were now only 49 percent of total fat supply. They were still high compared to values for Europe in general (48g and 37 percent).[30] In 2016, the age-adjusted mortality (per 100,000) from heart disease was 6 for Israel and 36 for Europe in general.[31]

According to a leading Israeli cardiologist, this dramatic decline has been due to a wide range of measures; including very early management of acute heart attacks, insertion of improved stents, use of more effective anti-coagulants, extensive use of emergency ambulance services, specialized intensive care units in hospitals, and other activities.[32] Like many other high-income countries, the decline in mortality from cardiovascular disease in Israel over the last couple of decades has been largely due to medical treatments rather than changes in diet.

So What Is the Cause of Coronary Heart Disease?

The "diet-heart" hypothesis proposes that saturated fat in the diet is the cause of heart disease, and it has become one of the most influential hypotheses in modern health. It is central to much official dietary advice, as well as being the basis for the considerable production and marketing of "fat-free" or "reduced-fat" foods.

A *paradox* is a finding contrary to accepted belief; if a belief is especially strong, the response to a paradox is to search for a different special explanation. One paradox can be reasonably accepted, but if there are several paradoxes, it is likely best to face the facts and challenge the belief. The Inuit Paradox, the French Paradox, the Israeli Paradox, and the several trials in which dietary saturated fat reduction has not reduced coronary heart disease mortality are enough for me to reject the "diet-heart" hypothesis. So, let me state my opinion: *dietary saturated fat is not the cause of coronary heart disease.* This does not, however, negate the proposition that other fats may be involved. So what is the cause of coronary heart disease?

The formation of plaques in the arteries supplying heart muscle is the cause of much coronary heart disease, and the high content of fats, especially cholesterol, in atherosclerotic plaques was instrumental in the belief for many years that atherosclerosis was a cholesterol storage disease.

Cholesterol and other fats are not soluble in water and are carried in the blood as complex "lipoprotein" particles, made of many different fat molecules in various proportions and in combination with proteins. They have different densities, with the more fat in the lipoprotein particle, the lower its density. The four types of lipoproteins in blood plasma are (1) chylomicrons, (2) very low-density lipoproteins (VLDL), (3) low-density lipoproteins (LDL) and (4) high-density lipoproteins (HDL). All are surrounded by a monolayer of phospholipid (membrane fat) molecules and, as explained earlier, a single layer of membrane fat molecules surrounding a globule of fat molecules with all the "water-loving" ends of the membrane fat molecules on the outside will make the fat globule "soluble" in water. Only two lipoprotein particles will concern us here; LDLs (responsible for transport of cholesterol from liver to tissues) and HDLs (responsible for cholesterol transport from tissues to liver). Cholesterol that is part of LDLs is called "bad" cholesterol, while the cholesterol of HDLs is called "good" cholesterol. It seems to me that it is not the cholesterol that is either "good" or "bad"; rather, it is the package that contains the cholesterol that is either "good" or "bad."

An "average" LDL particle has been calculated to consist of one protein molecule (ApoB), 180 storage fat (triglyceride) molecules, 700 membrane fat (phospholipid) molecules, 600 "free" cholesterol molecules, and 1,600 "cholesterol ester" (a single fatty acid attached to each cholesterol) molecules.[33] Thus an "average" LDL particle will have about three times the number of fatty acids as cholesterol (3,540 fatty acid chains versus 1,200 cholesterols). Using published data for the fatty acid composition of human plasma lipids, it can be estimated that an "average" LDL particle has about 115 omega-3 and about 1,400 omega-6.[34]

Atherosclerosis has three stages: initiation, progression, and rupture. Inflammatory processes are strongly involved in each stage.[35] All blood vessels have an inner layer of endothelial cells, and when stressed they produce adhesion molecules in their cell membrane. The stress can range from biological (attack by a pathogen) to physical (non-laminar blood flow).[36] For example, periodontal pathogens are often found in atherosclerotic plaques,[37] and of all blood vessels, those in the heart will experience both the highest and most fluctuating blood pressure. Once the endothelial cells have such adhesion molecules in their cell membranes, white blood cells attach to them, slowly move along the endothelial cells, and squeeze into the gaps between endothelial cells to enter the space between the endothelial cells and the muscle in the blood vessel wall. This is a normal part of the inflammatory process. Once in the wall of the blood vessel, the white blood cell matures into a macrophage (= big eater), producing "scavenger" receptors in its cell membrane that allow the macrophage to engulf foreign molecules. Once activated, macrophages also have other activities: (1) they produce and secrete a variety of chemical signals (cytokines) that attract other white blood cells to the site, and (2) they produce large amounts of powerful oxidants (including superoxide and hydrogen peroxide) that damage other molecules and kill any pathogen intruders. These activities are also part of the normal process of inflammation.

In the case of atherosclerotic plague formation, LDL particles are engulfed by the macrophages in the growing plaque, and it is this continual uptake of LDL particles that is predominantly responsible for the very large accumulation of cholesterol and other fat molecules and eventually leads to the transformation of a macrophage cell into a foam cell. These are characteristic of atherosclerotic plaque, and as the plaque grows, they become more inflamed and eventually die, forming a necrotic lipid-filled center of the atherosclerotic plaque. If the plaque ruptures, it can release its contents into the blood vessel and initiate the formation of a blood clot. The blood clot can remain in the coronary artery and stop blood flow to the downstream heart tissue, thus causing a heart attack (myocardial infarction), or it can become dislodged, travel through the circulation and interfere with blood flow in a different body organ. If it interferes with blood flow in the brain, it can cause a stroke. It is this final step of forming a blood clot that is the most dangerous part of atherosclerosis and sometimes results in sudden death.

There is something special about the LDL particles taken up by macrophages in atherosclerosis; they are *not* normal. About three decades ago, some investigators observed that normal LDL particles did not result in macrophages becoming foam cells, but if the LDL particles are "oxidatively damaged" (oxLDL), then massive uptake via the scavenger receptors of the macrophages ensues, and foam cells are formed. This observation led to the "oxidised LDL hypothesis of atherosclerosis"[38] and is significant because it shifts the emphasis from the cholesterol component of LDL particles to the fatty acids that are part of the LDL particle and more specifically to the polyunsaturated fatty acids in the LDL particle; unlike saturated and monounsaturated fats, polyunsaturated fatty acids are extremely susceptible to oxidative damage.

Undamaged "native" LDL particles bind to receptors on the surface of normal tissue cells (to be taken up by the cell); oxidatively damaged LDL particles, however, are avidly bound by scavenger receptors on the surface of macrophages. Much additional oxidative damage to LDL particles actually occurs in the macrophage-dominated environment of the atherosclerotic plaque, where the macrophages secrete powerful oxidants that cause considerable oxidative damage. Many of the products of oxidatively damaged fats stimulate the production of inflammatory attractants by both macrophages and endothelial cells associated with atherosclerotic plaques (see note 33).

The concept of "bad" cholesterol (LDL cholesterol) finally makes sense. It is *not* the cholesterol that is "bad" but rather it is its travelling companions in the package containing the cholesterol. It is the $18{:}2\omega{-}6$ and $20{:}4\omega{-}6$ (which are very abundant in LDL particles) that are capable of becoming "bad" (by being oxidatively damaged) and initiating processes common to inflammation. It may be that mea-surement of "LDL cholesterol" is primarily useful because it is a sur-rogate measurement of LDL particles *per se*. Similarly, it is likely that statins (a class of drugs with the primary action of inhibiting choles-terol synthesis in the liver) and one the most commonly prescribed drugs, exert their beneficial effects by lowering the production and secretion of LDL particles rather than by lowering cholesterol pro-duction *per se*. In light of this, it is interesting that studies show that the actual number of LDL particles is a better discriminator of risk for cardiovascular disease than is measurement of the amount of cho-lesterol associated with LDL particles.[39] Atherosclerosis, and the de-velopment of plaque, is not a disease of malfunctioning lipid storage but primarily a disease of chronic inflammation.

Inflammation: The Role of Omega-6 PUFA

Classically, inflammation was characterized by heat, pain, redness, and swelling. It responds to both injury (such as trauma, burns, or surgery) and pathogens by increasing blood flow to the area of damage, coupled with increased leakiness of capillaries, allowing passage of plasma and white blood cells into the spaces between cells. It is a complex regulatory response involving blood vessels, white blood cells, and many molecular mediators. The aim is to kill and remove damaged cells and pathogens and initiate tissue repair. Inflammation is a general response, not specific to a particular patho-gen or irritant. Although inflammation is often described as part of the immune system, in many ways it is more than that. When we say a person is immune, we are normally saying the person has the ability to defeat a foreign organism—a pathogen. This involves the "adaptive immune system" and the production of antibodies. Inflam-mation does not require an attack by a pathogen but is a response to damage. It is sometimes called the "innate immune system" and is an essential part of the defense process being recruited when needed by the adaptive immune system.

The inflammatory response needs to be fast and recruit its various actors quickly; once it has finished the job, it needs a return to normal, to be resolved. Inflammation involves a large number of molecular mediators that act as chemical signals between cells and chemo-attractants, and these signaling molecules are either modified fatty acids or peptides. The modified fatty acids include some of the first responders and are predominantly made from the 20:4ω-6 in membrane fats. As a group, these inflammation mediators made from 20:4ω-6 in membranes are called "eicosanoids" (eicosa = Greek for "twenty").

The first eicosanoid was called "prostaglandin" because it was isolated from semen in 1935 and initially was thought to be a product of the prostate gland. Later, many different types of prostaglandins were discovered, and many tissues were found to secrete prostaglandins for various functions.

The first step in the synthesis of eicosanoids is the release of 20:4ω-6 from a membrane fat molecule by a specific phospholipase enzyme (called PLA2).[40] I earlier introduced phospholipase enzymes as an important part of *membrane remodeling* (see chapter 5). Once released from a membrane fat, 20:4ω-6 can be metabolized by enzyme pathways that add oxygen atoms to the fatty acid chain. There are three pathways, each named after the first enzyme in the pathway. The COX (cyclooxygenase) pathway produces prostaglandins, prostacyclins and thromboxanes, while the LOX (lipoxygenase) pathway produces leukotrienes and lipoxins, the CYP (cytochrome P-450) pathway produces a series of complicated molecules I will just call EETs and HETEs. Some eicosanoids can even be synthesized by oxidative mechanisms that do not involve enzymes.[41]

The eicosanoids exert their effects by binding to specific receptors on target cells. There are a huge number of different types of receptors, and each produces a different effect. Most of the receptors are membrane-bound "G protein-coupled receptors," but some are nuclear receptors. The combination of a range of different eicosanoids produced by a range of different cell types, in turn acting through a range of different receptors, results in a huge diversity of complex effects. For example, prostaglandin PGE2 is a relatively common prostaglandin that can be produced by most cells. It acts through four types of receptors (called EP receptors). It can act as a constrictor of smooth muscle (through the EP1 receptor) in the trachea and parts of the gut but as a relaxer of smooth muscle in the walls of arteries and veins (through the EP4 receptor), thus causing vasodilation and facilitating the influx of white blood cells to the site of tissue injury or infection. It will produce a "pain" response when it acts through the EP1 receptor on spinal neurons, and will result in a "fever" response when it acts through the EP3 receptor on specific neurons in the brain. When it acts through the EP2 receptor, it plays an important role in uterine implantation as well as a relaxant role in bronchioles.[42] Paradoxically, PGE2 also exerts control over a number of mechanisms that lead to the resolution of inflammation and tissue repair.[43] A different prostaglandin, PGI2 , produced by endothelium cells lining blood vessels will cause vasodilation when acting though an IP receptor on smooth muscle cells of blood vessels, and will also cause aggregations when acting through the TPα receptor on blood platelets (see note 40).

Enough already! It's too complicated to describe here. To summarize: at the very beginning of the inflammatory response, there is an "eicosanoid storm" through which these lipid inflammation mediators, together with non-lipid signals, stimulate and coordinate various activities required for the rapid inflammatory response (see note 41).

Another part of the inflammatory response is called the *acute phase* response. This involves the liver, which, in response to inflammatory cytokines, increases its production and secretion of certain proteins while decreasing the production of others. Only one acute phase protein will concern us here: it is called *C-reactive protein* (CRP) and is important because it is used as a common marker of the degree of inflammatory stress. In healthy adults, the CRP concentration in the blood is about 0.8mg per L, but it can rise dramatically with inflammation, reaching levels as high as 500mg per L. Because it has a relatively short half-life (which is constant during both health and disease) the serum CRP level is a reflection of its rate of production.[44] CRP is involved in the removal of damaged membrane fats, binding to the head-group of a specific type of membrane fat when the fatty acid chain of the membrane fat molecule is oxidatively damaged.[45] It has also been shown to bind to oxidized LDL particles.[46] Interestingly, elevated serum CRP levels (which indicates high levels of inflammation) are associated with higher risk of atherosclerosis and coronary heart disease (see note 44).

Drugs can be used to inhibit inflammation, and they include both non-steroidal anti-inflammatory drugs (NSAIDs) and steroidal anti-inflammatories. In 1971, aspirin (the first NSAID) was discovered to stop the production of prostaglandins by inhibiting the COX enzyme. Medicines made from willow bark extract (which contains the active ingredient of aspirin) have been used for a long time to reduce fevers, pain, and inflammation and are mentioned in clay tablets from ancient Sumer as well as in an ancient medical papyrus from Egypt.[47] There are many types of NSAIDs available nowadays, and while most inhibit the COX enzymes unselectively, there are some that only inhibit a particular form of the COX enzyme. Because they only inhibit the COX pathway, NSAIDs do not inhibit the production of leukotrienes, which are made by the LOX pathway.

Glucocorticoids are potent steroidal anti-inflammatories and act by combining with receptor proteins, which in turn stimulates the production of some proteins and inhibits the production of others. One of the proteins produced suppresses PLA2, the enzyme responsible for releasing $20{:}4\omega{-}6$ from the membrane fat. Consequently, glucocorticoids also suppress the production of eicosanoids, but unlike the NSAIDs, they also suppress the production of leukotrienes as well as prostaglandins.

The importance of $20{:}4\omega{-}6$ in the inflammatory process is highlighted by the fact that the main anti-inflammatory drugs act by inhibiting enzymes responsible for early processes of eicosanoid production from this membrane omega-6 fatty acid.

The Influence of Diet Omega Balance on Inflammation

Although there is a negligible amount of 20:4ω-6 in a normal diet, studies in animals show that this important fat is often the most abundant omega-6 fat in cell membranes and shows the greatest response to diet. Furthermore, the most accurate predictor of its abundance in membranes is diet omega balance (better even than diet omega-6 content).[48] Diets with a low omega balance (low omega-3 but high omega-6) will result in cell membranes with a high 20:4ω-6 content, and because this omega-6 is the source of inflammation mediators, then such diets will favor the development of inflammation. A schematic describing this process is presented in figure 7.1 (the numerical values in this figure are from the twelve-diet rat described in chapter 5). There is good evidence of diet omega balance influence on inflammatory processes in both rats and humans.

Although there was no measure of the membrane fatty acid composition of white blood cells in the twelve-diet rat experiment discussed in chapter 5, a different rat experiment provides experimental proof of such a connection. Rats were fed one of five diets with the same fat content but different fatty acid compositions and

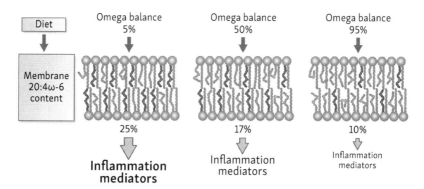

Figure 7.1 Schematic describing the effect of diet omega balance on membrane content of 20:4ω-6 and the consequent production of eicosanoid "inflammation mediators." The shaded parts of membrane fats are 20:4ω-6 fatty acid chains. The lower the diet omega balance, the greater the production of inflammation mediators.

their white blood cells isolated. Membrane 20:4ω-6 content of these cells varied twofold (from 12 to 24 percent), and when production of an eicosanoid (PGE2) was measured, there was a fivefold difference, with white blood cells with more membrane 20:4ω-6 producing more PGE2.[49]

Although diet omega balance can influence an inflammatory response in laboratory rats, what about humans? We cannot perform the biochemical experiments on humans that we can on rats, but we can examine the effect in humans of diet omega balance on CRP (C-reactive protein), a marker of inflammation. Serum CRP concentration for a healthy adult is about 0.8mg per L; values greater than 10mg per L are indicative of acute inflammation, while values in the 1–10mg per L range are considered indicative of chronic inflammation.

Several studies have shown that higher plasma omega-3 levels are associated with lower CRP concentrations. This has been observed in a US study of patients diagnosed with stable coronary artery disease,[50] as well as in healthy Australian adults,[51] healthy Greek adults,[52] healthy Italian adults,[53] and healthy Finnish adults.[54] The higher the daily fish intake by healthy elderly Japanese, the lower was their plasma CRP.[55] Because many of these studies are correlations, they do not provide direct evidence of a cause-effect relationship between increased diet omega balance and lowered inflammation. Such evidence needs to come from experiments of diet manipulation.

A meta-analysis of 15 randomized controlled trials as to whether increased omega-3 intake is beneficial after gastrointestinal surgery showed that increased omega-3 intake reduced plasma CRP levels by about 4mg per L, reduced the duration of systemic inflammatory response, and also reduced the hospital stay.[56] Similarly, provision of omega-3 to a group of US patients with CRP levels indicative of chronic inflammation resulted in a significant decrease in their CRP levels compared with a placebo group.[57] Addition of fish oil to the normal diet of patients with fatty liver disease and plasma CRP levels of about 10mg per L (strong chronic inflammation) resulted in reduced CRP levels compared with a control group.[58]

When plasma CRP is low (which can indicate no inflammation), then increased dietary omega-3 will have no influence. A study of adult male Greeks is indicative in this respect.[59] Half consumed a traditional Mediterranean-Cretan diet, while the other half consumed a Westernized-Greek diet. Both groups were provided with flaxseed oil (15ml; 8g of 18:3ω-3 and 2g of 18:2ω-6 per day) to add to their normal diet for twelve weeks. At the beginning, the plasma CRP was 1mg per L in the Mediterranean-Cretan diet group and 2mg per L in the Westernized diet group, indicating a slightly greater degree of mild chronic inflammation in the Westernized diet group. While there was no change in plasma CRP of the Mediterranean-Cretan group (1mg per L), the plasma CRP levels of the Westernized diet group significantly declined to 1mg per L. This study is of interest for two reasons. First, the treatment was not fish-oil capsules but was 18:3ω-3, which is the dominant omega-3 in the normal diet. Second, it suggests that the Westernized-diet produced a mild level of chronic inflammation that was returned to a state of no chronic inflammation by simply increasing diet omega balance.

Another study also deserves special comment.[60] This study involved US adults who volunteered for a controlled, three-diet, three-period crossover study. All diets had the same protein, carbohydrate and total fat content but differed in fatty acid composition. The control diet was an average American diet, which had an omega balance of 9 percent, while the other two diets had some of the saturated fat replaced with different polyunsaturated fats. The two experimental diets that had the same total polyunsaturated fat content, and as is typical for most normal human diets, the omega-6 in all diets was 18:2ω-6, while the omega-3 was 18:3ω-3. One of the experimental diets had an omega balance of 22 percent, while for the other it was 38 percent. The median CRP levels were 1.5mg per L on the average American diet, 0.8mg per L on the 22 percent omega balance diet, and 0.4mg per L on the 38 percent omega balance diet. These differences show that an increased dietary omega balance will result in a lower level of chronic inflammation and that the increased diet omega balance need not involve increased consumption of fish or fish oils.

While I have concentrated on changes in membrane 20:4ω-6 content as an explanation of why an increased diet omega balance reduces the inflammatory state, there is an extra mechanism that is also likely involved. An increase in diet omega-3 relative to omega-6 will also result in an increased omega-3 content of membrane fats. The enzymes that act on 20:4ω-6 (and produce omega-6 derived eicosanoids) can also act on omega-3, and the molecules produced by this process are called resolvins, protectins, and maresins.[61] These generally act to diminish or resolve the inflammatory response, and they consequently also reduce the chronic inflammatory condition.

So far, I have only considered the influence of diet omega balance on the eicosanoid inflammation mediators. Does diet omega balance also affect the other inflammation mediators, those *not* made from membrane 20:4ω-6, the non-eicosanoid mediators? Important non-eicosanoid inflammation mediators include *tumor necrosis factor* (TNF) and a number of *interleukins* (ILs). Insight is provided by a study that examined the effect of fish-oil consumption (18g per day for six weeks) on the membrane composition of white blood cells as well as on their twenty-four hour production of both eicosanoid and non-eicosanoid mediators.[62] Blood samples were taken before and at the end of the treatment, as well as 10 and 20 weeks after the treatment ended. The omega-3 treatment reduced the 20:4ω-6 in the membrane fats by 38 percent, which was still reduced by 31 percent 10 weeks later but had returned to pre-supplement levels by 20 weeks. The production of the eicosanoid PGE2 showed a similar pattern, reduced about 50 percent at end of supplementation, still reduced by 31 percent 10 weeks later but slightly above the pre-supplement level 20 weeks later. The omega-3 supplementation also affected the production of the non-eicosanoid inflammation mediators (TNF and three ILs). The production of these non-eicosanoid mediators was reduced by 20–45 percent at the end of the treatment period, reduced by 40–65 percent 10 weeks later and returned to pre-supplement levels after 20 weeks. This experiment demonstrates that the influence of dietary omega-3 PUFA is not *limited* to eicosanoid production but is also observed for other non-eicosanoid inflammation mediators.

Chronic Inflammation: Linking the "Modern Epidemics"

In earlier times, before the knowledge of microbes, "epidemics" would have been acknowledged without knowing the precise cause. So, it is today. Although we know they are not due to infectious pathogens, we do not agree as to the underlying cause of many chronic diseases that are increasingly more common. We often describe them as "epidemics" and they include the "heart disease epidemic" discussed earlier in this chapter, as well as the "obesity epidemic," the "diabetes epidemic," and the "fatty liver epidemic" discussed in the previous chapter.

What has become apparent over the last couple of decades is that many of these diseases are associated with chronic inflammation. In the early 1990s, atherosclerosis was the first of these modern diseases to be associated with inflammation, followed by obesity and insulin resistance. Increasingly, more diseases are being associated both with inflammation and with each other, sometimes being grouped together as syndromes. One recent estimate proposed that in 2014, nearly 60 percent of Americans had at least one chronic condition, 42 percent had more than one, and 12 percent of adults had five or more chronic conditions.[63] In its December 17, 2010, issue, the magazine *Science* featured what it regarded as the most important insights of the first decade of this millennium. Among them was that "inflammation is a driving force behind chronic diseases that will kill nearly all of us."[64]

The Framingham study identified statistical correlates of heart disease and renamed them "risk factors." This new name implies a cause-and-effect relationship. However, we should remember that many are really just statistical correlates. For example, it is increasingly common to see "obesity" referred to as a risk factor for other diseases, but, it is hard to envisage a mechanism as to how obesity might cause many of these other diseases.

Chronic inflammation has been associated with many of the modern epidemics. There are also several conditions for which although inflammation is not the cause of the disease, the inflammatory response is responsible for much of the ill-health associated with the condition. Many of these have also increased in recent times. The next chapter will examine whether the change in omega balance of the modern human food chain and diet is also involved with increased prevalence of these disease conditions.

CHAPTER 8

ALLERGIES, AUTO-IMMUNE DISEASES, AND CANCER

Diseases Associated with Chronic Inflammation

Just as chronic inflammation was found to accompany obesity, insulin resistance, and fatty liver (chapter 6) as well as cardiovascular disease (chapter 7), inflammatory processes also are essential parts of other diseases and conditions whose prevalence has increased in recent times. This chapter will investigate whether the decreased omega balance of the modern food chain is involved in such changes.

Diseases associated with chronic inflammation are diverse and include some associated with antibody production by the immune system, as well as some not associated with antibody production. Chronic inflammation diseases include allergies responsive to environmental factors (asthma, eczema, and food allergies) while others are autoimmune diseases where the immune system is responding inappropriately to one's own body (rheumatoid arthritis, Type 1 diabetes, and multiple sclerosis). Some seem to involve only chronic inflammation rather than the specific immune system and include inflammatory bowel diseases, chronic obstructive pulmonary disease, and macular degeneration. I will briefly describe each of these diseases and examine whether they have become more common in recent times, before considering the influence that diet omega balance may have on each of them. But first some general comments on chronic inflammation.

The *prevalence* of a disease is the number of individuals with the disease in a specific population at a specific time. It can be dependent on the criteria used for diagnosis of the disease. For example, when the "skin prick test" is used to measure allergies, what is actually being measured is the "inflammation response" induced by the food. Whether an allergy is identified or not, will in part be determined by the intensity of the inflammatory response. An inflammatory hyper-response will thus affect the measured "prevalence" of the allergy. While allergies are caused by the immune system responding to partic-ular molecules (allergens) from the environment and can sometimes be relatively innocuous, others, such as bee stings, can be painful. However, it is often the uncontrolled inflammatory response to insect stings that is the likely danger, rather than the sting itself.

That diet omega balance likely influences such inflammatory diseases is illustrated by a comparison of their incidence among the Inuit of Greenland with the disease's incidence in Denmark. Records (1950–1974) from a hospital serving sealing and whaling populations of Greenland show that for Greenland Inuit the incidence of asthma was 4 percent of that observed in Denmark. Similarly, the incidence of myocardial infarction in Greenland's Inuit was 8 percent, of mul-tiple sclerosis was 0 percent, of diabetes mellitus was 11 percent, and of psoriasis was 5 percent of that observed in Denmark.[1]

Asthma and Allergies

Asthma (from Greek for *panting*) was recognized in ancient Egypt;[2] it is a chronic inflammatory disease of the airways characterized by reversible broncho-constriction, airway remodeling, and excess mucus secretion. During asthma attacks, the smooth muscle con-tracts around the bronchial tubes, the bronchial tube walls are thick-ened, and the air passages fill with mucus, making air movement and thus gas exchange very difficult. The inflammation mediator responsible is a leukotriene, made from 20:4ω-6 through the LOX pathway. Aspirin, which inhibits the COX pathway, will thus *not* stop broncho-constriction and can, in fact, *cause* an asthma attack because a much *greater* amount of 20:4ω-6 will be available for leukotriene

production from the LOX pathway. Other eicosanoids can also participate in asthma, by stimulating the migration of cells that collect and
present allergens to other cells and thus promote the development of
allergic asthma.[3] Asthma can be initiated by an allergic response to
environmental allergens and can also be nonallergic. Most childhood-
onset asthma is of the allergic type, while adult-onset asthma includes both types, with nonallergic asthma being more prevalent in
females than males and also more prevalent in older than younger
adults.[4]

Over the last half-century, many countries, including the United
States have reported dramatic increases in the prevalence of asthma.[5]
There is no clear difference in trends between children and adults,
between severe and mild asthma, or between developed and developing countries. When allergic and nonallergic forms of asthma have
been differentiated, there are essentially no differences in the trends.
The increased asthma prevalence is often associated with an increased prevalence of other allergic conditions such as hay fever and
eczema.[6] Several studies have examined whether the diet of individuals with allergy-related diseases (such as asthma) differs from that
of individuals without such diseases. Two US studies found that
higher intake of omega-3 was associated with a decreased incidence
of asthma in adults.[7] An Australian study compared the diet of asth-
matic and nonasthmatic adults, and although it found no difference
in daily fish intake, when "fried" and "non-fried" fish were differentiated, they observed that daily intake of fish "fried" (in vegetable oil)
was associated with *greater* incidence of asthma. An interesting finding of this study was that daily intake of "whole milk" and "butter"
was associated with *lower* asthma but daily intake of "soy beverage"
was associated with *greater* incidence of asthma.[8] This is consistent
with a high diet omega balance being beneficial for allergy-related
diseases. An Australian study of schoolchildren reported that asthma
was found in 9 percent of children that ate "oily" fish, in 16 percent
of the children that ate "non-oily" fish, and in 23 percent of those who
never ate fish.[9] A survey of the parents of schoolchildren in Sweden

found that consumption of both fish and fresh milk was associated with less asthma.[10] A Portuguese study reported that a high diet omega balance was strongly associated with good control of asthma,[11] while a Dutch study of respiratory disease (including asthma) found that *increased* dietary omega-6 intake was associated with a significantly *reduced* pulmonary function.[12]

Comparison of diet omega balance of affected and nonaffected individuals are correlations, and manipulation of diet is necessary to prove a causal connection. Several studies have used fish-oil supplements as treatment, and I repeat my concern that such studies sometimes result in relatively trivial changes in diet omega balance because of the small amount of omega-3 in the supplement. A meta-analysis, combining data from nine randomized controlled trials[13] with omega-3 treatment ranging from 0.7 to 6 grams per day, found two statistically significant effects; (1) an increased pulmonary function, and (2) in crossover studies, a lessening of asthma symptoms after fish-oil supplementation. Another study compared the use of fish oil (5g omega-3 daily for 3 weeks) with an anti-asthma drug on exercise-induced broncho-constriction in asthmatics and found that the fish-oil treatment was as beneficial as the drug.[14]

Interesting effects have been reported when omega-3 supplementation is given before allergic disease becomes manifest. Several studies have investigated the effect of fish-oil supplementation in pregnant mothers on the emergence of asthma and allergies in their children. A Danish study showed a reduced occurrence of asthma in children whose mothers received fish oil during pregnancy compared with those receiving olive oil.[15] Swedish investigators extended the maternal fish-oil supplementation into the first few months of lactation and similarly found that the children of such mothers developed fewer allergies.[16] An Australian study of mothers with a history of allergy found that even small fish-oil supplementation (less than 1g daily) during the last half of pregnancy lowered occurrence of asthma, chronic cough, and recurrent wheeze in the children at 1 year old (but the results failed to achieve statistical significance).[17]

These studies suggest that an increased omega-3 intake very early (during intra-uterine development) is helpful in diminishing the development of allergies later in life.

Food allergies are also on the rise. They are difficult to diagnose, and many individuals mistake food intolerance for a food allergy. Food allergies are most prevalent in childhood, and their prevalence decreases with age. The gold standard for determination of a food allergy is the "oral food challenge," and there is a relative scarcity of such high-quality evidence regarding the prevalence of food allergies. Nevertheless, use of surrogate data such as (1) hospitalization rates for food allergy or food-induced anaphylaxis, and (2) outpatient presentations for food allergy have been used to demonstrate that the prevalence of food allergy has been increasing in recent times. Between 1997 and 2007 the prevalence of reported food allergy in US children under 18 years old increased by 18 percent, with approximately 4 percent of children reported to have a food allergy.[18] In Australia, admissions for food-induced anaphylaxis increased almost sixfold between 1994 and 2005, while in the United Kingdom admission rates for anaphylaxis due to a food trigger doubled between 1998 and 2012. Similar increases have been reported in other countries.[19] The increase is not restricted to the Western world. For example, a study examining prevalence of food allergy in Chinese babies (0–2 years old) found that between 1999 and 2009, food allergy doubled from 4 percent to 8 percent.[20]

When the pediatric allergist Susan Prescott wrote her book *The Allergy Epidemic* in 2011, she subtitled it *A Mystery of Modern Life*.[21] A well-known hypothesis to explain the allergy epidemic, the "hygiene hypothesis," was first proposed by David Strachan in 1989 and proposes that a lack of exposure to microbes and parasites in early childhood suppresses the normal development of the immune system, thus increasing later susceptibility to allergic diseases such as asthma. It has received much discussion, some supportive and some dismissive. For me, as an explanation it is insufficient. For example, its emphasis on the antibody production might explain the increased prevalence of allergic *asthma* but cannot explain the increased prevalence of nonallergic asthma (which does *not* involve antibodies).

For me, the "asthma epidemic," the "allergy epidemic," and the "obesity epidemic" are not separate events. Obesity is sometimes cited as a *risk factor* for asthma. What this really means is that it has been observed that many people who have asthma are also obese (more than expected by chance) and that many obese people also have asthma (more than expected by chance). The two conditions are correlated with each other. Does obesity result in asthma? Or does asthma result in obesity? Likely neither. More likely is that they have something in common, possibly the same cause, possibly diet?

Sometimes the immune system gets things wrong. In the case of allergies, it directs its attention to otherwise harmless foreign molecules, and sometimes it directs its attention to our own cells. While this is beneficial when some of our own cells have gone rogue and become cancerous, it is not beneficial if they are behaving normally. Such situations result in "auto-immune diseases," of which more than eighty have been identified, with most being relatively rare. Forty-five of the auto-immune diseases have been associated with specific molecules (auto-antigens) against which the immune system is producing antibodies. These are proteins specified by the human genome, and although it is estimated that about 33 percent of normal human proteins are membrane-associated proteins, this class of proteins constitutes almost 60 percent of auto-antigens.[22]

Auto-immune diseases vary in their age of onset. The five most prevalent are rheumatoid arthritis, Type 1 diabetes, celiac disease, and two thyroid-related autoimmune diseases. Both Type 1 diabetes and celiac disease have a mean age of onset of 0–9 years, while for rheumatoid arthritis it is 20–29 years. The next twelve most common auto-immune diseases include multiple sclerosis, and the mean age of onset for these diseases is 20–39 years (see note 22). For reasons of space, I will consider only three: rheumatoid arthritis, Type 1 diabetes, and multiple sclerosis.

Rheumatoid Arthritis

Rheumatoid arthritis is the most common auto-immune disease and is a chronic, progressive, inflammatory disorder of synovial joints. Generally, it affects the smaller joints first (those attaching fingers to the hand and toes to the foot) and can then spread to the wrists, ankles, elbows, knees, hips, and shoulders. It often develops symmetrically on both sides of the body and in some cases can affect other tissues (skin, eyes, lungs, and heart). If left untreated it can result in joint destruction. Genetic factors account for up to 60 percent of disease susceptibility, but it is not known what starts the destructive inflammatory processes. Intriguingly, it has some connections to atherosclerosis. Although not caused by an infectious organism, periodontal pathogens are often found in affected joints.[23] Sufferers have a greater prevalence of cardiovascular disease and accelerated atherosclerosis than nonsufferers. Oxidized LDL particles are also observed in rheumatoid arthritis as in atherosclerosis.[24] Prevalence (per 100,000 persons) varies between regions and cultures and is about 1,250 in the American region.[25] A comparison of the prevalence in North American Indigenous groups found it ranged from 5,000 in some Indian populations (including the Pima of Arizona) to about 600 among the Inuit.[26] In the United States, rheumatoid arthritis is the most common non-thyroid-related autoimmune disease,[27] and it has a prevalence greater than the global average; it also had an increased prevalence between 1990 and 2017.[28]

While several studies report that greater fish consumption is associated with a reduced risk of rheumatoid arthritis[29] or less disease activity,[30] other studies report a reduced risk but without statistical significance.[31] Other dietary factors have also been investigated. One study of diet revealed that *arthritis* patients consumed about 30 percent less fish, about 15 percent less dairy products, and about 15 percent less beans than healthy controls,[32] while another reported that when rheumatoid arthritis patients were asked whether certain foods make their symptoms worse, better, or unchanged, the foods most often reported to improve symptoms were fish, spinach, blueberries, and strawberries.[33]

A 2018 meta-analysis combined the data from twenty randomized-controlled trials in which the average omega-3 treatment involved receiving 3g per day for 21 days, and the majority of the placebo treatments involved vegetable oils.[34] The meta-analysis concluded that omega-3 supplementation resulted in (1) reduced joint tenderness, (2) reduced pain, (3) reduced "early morning stiffness" of joints, and (4) a reduced disability. It also resulted in a significant improvement in grip strength.

Type 1 Diabetes

Type 1 diabetes is a disease in which self-antibodies are produced against the insulin-producing cells in the pancreas, and they consequently destroy an individual's ability to secrete insulin. It differs from Type 2 diabetes, which involves insulin-resistance of target tissues (chapter 6). Type 1 diabetes has a strong genetic basis and has an early age of onset, often in the first decade of life;[35] it was previously also known as juvenile diabetes. The global prevalence of Type 1 diabetes is 480 (per 100,000 persons), approximately one-tenth the prevalence of Type 2 diabetes. There is an epidemic of both types of diabetes. A study of thirty-seven countries showed a significant increase from 1960 to 1996 that averaged about 3 percent per year, which is equivalent to a doubling time of approximately twenty years.[36]

Dietary studies concerning Type 1 diabetes have understandably concentrated on sugar, but examining other aspects of the diet has important implications. A study carried out from 1994 to 2006 in the Denver, Colorado, region recruited children known to be at high risk of developing Type 1 diabetes soon after birth; their diet was followed annually by a parent-answered food questionnaire.[37] Blood samples were also taken annually and tested for self-antibodies. When the diet of all children was examined, it was found that a high omega-3 intake was associated with a 65 percent *decreased* risk of developing auto-immunity while omega-6 intake was associated with a 68 percent *increased* risk of developing auto-immunity (although this was not statistically significant). The influence of omega-3 was due to 18:3ω-3, which constituted 87 percent of the total omega-3 intake. When these investigators used more stringent criteria, the influence of dietary omega-3 became even stronger (77 percent reduction in risk) and statistically more significant. In a separate study, they also showed that the omega-3 content of red blood cell membranes was strongly associated with a lower risk of risk of autoimmunity.

A Norwegian study contacted the families of Type 1 diabetics and control subjects and asked about the frequency of using cod liver oil and vitamin D supplements during their childhood. They found that use of cod liver oil during the first year of life was associated with a 26 percent lower risk of Type 1 diabetes and that this effect was likely due to the omega-3 in cod liver oil rather than its vitamin D content.[38] Damage to nerves (neuropathy) is a detrimental consequence of Type 1 diabetes, and omega-3 (seal oil) supplements have been shown to benefit some aspects of this neuropathy.[39]

Multiple Sclerosis

Multiple sclerosis is the most common auto-immune disease affecting the central nervous system. A group of specialized non-nerve cells in the central nervous system (oligodendrocytes) wrap closely around nerve fibers. There are many of these wrappings, and each can cover up to 1 mm of the nerve fiber, with a very small gap (a node) between each bit of wrapping. The wrapping is made up of the cell membrane of the oligodendrocyte and thus consists predominantly of membrane lipid. It is called the *myelin sheath,* and its function is to insulate and to increase the speed of the nervous impulse (which jumps from node to node). Because of its high fat content, myelin sheath is light-colored, and the "white matter" of the central nervous system is so-named because of the presence of myelinated nerves.

"Gray matter" lacks myelinated nerve fibers and is the location of the nerve-to-nerve connections.

Normally the endothelial cells lining the blood vessels of the brain and spinal cord are very tightly connected to each other and constitute the "blood-brain barrier." Multiple sclerosis occurs when white blood cells with antibodies against myelin break through this "blood-brain barrier," enter the brain and spinal cord, and initiate an inflammatory state, breaking down the myelin wrapped around the nerve fibers, destroying the oligodendrocytes and sometimes also the nerve fiber. This invasion and destruction, by white blood cells, causes "plaques" in the brain and/or spinal cord. These plaques contain large numbers of white blood cells (macrophages), which are often full of lipid derived from consumption of the myelin sheath. The plaques can be observed through postmortem tissue examination as well as by modern imaging techniques and give multiple sclerosis (= multiple scars) its name. An intriguing observation is that immune cells reactive to myelin are observed in the blood of both individuals with multiple sclerosis and those *without* the disease.[40] This suggests that the breaking-through the blood-brain barrier by white blood cells may be critical to the development of the disease rather than the development of the reactive immune cells themselves. The disabilities associated with multiple sclerosis will depend on in which part of the nervous system the breaking-through of the blood-brain barrier and development of plaque occurs. Multiple sclerosis has a variety of manifestations and can be thought of as a single disease existing in a spectrum ranging from relapsing ("inflammatory dominant") to progressive ("neurodegenerative dominant") types.[41] The prevalence of multiple sclerosis was shown historically to vary geographically, being more common the further the population was from the equator, and also to be more common in females than males. There has been an almost universal increase in the prevalence of multiple sclerosis in recent times, and although the geographic difference has diminished, the gender difference has increased over this period.[42] Among the largest studies investigating risk factors for the major chronic diseases of women are (1) The Nurses' Health Study, and (2) The Nurses' Health Study II. The initial study began in 1976, and the second in 1989. Both groups answered questionnaires about their medical history as well as their diet. Investigators using both studies showed that the highest intake of 18:3ω-3 was associated with a highly significant 39 percent reduced risk of multiple sclerosis.[43] While dietary 18:3ω-3 reduced the emergence of multiple sclerosis, a more recent study suggests it will also reduce the *activity* of the disease. New lesions were detected in about 90 percent of multiple sclerosis patients monitored over a two-year period, but those sufferers with high serum levels of 18:3ω-3 had a 40 percent lower risk of new multiple sclerosis lesions.[44]

The risk of multiple sclerosis in childhood and adolescence was reduced by use of cod liver oil supplements (which contain vitamin D as well as omega-3) in Norwegian studies. One study showed this effect was only apparent during adolescence,[45] while the other study found that, as well as cod liver oil consumption, the frequent consumption of fish was also associated with a 45 percent reduced risk of developing multiple sclerosis.[46] A Swedish study reported that frequent intake of oily fish is associated with a reduced risk of multiple sclerosis,[47] while a Canadian study reported a similar effect of fish intake but only for women.[48] An Australian study that recruited patients at their first clinical diagnosis of demyelination and assessed their diet for the previous twelve months found that higher omega-3 intake was associated with a lower risk of multiple sclerosis.[49]

A number of trials have tested whether fish-oil supplements are beneficial for multiple sclerosis with mixed results. One compared the effects of fish-oil supplements (2.9g omega-3 per day) on patients with relapsing multiple sclerosis to the effects of olive-oil placebo treatment. After two years, the fish-oil recipients reported better outcomes than olive-oil recipients (just failed to reach statistical significance).[50] Similarly, other trials testing similar doses of fish oil (1-3g omega-3 per day) for periods ranging from 12 weeks to 2 years either show no effect[51] or only small beneficial effects.[52] My consistent question is whether the treatment doses are large enough to adequately test for an effect.

Inflammatory Bowel Disease

The two most common inflammatory bowel diseases are ulcerative colitis and Crohn's disease. Both have been classified as autoimmune diseases but are possibly not strictly autoimmune diseases. Most of the antibodies elevated in the serum of patients are not antibodies against the self but are rather antibodies against gut microorganisms.[53] These antibodies may be a consequence of the disease rather than their cause. There is no serum antibody that can be used to diagnose either inflammatory bowel disease. Eicosanoids are elevated in both inflammatory bowel diseases, and it appears that the most important are those produced by the LOX pathway.[54] Use of nonsteroidal anti-inflammatory drugs (such as aspirin) that inhibit the COX pathway is listed as a risk factor for *inflammatory bowel disease*, which is similar to the situation with asthma, another inflammatory disease in which the LOX pathway is the most important source of eicosanoids.

Both inflammatory bowel diseases have shown dramatic increases in prevalence over recent times. The prevalence of inflammatory bowel diseases in the United States is predicted to exceed 600 (per 100,000) in 2025.[55] An example of the increase over the last half century is one county in Minnesota, which had a prevalence (per 100,000 persons) of Crohn's disease of 28 in 1965, 133 in 1991, and 247 in 2011 (see note 55). This represents an almost ninefold increase over 46 years. Since 1990, the incidence of these diseases has risen dramatically in many countries. After new cases of Crohn's disease in Japan went from less than 10 in 1966 to about 140 per 100,000 in 1985, investigators examined changes in the national diet over the same period and found that a decrease in diet omega balance was correlated with newly diagnosed cases of Crohn's disease.[56] This was one of the first examinations of any link between diet and inflammatory bowel disease. Analyzing the two Nurses' Health Studies in the United States, investigators found that a high diet omega balance was associated with a 30 percent lower risk of ulcerative colitis. They also observed a similar effect with Crohn's disease, but the effect was not statistically significant.[57] A UK study found that high omega-3 intake reduced risk of ulcerative colitis,[58] while a Canadian study showed that higher intake of fish and long-chain omega-3 was associated with a much reduced risk of Crohn's disease.[59] A large European-based study designed to investigate the influence of diet and lifestyle on cancer and chronic diseases found a high intake of 22:6ω-3 was associated with a *reduced* risk, and a high intake of 18:2ω-6 was associated with an *increased* risk of developing *ulcerative colitis*.[60] The same researchers found that individuals consuming milk had a 70 percent lower risk of Crohn's disease when compared to nonconsumers.[61]

A meta-analysis of six randomized placebo-controlled trials of Crohn's disease sufferers found fish-oil supplementation (1.8 to 5 g omega-3 per day) significantly reduced relapse at one year.[62] A Japanese study used "diet therapy" rather than "fish-oil supplementation" to treat inflammatory bowel disease.[63] Various drugs were used to induce disease remission in patients, and once remission was achieved, they were taken off the drugs and placed on dietary therapy to improve the omega balance of their tissues. The diet therapy treatment aimed for a diet omega balance of about 50 percent. After diet therapy, their red blood cell omega balance increased from 29 percent to 41 percent, and 63 percent maintained their remission from the disease compared to 37 percent that relapsed. The "relapsed" group had a significantly lower red blood cell omega balance than the "continued remission" group (35 percent versus 40 percent). These results suggest that a higher diet omega balance is beneficial for subjects with inflammatory bowel disease.

Chronic Obstructive Pulmonary Disease

Chronic obstructive pulmonary disease (COPD) is an umbrella term that describes a series of progressive diseases associated with chronic inflammation where breathing becomes difficult. It includes chronic bronchitis and emphysema, and about one-fifth of people with COPD also have asthma. The main causes are environmental and include smoking and breathing air with excessive dust or chemical fumes, and air pollution. Compared with non-COPD subjects, COPD patients have blood C-reactive protein levels indicative of chronic inflammation.[64]

COPD is more prevalent in older age groups, with a global prevalence (per 100,000 persons of more than 30 years old) of 10,670 in 1990 and 11,710 in 2010.[65] The region with the greatest prevalence is the Americas, where prevalence was 13,310 in 1990 and 15,190 in 2010. All regions of the world have shown an increase in COPD prevalence in recent times (see note 65). Some of the lung changes of COPD are irreversible, but if part of the ill-health is due to the chronic inflammation, it may be possible to lessen the severity of COPD and its ill-health by diet alterations.

COPD is strongly associated with smoking cigarettes, and a study of current and former smokers from four US communities found that a high dietary intake of omega-3 fats was associated with a much lower risk of developing COPD.[66] A Dutch study found that a high dietary omega-6 intake resulted in both a reduced lung function and a higher incidence of COPD.[67]

Some trials have investigated the effect of omega-3 supplementation on COPD. A Dutch study investigated the influence of omega-3 (2.6g per day) for eight weeks on the response to exercise rehabilitation of COPD patients and found a greater exercise capacity but no difference in blood inflammation markers, nor lung function compared to the placebo group.[68] A Taiwanese study examined the effect of fish-oil capsules (1.6g omega-3 daily) for six months on both exercise performance and lung function of COPD patients. Although there was no placebo group in this study, there was a 14 percent improvement in exercise capacity and a 9 percent improvement in lung function.[69] A review of twelve studies of the effects of omega-3 supplementation in COPD management found it resulted in reduced inflammation, enhanced exercise capacity, higher quality of life, and lower exacerbation occurrences but weaker influence on lung function.[70] These studies suggest a moderate beneficial effect of increased diet omega balance on COPD.

Macular Degeneration

The macula is the central area of the retina located directly behind the pupil and is responsible for high-resolution color vision. A single layer of cells behind the retina (the retinal pigment epithelium, RPE) is important in the normal functioning of the eye, and its degeneration plays a significant role in macular degeneration. In a healthy eye, the RPE maintains healthy photoreceptor cells, partly by consuming damaged sections of the photoreceptors. With age, extracellular material, called drusen, accumulates just outside the RPE; this is the first clinical sign of macular degeneration. Chronic low-level inflammation plays a role in drusen formation, and drusen itself is pro-inflammatory in the pathogenesis of macular degeneration.[71] This can lead to a vicious cycle, and during late-stage macular degeneration, fragile leaky blood vessels can invade the retina, resulting in permanent loss of vision in the macula. This is called "wet" macular degeneration, while late-stage disease without blood vessel invasion is called "dry" macular degeneration. Macular degeneration is irreversible (see note 71).

The global prevalence (per 100,000 persons) of early and late macular degeneration are 8,010 and 370, respectively.[72] However, these global prevalence values hide the influence of age: from 45 to 85 years of age there is a sevenfold increase in early macular degeneration and a thirty-sevenfold increase in late macular degeneration. Because of the powerful influence of age on the prevalence of macular degeneration, the age structure of the population needs to be taken into account when comparing prevalence between different populations. Consequently, it is difficult to ascertain whether the prevalence of macular degeneration has increased over recent times separate to changes in population structure. One study has examined this possibility in Britain by using the registration of blindness due to various causes between 1950 and 1990. These data relate to the very late stages of macular degeneration, and after controlling for changes in the age structure of the population, they estimate that late-stage macular degeneration in Britain has increased by 30–40 percent over this forty-year period. They also concluded that blindness due to cataract, glaucoma, and optic atrophy has decreased over this period.[73]

The Blue Mountains Eye Study is a large study of visual impairment and eye diseases of an older Australian population west of Sydney that began in 1992. At year five of the study, diets high in omega-3, especially from fish, were associated with a lower risk of developing both early and late macular degeneration.[74] After ten years, the same effect was observed, with the additional insight that the influence of omega-3 was statistically much more significant in those individuals who also had a low 18:2ω-6 intake.[75] This observation suggests that it is diet omega balance, rather than just omega-3 intake, that is important. A US study similarly showed that both high fish and high omega-3 intake was associated with a lower risk of macular degeneration and especially in individuals with a low intake of 18:2ω-6.[76] A separate US study has also found that higher daily intake of fish and long-chain omega-3 is associated with a reduced risk of late macular degeneration,[77] and a French study observed that high plasma omega-3 was associated with a low risk of late macular degeneration.[78]

Two randomized double-blind placebo-controlled trials have examined the influence of omega-3 supplements on macular degeneration and found no significant effect.[79] However, both used relatively low levels of omega-3 supplementation (about 1g per day), and the resultant changes in diet omega balance are not known.

Chronic Inflammation and Cancer

The idea that cancer and inflammation are linked is old. In 1863, Rudolf Virchow observed that macrophages were part of cancer tumors and furthermore proposed that chronic irritation and inflammation cause cancer. For many years, his theory was ignored, but in the past few decades the links between inflammation, the immune system, and cancer have become very active areas of research with exciting implications for prevention and treatment.

In the normal situation, most of our cells do not divide uncontrollably; this is mediated by a number of genes. It is the mutation of these genes that leads to uncontrolled cell division and in turn cancerous growth. While the basis of cancer involves genetic mutations, the microenvironment of the tumor is also a very important influence, and it is likely through such an effect that cancer and inflammation connect.

White blood cells are found in tumors and in some cases may account for as much as half of the total mass of the tumor.[80] It has been estimated that about 25 percent of cancers are associated with chronic inflammation (see note 80). Several diseases of chronic inflammation are associated with cancer. For example, having inflammatory bowel disease can dramatically increase the risk of later colorectal cancer.[81] Inflammatory cytokines are produced by both the cancer cells and inflammatory cells in tumors and have become a focus of development of some anticancer therapies.[82]

Macrophages are intimately involved in assisting the process of metastasis. Macrophages present in the tumor facilitate the growth of new blood vessels and the breakdown of the extracellular environment. By direct communication with the cancerous cells of the tumor, they assist the entry of cancer cells into blood vessels and their consequent spread to other parts of the body. Macrophages are obligate partners for tumor cell migration, invasion, and metastasis,[83] and the fats in their cell membranes are important contributors to the production of the inflammation mediators involved in this activity.

The enzymes responsible for production of eicosanoids (from 20:4ω-6) are elevated in several types of tumor, and the prostaglandins produced enhance the spread of cancer cells (see note 82). Aspirin and other NSAIDS that inhibit these enzymes have been shown to reduce both the risk of developing cancer and the growth of a number of cancers (see note 82) Many inflammation mediators are also elevated in cancer. Paradoxically, although tumor necrosis factor (TNF) was initially named because of its antitumor activity, its serum concentration is elevated in many cancer patients, and it is associated with tumor cell growth, survival, and invasion of tumor cells as well as the growth of new blood vessels in tumors (see note 82).

An often-used marker of inflammation is the plasma concentration of C-reactive protein (CRP). The Copenhagen City Heart Study, started in 1976–78, measured plasma CRP in adults who did not have cancer. It found that 14 percent had no inflammation (less than 1mg per L), 61 percent had mild chronic inflammation (1–3mg per L), while 25 percent had moderate chronic inflammation (more than 3mg per L). During the followup of this population, 17 percent developed cancer, including 10 percent who died of cancer. The greater the degree of chronic inflammation (as measured by CRP), the greater the risk of developing cancer.[84]

Of three large US observational studies, one found no significant associations between fish or omega-3 intake and colorectal cancer.[85] Another found a greater risk of colorectal cancers with both increased omega-6 and omega-3 intakes,[86] while the third found that an increased fish intake and an increased omega-3 intake were associated with a reduced risk of both colon and rectal cancers.[87] A Japanese study found that intake of fish and of omega-3 was associated with a reduced risk of liver cancer, and increased omega-3 intake was associated with a lower risk of colorectal cancers in women but only proximal colon cancer in men.[88] Another US study found that fish-oil supplementation had no beneficial effect on the incidence of cancer.[89] Unfortunately, the additional omega-3 taken daily was 0.84g, and from a whole-of-diet perspective likely made minimal difference to the diet omega balance. A meta-analysis of observational studies con-cluded that omega-3 was associated with a 14 percent reduced risk of breast cancer.[90] Of thirty-one studies that investigated prostate cancer, ten studies found a statistically significant reduced risk of prostate cancer with increased fish or omega-3 intake, two studies observed that greater fish intake was associated with less "aggres-sive" prostate cancer, and all three studies that investigated pros-tate cancer mortality found a reduced mortality with increased fish consumption.[91]

Summing Up

This chapter has considered a wide variety of diseases associated with chronic inflammation. They have included allergies, autoimmune and other chronic diseases as well as some cancers. To varying degrees, the prevalence of several have increased in recent times. There are two types of studies that can examine the connection between the specific diseases and diet omega-3 and omega-6. The first are obser-vational studies, in which associations between the diet and disease occurrence are examined, while the second type are intervention studies, where it is determined whether altered diet changes disease occurrence. The results from both types of studies are limited by the capacity and accuracy of the research techniques involved.

For most observational studies, diet is determined by "food fre-quency questionnaires," and these are limited by the memory of the subjects and truthfulness of their answers. In many studies, the diet is determined at a very different time from the development of the disease and sometimes many years distant. The ability of "food frequency questionnaires" to determine the intake of specific fatty acids is also influenced by the accuracy of food composition databases. The classification of "fish" is often circumspect in these questionnaires (whether it is fried, canned in oil, and so on), and generally no attention is paid to any omega-6 intake associated with the fish intake.

The majority of the *intervention* studies have altered diet by use of fish-oil supplements. As I have commented previously, this emphasis on fish-oil supplementation in intervention studies (rather than in "whole-of-diet" perspective) has the consequence that many intervention treatments involve minimal, almost trivial, dietary modification.

It is understandable, in view of these technical limitations, that while many studies have found there are significant beneficial effects of an increased diet omega balance that some studies have found beneficial effects that just fail to reach statistical significance. To my knowledge, no studies have observed detrimental effects and future studies will be hopefully, better designed to overcome some of the technical limitations described above. This chapter has considered a diverse range of inflammation-related diseases/conditions of a wide variety of tissues. The next two chapters will consider the role of diet omega balance on the composition and function of a single tissue; namely nervous tissue and especially the brain.

CHAPTER 9

ON THE BRAIN
AND ON PAIN

Let's return to the beginning of this book—to Shawna Strobel, who because of intestinal surgery in 1978, was fed an intravenous food that had plenty of omega-6 but was devoid of omega-3. She consequently developed symptoms that had no ready explanation but went away when her intravenous food was changed to one with both omega-6 and omega-3. Many symptoms associated with Shawna Strobel's omega-3 deficiency were neurological. They included both a tingling sensation and numbness in her limbs accompanied by a vague pain and inability to walk. Periods of visual blurring also occurred, and the speed of her nerve impulses was slowed. The fact that all these symptoms disappeared when Shawna started receiving omega-3 in her intravenous food emphasizes the important effects that omega-3 have on the nervous system separate from any effects due to omega-6 fats.

The Importance of Membrane 22:6ω-3 in Brain Function

The omega-3 in the brain is predominantly 22:6ω-3 (docosahexaenoic acid), and if 20:4ω-6 played a substantial role in the previous chapter, then 22:6ω-3 will be the "star" (but not the sole actor) of this chapter on the brain. Early animals had a simple nerve net processing information, and over evolutionary time both the "processor," and key sensors became concentrated in the front part (or "head") of animals. In our species, this information processor is large relative to our body size. At birth it is about a quarter of its final adult size and has become a limiting factor for birth of young humans. Our evolutionary response has been to give birth at a very early stage of development. Compared with other mammals, newborn humans are extremely immature that then have an extended period of postnatal learning and development.

Although all our organs are important for our existence, the brain is especially so for our "being." It is the source of our self-awareness, our mind, our instincts, our drives, and our emotions. It receives and responds to information from both inside and outside the body. It initiates most body movement; it coordinates our muscles to perform fine movements and maintain our posture. It is the location and source of our understanding, our language, our music, and other creative pursuits. Its operations are both a mystery and a frontier. Our communal brains and the passing of information between generations are responsible for culture. The brain is an information processor and an information store, and all these wonderful properties emerge as the products of the cells that make up the brain.

These cells fall into two groups: (1) cells that transmit "nervous impulses" (neurons), and (2) various cells that don't transmit nervous impulses but that perform many functions the details of which need not concern us here. I will call them "non-nerve" cells. Both types are essential for normal brain function. The neurons transmit nerve impulses and are responsible for processing information. They consist of a cell body (containing the cell nucleus) and two types of projections from this cell body called neurites (axons and dendrites). The mature human brain contains more than 100 billion neurons, and since each neuron can make connections with more than 1,000 other neurons, it is estimated that the brain has more than 60 trillion neural connections.[1]

Although a nerve impulse is sometimes loosely referred to as an electrical signal, it is not electricity. Nerve impulses travel at speeds ranging from about 1 meter per second to about 120 meters per second depending on the nature of the neuron. Electricity travels at speeds of about 280,000 kilometers per second—a huge difference!

In chapter 5, I described how living cells have different distributions of ions inside and outside the cell and that this means there is an electrical potential difference across the cell membrane. In nerve cells, this is equivalent to about -90 millivolts (inside relative to the outside) and is fundamentally due to a low concentration of Na^+ inside the cell. A nerve impulse (an *action potential*) is a wave of change in the charge across the cell membrane that passes along the cell membrane of the nerve cell. It is due to a temporary inflow of Na^+ across the cell membrane through a specific membrane protein, followed by a temporary outflow of potassium ions (K^+) across the cell membrane through a different specific membrane protein. It is a membrane event, an "all-or-nothing" response and, in a way, is a digital piece of information that passes along the nerve cell membrane. An action potential in one part of the cell membrane initiates an action potential in an adjacent part of the membrane. As described previously, the axons of nerve cells are sometimes wrapped by myelin sheath with gaps (nodes) between each wrapping. Action potentials are not possible in the wrapped parts of the axon and can jump from node-to-node, which results in a much faster nervous impulse. White matter of the nervous system is the area of myelin-sheathed axons and is an area of fast transmission of neural messages.

The communication between an axon of one neuron to the dendrites of the next neuron takes place at the synapse. This is a very organized structure that upon the arrival of a nerve impulse causes membrane-surrounded vesicles to release their contents (neurotransmitter) into the gap between the two neurons. The neurotransmitter molecules then diffuse across the gap and bind to receptors (membrane proteins) on the receiving neuron's dendrites. These then interact with other proteins in the membrane and in turn cause changes in the passage of ions across the dendrite membranes. Such changes can either stimulate or inhibit another nerve impulse in the receiving neuron. Other synaptic membrane proteins are responsible for either destruction or reuptake of the neurotransmitter after its release. Synaptic transmission involves several membrane-associated processes and is where most neural processing occurs. Many of the receptors are "G-protein-coupled" systems, and I have previously described the dramatic influence of 22:6ω-3 on such a system in retinal membranes (chapter 5). Synapses are very dynamic structures, with new synapses being formed and old synapses disassembled, while existing synapses can also be modified, either becoming stronger or weaker. This is called *synaptic plasticity* and is essential for memory formation.[2] It is at the synapse that many drugs exert their effects. Synapses occur predominantly in the *gray matter* of the brain and spinal cord.

The most abundant polyunsaturated fat in synapse membranes is 22:6ω-3.[3] In the human brain, 22:6ω-3 is especially high in gray matter, where it is essentially the only omega-3.[4] Its abundance in brain membrane lipids increases during intrauterine development and childhood and then remains relatively constant throughout adult life from about age 20. When neurons are grown in cell culture, it is observed that 22:6ω-3 (but not 20:4ω-6 or 22:5ω-6) stimulates the growth of neurites, resulting in both longer and a greater number of neurites.[5] This is important because it is the neurites that go on to become the axons and dendrites of mature neurons, and by this pathway omega-3 PUFA will significantly influence brain function. Furthermore, this very significant influence was observed not only when cells were grown in test tubes but also when brains from rats fed omega-3–deficient diets are analyzed (see note 5). Rats fed a diet with only omega-6 have less 22:6ω-3 in their synapse membranes and also show less exploratory behavior in a novel environment than those fed a diet with both omega-3 and omega-6. Many studies have shown that mice and rats fed diets containing omega-3 fats have improved learning and memory compared to those fed diets with only omega-6.[6] Intriguingly, even in honeybees, omega-3 in the diet increases learning ability, and it is the balance between omega-3 and omega-6 that is more important than the absolute amount of omega-3 in the honeybee diet.[7]

In order to understand whether the changes in the omega balance of the human food chain have implications for our mental abilities, health, and happiness, let's start at the beginning—the beginning of the brain, that is—and examine the role of dietary fat composition in the development of the brain and its function.

The Beginning: Early Fatty Acid Nutrition and Brain Development

Production of neurons begins after week 6, is largely complete by mid-gestation, and about 50 percent of neurons are lost in the second half of gestation (see note 1). In the week-12 human brain, about 90 percent of the omega-3 in neuronal membranes is 22:6ω-3. As they are produced, neurons migrate to different regions of the brain, where they make synaptic connections with other neurons. This *synaptogenesis* involves a structure at the front of the migrating neuron called the "growth cone," in which 22:6ω-3 is an important membrane component. When rats are fed diets without omega-3 (but with adequate omega-6), they substitute 22:5ω-6 for the normal 22:6ω-3 in growth cones,[8] which hinders growth of dendrites and axons as well as synaptogenesis.[9]

At birth, the normal human brain weighs about 350g, and at one year of age, it is already approximately 70 percent of its adult mass. Not only is there dramatic growth in the total brain size during this period, but there is also an exuberant increase in the density of synapses. At the end of the second trimester, there are about 100 billion synapses per g in the visual and auditory cortex of the brain and about 30 billion per g of prefrontal cortex. This density dramatically increases to 600 billion per g for all three areas during the first years of postnatal life before declining to about 350 billion per g in the adult brain.[10] An early exuberant production of synapses from just before birth and during the first years of postnatal life is followed by a pruning of almost half of these synapses.

The dramatic increase in brain size and density of synapses during early development is associated with an equally dramatic need for 22:6ω-3 in the developing human. From week 12 to week

40 (normal time of birth), the percentage of 22:6ω-3 in brain gray matter membranes doubles, and by birth it is 96 percent of the omega-3 in brain (see note 4). During intrauterine development, all nutrients come from the mother, and it is noteworthy that during pregnancy there is a twofold increase in the concentration of 22:6ω-3 in the maternal blood,[11] as well as preferential transport of 22:6ω-3 across the placenta to the fetus.[12] Values averaged for five countries found that 22:6ω-3 was 89 percent of all omega-3 in umbilical blood compared with 77 percent in maternal blood, and the omega balance of umbilical blood was 18 percent compared with 14 percent in the maternal blood.[13]

Observational studies of the diet of pregnant women in the United States, Denmark, and the United Kingdom have shown that higher fish consumption by mothers is associated with greater cognitive development of their children in early childhood.[14] A French study of mother-child pairs examining the diet during pregnancy and the psychomotor development of the child found a higher omega balance of the mother's diet was associated with an enhanced cognitive development of the two-year-old child.[15]

One Australian study that provided 22:6ω-3 (0.8g per day) to mothers showed no significant effect on child development level at age 1.5y compared with placebo,[16] while a different Australian study that provided a greater dose of fish oil (3.3g omega-3 per day) showed significantly improved eye-hand coordination in the children at two and a half years of age.[17] A Danish study that supplemented the mother's diet with cod-liver oil (22:6ω-3: about 1.2g per day) from week 18 until three months after delivery, found their children had higher mental processing abilities at age 4 and that the children's scores correlated significantly with the mothers' 22:6ω-3 intake during pregnancy.[18]

Birth is a time of dramatic change in diet. The first milk (colostrum) has more protein and less fat than later milk and also has less omega-6 but more long-chain omega-3.[19] There is relatively little change in milk polyunsaturated fat composition from post-natal week 6 to week 30.[20] Breast milk samples collected from mothers from nine countries varied more than twofold in omega balance: it was lowest in milk from US mothers (about 8 percent) and highest in milk from Japanese mothers (about 18 percent). The 22:6ω-3 content of the milk varied fivefold, from 0.2 percent (United States and Canada) to 1 percent (Japan). In contrast, there was very little variation in milk 20:4ω-6 content, which ranged from 0.4 to 0.5 percent.[21] Similarly, another study reported a 23-fold range in 22:6ω-3 content but only a fourfold difference in 20:4ω-6 content.[22] These differences are likely due to dietary differences among countries.

Since plants provide solely 18-carbon omega-3 and omega-6, vegans will *not* consume preformed 20:4ω-6 or 22:6ω-3. A comparison of milk from vegan and omnivore mothers from the United Kingdom shows that 22:6ω-3 content in breast milk from omnivore mothers was 0.6 percent but only 0.2 percent in the breast milk from vegan mothers. The omega balance of the milk from omnivore mothers was 21 percent compared with 6 percent in milk from vegan mothers, and when the fatty acid composition of red blood cells from the babies was measured, those with omnivore mothers had an omega balance of 27 percent compared to 11 percent in the babies with vegan mothers.[23] A mother's diet will affect the omega balance of her breast-fed baby.

For a variety of reasons, not all children can be breast fed by their mother. In the mid-1800s, breast-milk substitutes were introduced, but the composition of many infant formulas did not match that of human breast milk. In 1981 Bob Gibson and a colleague compared the fatty acid composition of twenty-six infant formulas available in Australia with that of human breast milk.[24] The source of fats in several infant formulas were vegetable oils, and although human breast milk had a quarter of its omega-3 as 22:6ω-3, this important fatty acid was *absent* from all of the infant formulas. Because long-chain polyunsaturated fats have significant influence on early neural and cognitive development, it has been an important change that modern infant formulas are now required to contain (added) 22:6ω-3.

This previous use of infant formula without 22:6ω-3 has emphasized the relative importance of preformed 22:6ω-3 in a baby's diet. A 1992 study compared full-term infants either breast-fed, or bottle-fed one of three infant formulas (with different amounts of 18:2ω-6 and 18:3ω-3 but *no* long-chain polyunsaturated fats). The absence of 22:6ω-3 resulted in a much reduced 22:6ω-3 content in both red blood cells and plasma of formula-fed infants compared with breast-fed infants. The omega balance of the three infant formulae varied from 5 to 24 percent, and those infants fed the high omega balance formula had approximately one-third more 22:6ω-3 in their red blood cells and plasma than those fed the low omega balance infant-formula.[25] A later study from the same laboratory compared the composition of the brain cortex of breast-fed and formula-fed infants.[26] There was no difference in 22:6ω-3 content of brain cortex (7 percent of total fat) during the first weeks of postnatal life, but in breast-fed infants, brain cortex levels of 22:6ω-3 continually rose to become more than 10 percent at 48 weeks of life, while the formula-fed infants showed no increase. A similar study from the United Kingdom has also shown that the formula-fed infants have a significantly lower level of 22:6ω-3 in brain cortex compared with breast-fed infants (7–8 percent versus 10 percent).[27] The infant formulas used in this study also differed in omega balance and the brain of infants fed the high omega balance formula (9 percent) had 14 percent more brain 22:6ω–3 than infants fed the low omega balance formula (2 percent). In all infants, 22:6ω-3 was the only omega-3 in brain membranes, and it is noteworthy that a low 22:6ω-3 content in the brain membranes is generally compensated by an increase in long-chain omega-6 content. In chapter 5, I described how long-chain omega-6 can result in dramatically slower membrane processes compared with long-chain omega-3.

For obvious ethical reasons, it is very difficult to determine the composition of human tissues. The studies cited above analyzed brain tissue from infants that died from "cot death," and I want to express gratitude to the parents of these children in allowing their tissues to be analyzed post-mortem.

Finding that the 22:6ω-3 content and the omega balance of the milk (or formula) that an infant consumes during its first year influences the composition of its brain membranes, the question becomes: Does it matter? Does it affect the sensory, motor, and cognitive development of the child?

The human brain weighs about 100g at the beginning of the third trimester and about 1,100g at age 2 (compared to 1,400g in the adult). The period from the beginning of third trimester to age 2 is very important in brain development, and it surprises many to learn that the huge increase in brain size (about 1kg) is *not* due to an increased number of neurons. The increase is, in part, due to more "non-nerve" cells, but a very large part is also due to an increase in neuron size, associated with growth of axons and dendrites and a dramatic increase in new synapses. A "back of the envelope" calculation[28] combining brain size and synaptic density suggests that at the start of the third trimester there are 10 trillion synapses in a human brain; 60 trillion are added in the last trimester; 390 trillion are added in the first year of life, and about 90 trillion more in the second year of life. Because of the high 22:6ω-3 content of synaptic membranes and its important role in synaptogenesis, it is understandable that intake of 22:6ω-3 by the growing infant in the period before and after birth will have a significant influence on brain development and consequently later brain function.

Babies born prematurely during the third trimester will be especially influenced by post-natal 22:6ω-3 availability. A study of pre-term babies born between 1982 and 1985 in the United Kingdom is of interest in this regard. Mothers were asked whether or not they wished to provide breast-milk for their pre-term infant, who were later tested for their level of mental development at 18 months of age[29] and for their intelligence quotient at 8 years of age.[30] At both ages, the individuals who received breast-milk were significantly more developed than those fed infant formula. At age 8, the IQ difference was more than 8 points. These differences were not due to other factors associated with breast-feeding, parenting skills, socio-economic status, or parental education.

Several studies have examined supplementation of long-chain polyunsaturated fats during the early postnatal life on neural or cognitive development of full-term infants, and while some have found no effect, others have demonstrated beneficial effects. A detailed consideration of these studies is beyond the scope of this book, but a few deserve comment. A UK study recruited full-term infants who were fed a formula, either without or supplemented with 22:6ω-3 during the first four months of postnatal life. At ten months their cognitive behavior was examined by problem-solving tests that required the intentional execution of three intermediate steps to achieve the goal of retrieving a toy. Those infants who received the formula with 22:6ω-3 had significantly better problem-solving scores.[31] Additionally, these children were also tested at 6 years of age, and those who received the formula with 22:6ω-3 for the first months of life were significantly faster and more efficient at processing information than those without 22:6ω-3.[32]

Before I consider the effects of diet omega balance on normal neural function in adults, I will first consider its role in neurodegenerative diseases. We jump from the beginning to the end of normal brain function.

Avoiding the End: Cognitive Decline and Dementia

Cognition might be considered the ultimate function of the brain. But what is it? It can be loosely described as the process of knowing and understanding through thought, experience, and the senses. An essential requirement is that "information" and "meaning" can be stored, and in its global sense this is what we call "memory." In many ways, cognition is a mysterious process that in ourselves is manifest as our "thoughts." It is what makes us human, and there is a large gap between ourselves and other mammals. During my teaching career, it seemed to me that this difference was the most common reason some students had problems initially accepting humans as products of evolution. It helped to remind them that this "gap" may have been created by our ancestors getting rid of closely related, presumably cognitive, competitors such as the Australopithecines and others.

This gap also imposes limits on our ability to understand cognition. While we can use experimental animals to understand the basics of how neurons and synapses work, much of our knowledge of the human brain comes from acute observation of the changes in behavior of other humans, especially after damage to their brain. Changes in brain structure, due to war wounds, accidents, or surgery increased our understanding, and in recent times, the era of sophisticated imaging technology has resulted in a dramatic increased understanding of brain function.

Henry Gustav Molaison has given us important insights. At age 10 he began having seizures that became increasingly more severe, such that by age 27 he was unable to work. In 1953, he was referred to a neurosurgeon who suggested removal of the part of the brain that was thought to be causing the seizures; because he was so incapacitated by his epilepsy, Henry agreed to undergo the procedure. The operation lessened his seizures, and Henry Molaison lived for another fifty-five years, dying at the age of 82 in 2008. However, the operation resulted in unforeseen immediate and dramatic effects. Soon after the operation, it became apparent Henry could no longer form new memories. Although he could recognize relatives, retained a good vocabulary, reasoning and perceptual capacities and an above-average IQ, and could recall historical facts (such as the stock market crash of 1929), he was now unable to convert short-term memory into long-term memory. His short-term memory span was limited to 30–60 seconds. The surgery performed on Henry Molaison involved the removal of a part of his temporal lobe, including most of a structure called the hippocampus, which is located beneath the cerebral cortex. After much research, the hippocampus has turned out to be very important in the formation of memory.[33]

After neuroscientists appreciated that the number of neurons in the brain did not change appreciably during postnatal life, they speculated that memory and the storage of information was likely associated with changes in synapses (nerve-to-nerve connections) rather than the number of neurons. It was proposed that synaptic connections are strengthened by continued use, and this was considered to be involved in learning, memory, and cognition.[34] Although new neurons are not produced in most parts of the adult human brain, a region of the hippocampus is one of the exceptions to this rule. The other exceptions are the amygdala and that part of the brain that makes neurons for the olfactory bulb. The production of new neurons from neural stem cells is called *neurogenesis* and has been most studied in laboratory rodents. There are dramatic decreases in the rate of neurogenesis during aging, and this is thought to be associated with cognitive decline. The process of creating new neurons is also associated with loss of neurons, and it is estimated that in rodents about 10 percent of neurons in the hippocampus are replaced per day. Neurogenesis also occurs in the adult human hippocampus, and the ^{14}C spike associated with atmospheric nuclear testing has been used to retrospectively birth-date hippocampal cells in postmortem subjects. It is estimated there is a turnover of 700 neurons per day in the human hippocampus. Although the decline in the rate of neurogenesis with age is more gradual in humans than in rodents, there is a gradual net loss of neurons in the human hippocampus during adult life.[35]

The dynamic nature of adult neurogenesis and its connection to memory and learning have suggested that its modulation will impact the cognitive decline observed during aging (see note 35). Studies have shown that 22:6ω-3 promotes neurogenesis, both when neural stem cells are isolated from the hippocampus of rats and grown in cell culture and also when the production of new neurons is measured in the intact hippocampus of living rats.[36] It also promotes the growth and branching of neurites and the formation of synapses by hippocampal neurons. Such stimulation is not manifest with other fatty acids and is unique for 22:6ω-3. When rats are deficient in 22:6ω-3, they display cognitive deficits.[37]

In order to test hippocampal function of healthy older adults, some Montreal researchers constructed a "virtual reality" town with eight landmarks to test spatial memory of subjects aged from 60 to 75. Additionally, their general cognitive abilities (attention, concentration, working memory, long-term memory, orientation language, and executive function) were assessed using a cognitive test. Their diet was determined by a food frequency questionnaire, and any association between cognitive abilities and intake of omega-3 and omega-6 analyzed. The investigators found a high diet omega balance was associated with better spatial memory and a higher score in the cognitive ability test.[38]

Normal aging is often associated with a degree of cognitive decline, and although this change is normally moderate, it can sometimes be substantial and lead to *dementia*. The term *dementia* was initially used to describe the cognitive and memory changes associated with both advanced age as well as psychoses and brain-destroying diseases. The dementia associated with advanced age was called senile dementia.

The disease most associated with dementia these days is Alzheimer's disease, but the name was originally applied only to what was thought to be a special case of pre-senile dementia. In 1901, the 51-year-old Auguste Deter was admitted to Frankfurt hospital, where she was examined by Alois Alzheimer. Her symptoms included reduced memory and comprehension, an inability to understand or produce speech, disorientation, unpredictable behavior, auditory hallucinations, paranoia, and pronounced psycho-social impairment. Alzheimer moved from Frankfurt to Munich, and when Deter died in 1906, he had her brain sent to the anatomy lab in Munich. There he examined her brain under the microscope and observed clumps of stained material outside the nerve cells and also unusual fibers inside the nerve cells. These are now known as the "plaques" and "tangles" distinctive for Alzheimer's disease. He wrote up his findings and in 1907 presented them to a psychiatric conference, where his talk received no questions and little interest. (It has been suggested that this might have been because the audience was keen to hear the following presentation, which was about compulsive masturbation.) Cases similar to that of Auguste Deter were described in the following years, and the condition was given the name *Alzheimer's disease*. For most of the twentieth century, the name of this disease was restricted to dementia in individuals between 45 and 65 years of age. At a conference in 1977, it was agreed that pre-senile and senile dementia were almost identical, and the diagnosis of Alzheimer's disease was, from then on, no longer limited by the patient's age. Nowadays, Alzheimer has a degree of name recognition that surely challenges that of the other famous psychiatrist, Sigmund Freud.[39]

The diagnosis of Alzheimer's disease was initially very difficult because there was no single test for it, and the presence of characteristic plaques and tangles could only be determined after death. Early diagnosis of Alzheimer's was based on the clinical recognition of memory loss and dementia coupled with clinical examinations that ruled out other causes of the diagnosed dementia. The development of modern scanning techniques and biochemical analyses that can either directly measure or imply the presence of plaques in living brain tissue has shown that the development of plaques may begin twenty years or more before the appearance of clinical symptoms of Alzheimer's. The revised diagnostic guidelines of Alzheimer's now identify three stages of the disease: (1) preclinical Alzheimer's disease, (2) mild cognitive impairment due to Alzheimer's disease, and (3) dementia due to Alzheimer's disease.

These days Alzheimer's is considered a slowly progressive neurodegenerative disease that begins well before clinical symptoms appear. Early symptoms of Alzheimer's may include difficulty remembering recent conversations, names, or events. Apathy and depression are also often early symptoms, while later symptoms include impaired communication, confusion, disorientation, poor judgment and, ultimately, difficulty in speaking, swallowing, and walking. The hallmark pathologies are the progressive accumulation of (1) amyloid-beta aggregations outside neurons (the plaques) and (2) twisted strands of the tau protein inside neurons (the tangles); these are accompanied by the progressive damage and death of neurons in the brain.

The pathogenesis of Alzheimer's disease is not fully understood. Related to this is the fact that there are no treatments for Alzheimer's dementia that have significant clinical effects. This may be due in part to the advanced stage of the pathological process when dementia is finally diagnosed. Once a substantial number of neurons are destroyed (as they will have been by the time dementia is apparent), they cannot be replaced. There is evidence that the pathogenic processes of Alzheimer's involve neuro-inflammation and some "non-nerve" brain cells. "Non-nerve" cells include the microglia, which are the resident macrophage cells of the brain. They take up residence in the brain during early development, are located throughout the brain and spinal cord for the rest of an individual's life, and account for about 10–15 percent of all brain cells. They are very important in brain maintenance and are constantly scavenging the brain for damaged or unnecessary neurons and synapses, as well as infectious organisms and plaques. Microglia are activated by amyloid-beta deposits, and in mouse models of Alzheimer's disease, individual microglia cells have been shown, by imaging techniques, to migrate toward amyloid-beta plaques. An increased activation of microglia, which parallels amyloid deposition, has been observed in patients with Alzheimer's.[40] It has been suggested that neuroinflammation is the pathogenic basis of many neurodegenerative diseases, with both the specific initial stimulus and the anatomical origin of the neuroinflammatory processes varying between the different types of neurodegenerative diseases. In Alzheimer's the amyloid-beta are the stimulus, and the hippocampus is the location of the origin of the neuroinflammation. A number of inflammation mediators have been shown to be elevated in brains from Alzheimer's sufferers.[41]

Consumption of anti-inflammatory medication has been shown to reduce the risk of developing Alzheimer's. The Rotterdam study invited all persons 55 years and older living in a suburb of Rotterdam between 1990 and 1993 to participate in a prospective study designed to investigate the occurrence of a range of diseases in the elderly. A total of 6,989 individuals, who were free of dementia, were followed up for an average of 6.8 years during which 293 developed Alzheimer's disease. A large number had consumed non-steroidal anti-inflammatory drugs (NSAIDs) during the follow-up period, mainly for arthritis, and those who had consumed NSAIDs for more than 24 months had an 80 percent reduced risk of developing Alzheimer's compared with those who had not consumed NSAIDs.[42] While other studies have also shown beneficial effects of NSAIDs in diminishing some aspects of Alzheimer's disease prevention, clinical trials of NSAIDs in Alzheimer's disease patients have not been successful, possibly because the disease is too advanced for NSAID therapy to be effective once dementia has been diagnosed (see note 41).

It is estimated that between 1990 and 2016 the global number of people with dementia more than doubled—from 20 million to 44 million—and that by 2050 it could affect around 100 million people.[43] The majority of the 1990–2016 increase was due to two factors; (1) an increased number of people on the planet (which increased by 40 percent from 5.3 billion to 7.4 billion), and (2) a change in the age structure of the population (the 65+ age group increased from 6.2 to 8.4 percent).[44] There was only a very small increase in the age-standardized prevalence, which went from 701 to 712 cases per 100,000 head of population. Age has a dramatic effect, with prevalence of dementia doubling for every five years over 50 years of age (see note 43).

There are two types of Alzheimer's: early-onset and late-onset. Interestingly, a variety of other diseases are statistically associated with late-onset Alzheimer's. They include many of the diseases discussed in earlier chapters: metabolic syndrome, Type 2 diabetes, obesity, and cardiovascular diseases.[45] It is possible, and I would suggest probable, that the associations between these diseases and Alzheimer's is related to the same imbalance between omega-3 and omega-6 in the diet.

Evidence that diet could be a factor in the development of Alzheimer's comes from comparison of its prevalence between cultures. The prevalence of Alzheimer's in Japan is generally much lower than it is in Europe and North America. The prevalence in Japanese Americans (living in the United States) is higher than the prevalence in Japan, being similar to that of Caucasian Americans living in the United States.[46] Similarly, a Japanese migrant community living in central Brazil has a higher prevalence of Alzheimer's, and eats less fish, than the Okinawan community from which it originates.[47] Sometimes, comparisons between communities will be limited by different methodologies used by the different investigators. However, in one comparison the same investigators, using the same methodology, measured the age-standardized prevalence of Alzheimer's in Africans living in Nigeria and also in African Americans living in Indianapolis. They found a value of 1.4 percent for the Nigerian Africans compared with 6.2 percent for the US African Americans.[48] These sorts of studies suggest that lifestyle, including diet, influences the development of Alzheimer's.

The Rotterdam study, mentioned earlier, also found that higher fish consumption was associated with a reduced risk of developing Alzheimer's.[49] A number of other studies have similarly shown that higher fish consumption is associated with a slower cognitive decline and reduced risk of dementia.[50] Two meta-analyses examining the diet of cognitively healthy adults concluded that higher fish intake was associated with slower cognitive decline and reduced risk of developing Alzheimer's.[51]

An interesting observation is that when the 22:6ω-3 content of different regions of the postmortem brains from Alzheimer's patients and age-matched controls are compared, the 22:6ω-3 content is consistently reduced in the hippocampus of Alzheimer's patients but not necessarily in other brain regions (see note 50).

Although observational studies have shown that diets with higher omega-3 are associated with slower cognitive decline and a reduced risk of Alzheimer's, only the random-control trial (RCT) is regarded as the gold-standard test to determine cause-and-effect. However, there are a couple of important considerations when considering the role of RCTs in determining the influence of diet omega balance on cognitive decline and dementia. The first is that, as with other disease states, most RCTs generally involve small amounts of additional omega-3, resulting in trivial changes to diet omega balance. The second consideration is that because dementia involves the loss of neurons in discrete parts of the brain, it is possible that omega-3 supplementation will have effects when taken before dementia appears but will *not* have an effect once moderate dementia has set in. A recent analysis combined the results from three RCT studies that examined the influence of omega-3 supplements on patients with mild-to-moderate Alzheimer's disease and found no statistical evidence of a beneficial treatment for dementia.[52] The additional 22:6ω-3 in these three studies ranged from 0.7g to 1.7g per day. The results from the study providing the highest daily dose of additional 22:6ω-3 are of interest. Although this study found no statistical difference between the omega-3 group and the placebo group in cognitive decline, when they analyzed a subgroup that had only very mild cognitive dysfunction at the beginning of the trial, this group had a significantly reduced rate of cognitive decline when supplemented with omega-3 compared to placebo treatment.[53]

The Middle: Diet Omega Balance and Normal Brain Function

There are three ways that diet omega balance might influence normal brain function. The first is that by influencing the fatty acid composition of neuronal and synaptic membranes, it consequently influences the speed of nerve impulses and synaptic transmission. The second pathway is that diet omega balance might influence the processes of synaptic plasticity and neurogenesis. The third is that diet omega balance might influence the production of a variety of mediators (chemical messengers) that in turn influence neuronal and synaptic function.

If the diet is deficient in omega-3 but has plenty of omega-6, then the less common 22:5ω-6 substitutes for the normally dominant 22:6ω-3 in brain membranes. As pointed out in chapter 5, such a substitution in retinal membranes halves the normal response of the G-protein cascade that converts the presence of light to nervous impulses. Most neurotransmitter receptors are also "G-protein-coupled" systems and thus are likely to also be affected by the fatty acid composition of the surrounding membrane bilayer and thus affect normal brain function.

In a study designed to determine whether there was an optimal ratio of omega-3:omega-6 for learning ability, rats were given daily injections of mixtures of 18:2ω-6 and 18:3ω-3. Seven different ratios of the mixture were tested, and those corresponding to an omega balance of 20–22 percent resulted in both the best learning performance and the highest pain threshold (to be discussed shortly).[54] Many other studies of laboratory rodents have shown that omega-3 deficiency hinders learning ability. What about humans? In the previous section, I presented studies that showed high omega-3 intake slowed cognitive decline in older humans, but does high omega-3 improve the cognitive performance of normal healthy adults?

A US study used a battery of psychological tests to assess five major dimensions of cognitive function and also measured the blood omega-3 levels of healthy adults. It found that higher 22:6ω-3 levels were associated with better working memory, better nonverbal reasoning, as well as better mental flexibility and vocabulary.[55] Similarly, a Japanese study found a significant correlation between performance on a mental arithmetic task and blood 22:6ω-3 and 20:5ω-3 levels in healthy adults.[56] A US study using neuro-imaging techniques observed a higher intake of long-chain omega-3 was associated with more brain gray matter (neurons and synapses) of three important brain areas,[57] and a Dutch study found that better cognition in healthy middle-aged adults was associated with higher oily fish intake.[58]

To test whether an increase in omega-3 intake can be used to improve cognitive performance, a number of random-controlled trials have been carried out in recent times. Most of these have used fish oil, and most suffer from my regular criticism that they lack a "whole-of-diet" perspective and the amount of omega-3 used as a treatment is very small. Seven such studies on healthy young adults found three resulted in improved cognitive function while four had no significant effect.[59] In the studies that showed improved cognitive function, the average daily supplement of 22:6ω-3 was 1.1g compared with an average of 0.4g in those studies that resulted in no statistically significant effect. The same publication included a compilation of ten studies on healthy school-age children; similarly, the average 22:6ω-3 supplement was 0.4g per day, and while five studies showed significantly improved cognitive function, the other five studies found no significant change.

A couple of other studies deserve comment. An Italian study of healthy adult volunteers using fish-oil supplements (2.8g omega-3 per day for five weeks) produced significant improvements in cognitive function as well as improved mood profile with significantly lower measures of anger, anxiety, fatigue, depression, and confusion and a significant increase in vigor.[60]

The DOLAB study in the United Kingdom was designed to investigate whether there are any associations between blood omega-3 levels and reading, working memory, and behavior of underperforming healthy 7- to 9-year-old schoolchildren. Low blood 22:6ω-3 was associated with poor reading ability and poor working memory performance, as well as higher oppositional behavior and very changeable emotions (as assessed by parents).[61] Following this initial analysis, children were randomly allocated to either placebo or 22:6ω-3 supplementation (0.6g per day for 16 weeks). Although the increased reading ability in the 22:6ω-3 treatment group was not statistically significant for the whole group of children, the reading improvement was greatest and statistically significant in the children with the very lowest reading abilities. Moreover, the 22:6ω-3 supplementation resulted in significant reductions in parent-rated behavior problems (ADHD-type symptoms).[62]

ADHD is the most common developmental disorder in children in developed countries,[63] and several studies have examined the relationship between omega-3 and ADHD. A 2018 meta-analysis found that children and adolescents with ADHD had lower levels of blood omega-3 (especially 22:6ω-3) compared with children without ADHD but no difference in omega-6 levels. Furthermore, this meta-analysis also concluded that supplementation with omega-3 (22:6ω-3 and 20:5ω-3) significantly improved ADHD symptoms.[64]

Research into the influence of omega-3 on brain function has been dominated by the use of fish-oil supplementation, and whether the most common omega-3 in the diet (18:3ω-3) affects normal brain function has essentially not been investigated. However, it is worth noting that serum level of BDNF (brain derived neurotrophic factor) which has a very important fundamental role in synaptic plasticity, was significantly increased in healthy adults after flaxseed oil supplementation (0.5g 18:3ω-3 per day for a week).[65] Whether an increased dietary consumption of this 18-carbon omega-3 fatty acid improves normal brain function (such as learning performance) is to my knowledge unknown.

Diet Omega Balance and Chronic Pain

Acute pain, the means by which our brain is informed of damage, is protective in that it motivates withdrawal from the damaging situation; the pain will often persist while healing takes place. Acute pain is one of the five cardinal signs of inflammation, and many of the inflammation mediators initiate pain by interacting with receptors on the cell membrane of sensory pain neurons. Non-neural cells, especially those associated with inflammation, can also, through the production of inflammation mediators, modulate the pain sensation.[66] One such effect of inflammation mediators is to heighten or amplify the sensitivity of pain neurons to noxious stimuli. You will have experienced this if you have suffered sunburn with its associated inflammation and then taken a warm shower or put on a shirt over your sunburnt skin. Such activities, which in the normal condition would not elicit any pain sensation, can be painful as long as the sunburnt skin remains inflamed. While the classic eicosanoids are involved in the hypersensitivity to pain during inflammation, it has become apparent in recent times that there are other lipid-derived molecules also involved. These additional pain mediators are varied and are also made from polyunsaturated fatty acids. They are a complex group of molecules that I will refer to as "oxy-PUFA" metabolites, because their production involves the oxidative modification of polyunsaturated fatty acids. Most of the oxy-PUFA pain mediators are made from both $20:4\omega$-6 and $18:2\omega$-6; as a generalization, oxy-PUFAs made from omega-6 fatty are pro-pain mediators while those made from omega-3 are anti-pain mediators.[67] Linoleic acid ($18:2\omega$-6) is the most abundant polyunsaturated fat in the human diet and also in the skin. As well as being pain mediators, oxidatively modified metabolites of $18:2\omega$-6 are involved in the "itch" sensation.[68] An exciting finding of recent years is that levels of the oxy-PUFA metabolites made from $18:2\omega$-6 in humans can be decreased by reducing the dietary intake of this common omega-6.[69] I will return to the implications of this finding shortly.

The two most common types of drugs used to treat pain are either the non-steroidal anti-inflammatory drugs (NSAIDs) or the opioids. The NSAIDs act by inhibiting the production of prostaglandins from $20:4\omega$-6 in membrane fats and consequently act to diminish the production of inflammation mediators involved in the first steps of pain sensation. The opioids act by reducing the excitability of neurons in the pathway transmitting the pain message. Both types of drugs are among the oldest drugs used to relieve human suffering.

Chronic pain differs from acute pain in that it is pain that persists beyond the normal time of healing. A commonly used definition for chronic pain is that it persists for a period of three months or longer. Chronic pain is a major cause of disability worldwide with, for example, "back pain and neck pain" listed as the leading global cause of disability in 1990, 2005, and 2015.[70] The prevalence of chronic pain has increased over recent years, and because the prevalence of chronic pain is higher in older age-groups, it is often believed that this increased prevalence of chronic pain is largely due to the change in age structure of human populations. However, because of its subjectivity and the consequent difficulty in measuring pain, such a conclusion is uncertain. The increased use of anti-pain medications (both NSAIDs and opiates) is consistent with the possibility that chronic pain has increased in recent times independent of the "aging" of the population.

Osteoarthritis is a disease associated with inflammation and chronic pain. The UPLOAD (Understanding Pain and Limitations in Osteoarthritic Disease) study recruited adults with knee osteoarthritis. Participants self-reported both their clinical pain, and their sensitivity to experimental pain as well as having their psychosocial symptoms and blood fatty acids measured. They were divided into four groups according to the ratio of omega-6 to omega-3 in their blood plasma (I have converted these ratios into omega balances), and compared the top and bottom quartile for the various pain measurements. The omega balance for these two quartiles were 9 percent and 17 percent. In general, the two groups were similar demographically, although the low omega balance group were more obese. The low omega balance group self-reported *more* knee pain, stiffness, and functional limitations. They also had *greater* sensitivity to the experimental pain (both when applied to the knee and when applied to the hand), and higher scores for perceived stress and more negative emotions.[71] Having a low blood omega balance was associated with greater chronic pain and a less enjoyable life.

For me, one of the most exciting random-controlled trials examining the dietary balance between omega-3 and omega-6 fatty acids is the Chronic Daily Headache (CDH) trial, carried out by a team lead by Christopher Ramsden from the US National Institutes of Health.[72] An important part of this trial was its "whole-of-diet" approach. The theme of this book is that the increase in omega-6 (relative to omega-3) in the modern food chain is of serious concern and involved in the increased prevalence of chronic diseases over recent times. While this change is happening in many countries, it is especially advanced in the United States, where the intake of 18:2ω-6 per person averages about 7 percent of food energy intake. This value compares to historic intakes of about 2.5 percent energy and to an intake of only about 0.5 percent energy needed to satisfy minimal requirements. The diets used in the CDH trial provided total protein, total carbohydrate, and total fat typical of the average US diet, but provided approximately 40 percent of the current average consumption of omega-6 (2.5 percent energy). The two diets were thus both "low omega-6" diets but while one (L6 diet) provided the average US omega-3 intake (about 0.6 percent energy), the other diet (H3-L6 diet) provided additional omega-3 (about 2.5 percent energy). Participants were intensely counselled by dietitians throughout the twelve-week study, provided with study foods, and six unannounced twenty-four-hour dietary-recall questionnaires were administered. The preintervention diet did not differ between the two groups and had an omega balance of 9 percent (typical of the average US diet) while the omega balance of the L6 diet was 23 percent and that of the H3-L6 diet was 49 percent. This latter value is essentially the same as the omega balance of the 1960s Inuit diet. As confirmation that the different diets influenced body composition, the omega balance values of red blood cells went from 13 to 14 percent before the study to 17 percent in the L6 group and 28 percent in the H3-L6 participants at the end of the intervention.[73]

The participants in the CDH trial were adults who experienced chronic headaches; after a four-week run-in period (during which their normal diet and headache history were recorded), they were randomly allocated to either the L6 or H3-L6 diet. Only the dietitian knew of their treatment, and all other investigators (including each participant's personal physician) were not informed of the intervention treatment. After twelve weeks on the L6 diet, there were significant decreases in the number of headache days per month, headache hours per day, and the use of acute headache medications. The changes were greater and more statistically significant on the H3-L6 diet. Similarly, plasma concentrations of oxy-PUFAs significantly decreased on the L6 diet and even more so on the H3-L6 diet (see note 73).

Endocannabinoids (whose appetite-enhancing effects were considered in chapter 6) diminish the transfer of pain signals to the central nervous system. Endocannabinoids seem to be important in pain associated with cancer, and their concentrations in tissues are determined by the relative rates of their manufacture and degradation. When one of the enzymes that degrades endocannabinoids is blocked, the local concentration of endocannabinoids remains elevated and fewer pain signals reach the central nervous system.[74] The importance of endocannabinoids in pain is highlighted by the observation that a 66-year-old woman who did *not* feel pain also had low levels of anxiety and was found to have a mutation in a gene responsible for an enzyme that degrades endocannabinoids and also to have elevated blood endocannabinoid levels.[75] The Chronic Daily Headache trial participants on the H3-L6 diet had a significant *increase* in blood endocannabinoids made from omega-3 fats and a significant *decrease* in those made from omega-6 fats. Furthermore, it was found that the greater the change in the level of endocannabinoids, the greater the *decrease* in severe headache hours per day.[76]

As well as measuring headache and blood metabolite levels in the CDH trial participants, Ramsden and colleagues assessed their health-related-quality-of-life (HRQOL) and their level of psychological distress. The questionnaire used assesses three symptom dimensions—depression, anxiety, and somatization (manifestation of psychological distress in physical symptoms)—which are then combined to give a global measure of psychological distress. The HRQOL questionnaire can separately assess physical and mental health. Although there was little change after twelve weeks on the L6 diet, participants on the H3-L6 diet had significant improvement in physical and mental health as well a significant reduction in psychological distress.[77]

Patients with chronic pain commonly have a greater prevalence of psychological disorders than found in the general community. For example, one study of patients with chronic lower-back pain found that 59 percent demonstrated current symptoms for at least one psychiatric diagnosis, with the most common being major depression, substance abuse, and anxiety disorders, with prevalence being significantly greater than that for the general population. The common assumption that the chronic pain is the *cause* of these conditions is challenged by a study that reported 36 percent of those with major depression, 89 percent of substance abusers, and 71 percent of those with anxiety disorders experienced these conditions *before* the onset of the chronic back pain.[78]

We have come to the stage where physiology meets philosophy. The next chapter will examine the relationship between the diet omega balance and mental health. We will see that depression and obesity are associated with each other (they are co-morbid). Over the years, I have found that while many individuals readily accept that diet can affect physical health, they are very reluctant to accept that it will influence mental health. Their standard responses to explain the associations of physical and mental health are: "If I was obese, I'd be depressed," "If I had chronic knee pain, I'd be stressed," "If I had chronic headaches, I'd be anxious and depressed." All these responses are strongly influenced by the belief that "mind" and "body" are separate entities. In philosophical circles, this is called "Cartesian dualism" and although associated with the French philosopher René Descartes, this "mind-body" dualism has a much older history. My problem is that it hinders consideration that diet omega balance might be a very significant influence on mental health.

CHAPTER 10

MENTAL HEALTH AND HAPPINESS

Diet Omega Balance and Emotion: Aggression and Violence

In 1973, it was not appreciated that omega-6 and omega-3 were separate essential fatty acids, and an experiment on capuchin monkeys used a diet that was believed to contain all the essential dietary requirements, with the essential fats being provided by corn oil (which is devoid of omega-3). Some of the monkeys self-mutilated and had to be euthanized. Analysis showed a deficiency of omega-3 fats, and when 18:3ω-3 (in the form of flaxseed oil) was added to the diet, complete recovery of the remaining monkeys ensued.[1] Later studies on laboratory rodents observed that diets deficient in omega-3 or with excess omega-6 increased both aggression and depression behaviors.[2]

Regarding humans, a 1990 review of the mortality statistics from six primary prevention trials of cholesterol reduction provided some unexpected findings.[3] The participants, who all lacked a history of coronary heart disease but were diagnosed with high blood cholesterol, were randomly allocated to either a control treatment or a "cholesterol-lowering" intervention. Two were dietary interventions, two were pharmacological interventions, while the remaining two combined pharmacological and dietary intervention. The average cholesterol reduction achieved by the interventions was about 11 percent. Unexpectedly, total mortality was greater in the cholesterol-lowering intervention treatments than in the control treatment. Although the interventions resulted in a 15 percent *lower* mortality from coronary heart disease, there was a 76 percent *greater* mortality from "accidents, violence and suicide" and a 43 percent *greater* mortality from cancer. Intriguingly, it was the trials using dietary interventions that showed the greatest effect on mortality due to "accidents, violence and suicide." This finding was linked to earlier reports from Finland of low blood cholesterol levels in men with antisocial personalities as well as in homicidal offenders with habitually violent tendencies.[4] The study provoked discussion within the scientific community about a possible connection between low blood cholesterol and mental health consequences. However, not all studies had shown a negative effect of low blood cholesterol on mental health. For example, the Family Heart Study found the lowering of blood cholesterol by dietary change resulted in reduced levels of depression and aggressive hostility.[5]

In 1995, Joseph Hibbeln and Norman Salem Jr. entered the discussion and suggested that it was not the lowered cholesterol per se that caused these changes but possibly the dietary intervention.[6] At the time, the dietary advice included substitution of polyunsaturated fats for saturated fats, and this often involved the increased consumption of omega-6 dominated vegetable oils. Hibbeln and Salem suggested that the source of polyunsaturated fats in the diet might explain the conflicting findings regarding blood cholesterol and aggression. They suggested that use of a high omega-3 diet intervention to lower blood cholesterol would have the opposite effect to the use of vegetable oils. They also pointed out that although low blood cholesterol was associated with higher mortality due to violence and accidents in eastern Finland, the *opposite* trend was observed in western Finland.[7] They suggested that this difference may be related to greater fish consumption in coastal western population compared to the inland eastern population. Hibbeln and Salem reviewed the relationship between diet polyunsaturated fats and depression (which will be discussed in the next section).

Several studies have demonstrated beneficial effect of dietary omega-3 on aggression and hostility. For example, a US longitudinal study of heart disease risk recruited young adults in 1985–1986, and later years involved assessments of both diet history and of "hostility" (a trait with components of cynicism and mistrust of others, anger, and aggression). Intake of omega-3–rich fish and 22:6ω-3 were associated with significantly reduced hostility scores.[8] Japanese researchers had recruited university students for a randomized double-blind trial in which half received fish-oil capsules while the other half received a placebo. The three-month trial ended in the middle of the stressful final exam period, and while the students taking the placebo showed increased aggression against others at exam time, the fish-oil group showed no increased aggression during this stressful period.[9]

Some of the studies have centered on populations with mental health issues. In one study of men seeking hospital treatment for cocaine addiction, one-quarter had a history of assaulting others and were assessed to be highly aggressive. The aggressive addicts had significantly lower blood omega-3 levels than the nonaggressive addicts but no difference in blood omega-6.[10] Another group of substance-abuse patients seeking outpatient treatment participated in a randomized trial in which half took omega-3 capsules (2.8g/day) and half consumed placebo capsules. The placebo group showed no change in anger or anxiety, while the omega-3 group showed a decline in both anger and anxiety over the three-month period. Interestingly, the study found that blood omega-3 differed in their associated effects. Increased blood 22:6ω-3 was associated with a reduced anger, while an increased blood 20:5ω-3 level was associated with a reduced anxiety.[11] A study of an Australian prison population found that the higher their blood omega-3 index, the lower their level of aggression and attention-deficit disorder.[12]

Although not perfect, "homicide" is likely some sort of measure of "anger and hostility" at a national level. It is of interest that Joseph Hibbeln[13] showed there was a significant relationship between homicide in twenty-one countries and their apparent seafood consumption. The greater the seafood consumption (per person) the *lower* the homicide mortality (per 100,000 persons).[14] In 2004, Hibbeln and colleagues published an even more provocative graph that plotted the homicide mortality (per 100,000 persons) for Argentina, Australia, Canada, the United States, and the United Kingdom for each year from 1961 to 2000 against the apparent consumption of 18:2ω-6 (as percent energy intake per person) in each of these countries for each of these years.[15] The authors demonstrated that for each country, independently, there were highly significant relationships such that greater homicide mortality was associated with higher 18:2ω-6 consumption. They also appropriately pointed out that for each country they were plotting a "correlation," not necessarily a "cause-effect" relationship. This is important, as when two things that both increase with time are plotted against one another, they will almost certainly show a correlation. For example, if the "size of television screens" was plotted against the "miles of freeways" for the period 1960–2000, it is likely we would also observe a significant "correlation" between these two variables. However, the size of television screens does not determine the amount of freeways, nor do freeways determine television screen size. It is obvious there is no "cause-effect" relationship between them, even though they show a correlation because they both increased with time. If Hibbeln and his colleagues had left their analysis to only showing correlations for the five individual countries, the paper would not have impressed me. However, when the data for the five individual countries were all plotted on the same graph, they belonged to a single relationship. Considering the many societal factors that will influence national homicide rates, there was no intrinsic reason why there should be a single association for these five countries, and to me, a single relationship implied there may be something significant underlying it. While a "correlation" cannot prove a "cause-effect" relationship between the two variables, it should be remembered that a "correlation" is a *necessary* requirement for "cause-effect" relationships. If you can show there is *no* correlation between two variables, you can rule out a "cause-effect" relationship. If there is a significant correlation between the two variables, it means they share something in common. It may mean that one variable is "cause" and one is its "effect," or it may mean that neither is the "cause," but that they have a common "cause."

In his 2002 film *Bowling for Columbine,* Michael Moore examined gun violence in the United States and noted that while Canada had a high level of gun ownership, it had a much lower level of gun violence than the United States. Moore did not resolve the paradox to my satisfaction, and I wondered whether this graph presented at least part of the answer. To myself, I speculated that part of the reason for the high rate of homicide in the United States (as well as gun ownership) might be related to the national diet, namely an imbalance between omega-3 and omega-6 fats in the US diet. The Hibbeln graph stimulated quite a provocative idea.

Impulse control, an individual's ability to inhibit his/her actions, is an executive function important for normal development and is diminished in some behavioral conditions. A study of adolescents found a significantly greater impulse control with greater omega-3 intake.[16] In adolescent boys (with ADHD) it has been shown that lower blood omega-3 is associated with greater callous and unemotional traits,[17] and another study by the same investigators, measuring brain electrical patterns in response to pictures of faces expressing various emotions (for example, fear, sad, happy, angry, and so on) found that boys with ADHD had deficits in emotional processing and furthermore the lower the level of blood omega-3 fatty acids, the greater the impairment.[18]

A continuing study of child health and development, the Mauritius Child Health Project was set up in 1972 and aimed to identify early risk factors for later psychopathology, focusing on outcomes for antisocial/violent behavior. This study has produced more than 63 journal articles and book chapters with many significant findings, including that early enrichment (nutritional, educational, and physical) at 3–5 years results in reduced conduct disorder and criminal offending in later years.[19] One of the later studies was an omega-3 supplementation trial on children randomly allocated to either a treatment group that received a daily fruit drink containing 1g omega-3 for six months or a placebo of the same fruit drink but without added omega-3. Parents administered the drink, and all children, parents, and research assistants were blinded as to their treatment group. The omega-3 supplement significantly reduced aggressive and antisocial behaviors, including reduction in callous-unemotional traits. Interestingly, parents had been informed at the beginning of the study of the hypothesis being investigated (namely "omega-3 supplements may improve behavior") and when asked, at the end of the experiment, the treatment they thought their child had received, as expected about a half of the placebo-group parents said their child received omega-3, while 97 percent of the treatment parents correctly guessed their child had received omega-3. The improved behavior must have been very obvious to the parents! Another interesting finding was that the parents of those children who took omega-3 also showed significant post-treatment improvements in their own antisocial and aggressive behavior. Indeed, the investigators estimated that the improvements in parental behavior accounted for 60 percent of the improvement in child antisocial behavior.[20] This study showed that improving child behavior through omega-3 supplementation also resulted in reduced psychological aggression between intimate adult partners and that this can have long-term benefits to the family system as a whole.[21]

Diet Omega Balance and Depression: "The Inflamed Mind"

I have taken the title for this section from the book by Edward Bullmore, a professor of psychiatry at the University of Cambridge. The book is an account of Bullmore's journey from physician to psychiatrist and the emerging evidence of how medical depression is related to inflammation.

We all likely experience sadness at times, but when this low mood continues and is associated with the inability to experience pleasure from normally enjoyable activities, the condition is called depression. It can often also be associated with other conditions: feelings of worthlessness and guilt, fatigue, loss of appetite, insomnia, reduced ability to think or concentrate, indecisiveness, and pain without a clear cause and sometimes thoughts of death or suicide. Between 2 and 8 percent of adults with major depression die by suicide, and about half of the people who die by suicide had depression or a similar mood disorder.[22] The diagnosis is normally determined by a series of standardized checklists: major depressive disorder (MDD) is when five or more symptoms are present nearly every day during a two-week period. MDD can vary in severity, in pattern, onset, and remission and can include other conditions. For example, although anxiety can be diagnosed as a separate psychiatric condition, it is commonly associated with depression (almost two-thirds of patients), and anxiety symptoms can often appear one to two years ahead of the onset of major depression.[23] There is no biomarker for depression. The cause of MDD is unknown. There can be a genetic contribution, but while many gene variants have been linked to an increased risk for MDD, it is calculated that even combined they explain only a small proportion of risk for MDD. Stressful life events are strongly associated with major depression, but individuals differ in their sensitivity or resilience.[24]

Depression co-occurs especially with those diseases that involve chronic inflammation, the same diseases discussed in earlier chapters. For example, the 2003 World Health Survey, involving sixty countries in all world regions, found the prevalence for depression alone was 3 percent, while it was 11 percent among individuals with arthritis, 18 percent among individuals with asthma, 15 percent among individuals with angina, and 9 percent among those with diabetes. Among individuals with two or more of these chronic diseases, the prevalence of depression was 23 percent.[25] The 1999 US National Health Interview Survey produced similar results about the co-occurrence of chronic diseases and depression. The prevalence of depression was 9 percent in adults with diabetes, 15 percent in chronic obstructive pulmonary disease sufferers, 9 percent in adults with coronary artery disease, 11 percent in adults with stroke or cerebrovascular accidents, but only 5 percent in adults without any of these chronic diseases.[26]

Obese individuals have an increased risk of depression. Obesity itself is a mixed condition in that some "unhealthy obese" individuals also have other metabolic complications (such as high blood pressure, high blood triglycerides, elevated inflammatory markers), while "healthy obese" individuals lack such complications. Both types are associated with a greater risk of depression: "unhealthy obese" adults have an approximately 60 percent greater risk, while "healthy obese" adults have an approximately 30 percent greater risk of depression than nonobese adults.[27]

The initial response to learning of the co-occurrence of depression with these other chronic diseases is the standard "well, you would, wouldn't you? If you had rheumatoid arthritis (or obesity, . . . chronic obstructive pulmonary disease, . . . coronary artery disease, . . . diabetes . . .), you'd be depressed." This is the response when mind-body dualism dominates. But what if the depression is not a psychological response to having a chronic disease but is rather another manifestation of the chronic inflammation associated with the co-occurring disease? Neuro-inflammation has increasingly become an explanation of the pathophysiology underlying MDD.

Probably the dominant mechanistic explanation of MDD has been the "monoamine hypothesis" which posits that MDD is due to a decrease in the monoamine neurotransmitters (serotonin, noradrenaline, and dopamine). It is the basis of most of the antidepressant drug treatments, but it does not fully explain the variability in clinical presentation of major depressive episodes nor why some patients respond to particular antidepressants but others do not, and, importantly, it also does not explain why antidepressants often take weeks to work. Inflammatory mediators, as well as both neurogenesis and neuroplasticity have been linked to MDD. A key regulatory molecule in neuroplasticity, BDNF (brain-derived neurotrophic factor) is diminished in major depression and antidepressant treatments can restore BDNF levels, as can dietary 18:3ω-3.[28] Antidepressants increase neurogenesis in the adult brain.

If inflammation causes depression, it is likely present before the depressive episode. One longitudinal study found higher levels of a blood inflammatory marker in blood of children (9 years old) was associated with an increased risk of developing depression and psychosis in young adulthood.[29] Another longitudinal study of adults found a similar relationship in that participants with high levels of inflammatory marker in their blood measured in 1992 and 1997 had a significantly greater risk of a mental disorder in 2003-2008.[30]

Other important evidence of a link between inflammation and depression was the finding that use of an inflammatory mediator (α-interferon) could produce psychiatric symptoms, including fatigue, lack of concentration, anxiety, and depression.[31] Interferons activate immune cells such as macrophages and natural killer cells and produce an inflammatory response, and interferon treatment is used to fight various cancers and viral infections. A controlled-trial on chronic hepatitis-B patients compared interferon treatment for 3 to 6 months with a control treatment; although they were not depressed before their treatment, the patients receiving the interferon developed psychiatric symptoms (including depression), unlike the control group. Three months after the treatment finished, the symptoms had disappeared (see note 31). Similarly, a study in which lung cancer patients were given interferon treatment reported that although they were all mentally healthy at the beginning, six days later a majority of the patients developed symptoms indicative of a major depressive episode and five developed a severe depressed mood. All symptoms disappeared within two weeks of stopping treatment.[32] Since these early studies, it is now well established that a number of different pro-inflammatory mediators can induce true major depressive disorder in patients with no prior history of mental disorders.[33] Furthermore, in clinical trials where therapies directed against inflammatory mediators have been used to treat chronic inflammatory diseases (including Crohn's disease and rheumatoid arthritis) have also produced significant antidepressant effects.[34]

In view of the influence of omega-3 on diseases associated with chronic inflammation (chapters 6–8) and the importance of omega-3 in neurogenesis, neuroplasticity, learning, and cognitive function (chapter 9) it is worthwhile to examine the influence of omega-3 on depressive illness. But first, let's consider an early suggested cure. In the seventeenth century, Robert Burton, author of the multivolume *The Anatomy of Melancholy* presented a particular cure for head melancholy. He wrote:[35]

> Take a ram's head that never meddled with an ewe, cut off at a blow, and the horns only take away, boil it well, skin and wool together; after it is well sod, take out the brains, and put these spices to it, cinnamon, ginger, nutmeg, mace, cloves . . . stirring them well. . . .
>
> Keep it so prepared, and for three days give it the patient fasting, so that he fast two hours after it. It may be eaten with bread in an egg or broth. . . . For fourteen days let him use this diet, drink no wine.

Although at the time he didn't know of 22:6ω-3 and its high concentration in the brain, he may have been on the mark. The logic that brain tissue contains important ingredients required for normal brain function certainly appeals to me—although I'm not enamored with his suggested method of preparation and cooking.

Three and a half centuries later, Italian researchers compared the effect of a placebo treatment with that of cattle brain lipid extracts on elderly women with depressive disorders. They found that the marked depressive symptoms in their patients before treatment did not change with placebo treatment, but after 30 days of treatment with the cattle brain lipid extract, the depressive symptoms were significantly improved,[36] which supports Burton's suggested treatment.

Several studies have compared the fatty acid composition of postmortem brains from MDD subjects with control postmortem brains. Most report a lower 22:6ω-3, but some have not reported differences.[37]

Postmortem brain comparisons need to be considered carefully, especially the "control" brains. For example, one study found the postmortem brains of adult MDD suicide victims had lower 22:6ω-3 levels compared with controls, but the difference was not statistically significant. However, when individuals who had died from cardiovascular disease were excluded from the control group, the reduction in 22:6ω-3 brain content between MDD sufferers and controls was both greater and statistically significant.[38]

Is depression associated with low tissue levels of omega-3? A meta-analysis that compared blood polyunsaturated fatty acid composition in depression patients with control subjects found that blood levels of 22:6ω-3, 20:5ω-3, and total omega-3 were significantly lower in patients with depression but that there was no difference in blood omega-6 levels between the two groups.[39] A different study similarly reported a significantly reduced 22:6ω-3 in red blood cells of MDD adolescents compared with healthy controls but no reduction in omega-6 levels.[40] When plasma fatty acid composition was measured in adults prior to receiving interferon treatment for hepatitis C, it was found that low omega-3 and elevated omega-6 were associated with greater risk of developing depression.[41]

An indication that diet omega balance and major depression were likely connected was illustrated when Joseph Hibbeln demonstrated that the prevalence of major depression in nine countries was significantly correlated with their annual fish consumption (per person).[42] The greater the apparent fish consumption, the lower the prevalence of major depression. In the same year a UK study reported that among severely depressed adults, the lower their diet omega-3 intake, the greater the severity of their depression.[43] A meta-analysis of thirty-one observational studies published over the period 2001–2015, estimated that (1) fish intake of 125g per day was associated with a 22 percent lower risk of depression; (2) omega-3 intake of 2g per day was associated with a 70 percent reduced risk of depression; and (3) a daily intake of 1.2g of combined 22:6ω-3 and 20:5ω-3 was associated with a 40 percent lower risk of depression.[44]

This meta-analysis did not consider omega-6 intake, but a Japanese longitudinal study later examined correlations between dietary intake of both omega-3 and omega-6 fats by Japanese adults from 1997 to 2012 and the development of depression.[45] Furthermore, the dietary omega-6 to omega-3 ratio was calculated for each individual, and (after converting omega-6/omega-3 ratios to omega balance values) when the population was divided into thirds, the third of the population with the lowest diet omega balance (median of 14 percent, range of 6–16 percent) had a significantly greater risk of developing depression than did the third of the population with the highest diet omega balance (median of 24 percent, range of 20–55 percent). This study confirmed that diet omega balance significantly influenced the risk of depression.

These observational studies of links between diet and depression are correlations, and consequently, although compatible with it, they do not prove a "cause-effect" relationship, which requires consideration of randomized-controlled trials. There have been such trials, and although several show significant beneficial effects of omega-3 supplements on depression, others fail to show statistically significant effects. A 2014 meta-analysis considered 19 such trials, most of which examined the effect of supplements of 22:6ω-3 and 20:5ω-3 combined, while the others examined the influence of only one of these omega-3 fatty acids. The average daily dose of 22:6ω-3 was 0.9g, and for 20:5ω-3 it was 1.2g, with an average duration of 10 weeks. The conclusion from this meta-analysis is that increased intake of long-chain omega-3 fatty acids reduced the risk of depression.[46] Of two later meta-analyses, one concluded that omega-3 supplements were beneficial but mainly those supplements that emphasized 20:5ω-3.[47] The other found a significant overall beneficial effect of omega-3 supplementation on major depressive disorder in adults, but its authors concluded that they did not have sufficient evidence to determine the effects of omega-3 as a treatment for MDD and that further research was required.[48] Ambivalence is not uncommon in many meta-analyses of omega-3 supplementation trials, and such ambivalence is strongly influenced by the fact that *some* trials fail to show a statistically significant beneficial effect. My opinion, already expressed in previous chapters, is that a large number of these trials lack a whole-of-diet perspective and consequently test very small doses of omega-3 supplements for a relatively limited period of supplementation. Sometimes even a positive (beneficial) effect that did not reach statistical significance has been described as a "negative" finding. To me a "negative" trial would be one in which omega-3 supplementation is detrimental to the condition being examined, not the situation of a statistically nonsignificant positive effect on the condition!

What about studies examining other types of patients suffering depression? The Vienna omega-3 study was a longitudinal study in which young people at ultra-high risk for psychosis were enrolled in a randomized double-blind placebo-controlled trial in which the treatment group received fish oil (1.2g per day) and the placebo group received coconut oil for 12 weeks. At the seven-year follow-up, only 10 percent of the omega-3 treatment group had progressed to psychosis compared with 40 percent of the placebo group.[49] Importantly for our consideration, when blood fatty acid composition was measured, it was found that a low blood omega balance at the beginning of the study was significantly associated with a depressive mood disorder during the following seven years.[50]

Interferon treatment has become a standard therapy for chronic hepatitis-C infection, and because of the high rate of side-effects such as depression and sickness behavior during such therapy, omega-3 supplementation has been examined as a prophylactic treatment to possibly reduce the depression side-effects. A two-week randomized, placebo-controlled trial showed that treatment with 20:5ω-3 (3.5g/d) both decreased the incidence of interferon-induced major depressive episodes and delayed its onset, while treatment with 22:6ω-3 (1.8g/d) delayed the onset but did not significantly reduce the incidence of interferon-induced major depressive episodes.[51]

A form of depression, postnatal depression, is the most common complication related to child-bearing. In view of the mother's provision of 22:6ω-3 to both the developing fetus and the newborn baby, the relationship between omega-3 and postnatal depression has been investigated in recent times. The prevalence of postnatal depression varies among countries and is inversely related to the apparent fish consumption of the particular country.[52] Those countries with low fish consumption have high rates of postnatal depression. The same publication showed that there was also an inverse relationship between the average 22:6ω-3 content of mothers' milk and the prevalence of postnatal depression among a number of countries. A low 22:6ω-3 content of mothers' milk was associated with a greater prevalence of postnatal depression.

A meta-analysis of observational studies in which the blood fatty acid composition has been compared between mothers with and without postnatal depression confirmed a connection between blood fatty acids and postnatal depression. Specifically, it found that it was blood omega balance that had the strongest relationship. The lower the blood omega balance, the greater the prevalence of postnatal depression.[53] Similarly, a Belgian study that examined the relationship between blood fatty acid composition of mothers in early pregnancy on the later development of postnatal depression following childbirth, found the strongest relationship was with blood omega balance. Again, the lower the blood omega balance, the greater the risk of postnatal depression.[54] A number of fish-oil supplementation trials have been carried out, and a meta-analysis of these studies that found some had statistically significant beneficial effects on postnatal depression while others did not. The average dose of fish oil for all these studies was about 1.5g per day.[55]

Suicide is sometimes a sad consequence of major depression. A US study of unmedicated depressed subjects monitored for suicide attempt over a two-year period found that low omega balance of plasma fatty acids was a predictor of suicide attempt.[56] A Japanese-Chinese study compared the red blood cell fatty acid composition of suicide-attempt patients with matched controls. The suicide-attempters had been referred to a hospital because of acute deliberate self-harm but were excluded if they were under the influence of alcohol or drugs, had delusions, hallucinations, dementia, or disturbed consciousness. The control subjects were general trauma patients (injured at construction sites, factories, at home or in car accidents) from the same hospital as the suicide-attempters and were matched by gender, age, and smoking status. The red blood cells of the suicide-attempt group had a significantly lower omega balance. When all subjects were combined and divided into quartiles according to blood cell fatty acids, the suicide risk was eight times higher in the lowest quartile than in the highest quartile of 20:5ω-3 content. A fivefold greater risk was calculated when the lowest and highest quartile of 22:6ω-3 were compared.[57]

The largest study examining suicide and omega-3 fatty acid status is one involving active-duty US military personnel. The Armed Forces Health Surveillance Center (AFHSC) is a repository of more than 40 million serum samples with matched health data from US military personnel. Sera and data were obtained for eight hundred active-duty military personnel who had died by suicide between 2002 and 2008. Control participants (800) were randomly selected by the AFHSC and matched by age, gender, rank, and availability of both health data and time when the serum sample was taken. The suicide-death group had a significantly lower serum 22:6ω-3. More significantly, when the data for the suicide group and the control group were combined, it was possible to determine the risk of suicide with respect to serum 22:6ω-3 level. The range of 22:6ω-3 levels varied from 0.3 to 4.5 percent of total fatty acids, and the risk of suicide-death was highest in those personnel with the lowest 22:6ω-3 levels. For example, the risk of suicide was 62 percent greater in military personnel with serum 22:6ω-3 levels below 1.75 percent compared with those above this level.[58]

Obviously, the risk of suicide is due to multiple social, psychiatric, environmental factors, and war experiences. Diet is not normally considered a significant factor for suicide risk, but the 62 percent increased risk associated with a low 22:6ω-3 shows it to be more significant than some other factors. For example, personnel who answered "yes" to the question "Did you see wounded, killed, or dead coalition during deployment?" had a 54 percent increased risk of suicide death. As pointed out in this study, these military personnel had a serum omega balance of only 6 percent, which is low compared with general North American, Australasian, Mediterranean, and Asian populations (see note 58). The relatively cheap nonpsychological approach of improving the omega balance of the diet of military personnel, as proposed by Joseph Hibbeln,[59] could have a significant influence in reducing military psychiatric distress, likely including posttraumatic stress disorder and its consequences.

From a "Traditional" to a "Modern" Diet: The Inuit Example

The theme of this book is that there has been a dramatic change, especially over the last half-century, in the balance of omega-3 and omega-6 fats in the modern food chain. This change is most pronounced in many developed countries, and the general population of these countries is essentially ignorant and unaware of the change. This imbalance affects the composition of cell membranes of a number of human tissues, which is associated with a number of chronic diseases. The Inuit of Greenland have been significant in the evolution of this perspective because it was the absence of cardiovascular diseases in the traditional Greenland Inuit that, in the 1960s, attracted the attention of two Danish physicians. Hans Bang and Jorn Dyerberg discovered that the absence of cardiovascular diseases in the Inuit was associated with a high blood concentration of omega-3 fatty acids, and this discovery marked the beginning of our awareness of the importance of omega-3 for human health.

Following Danish colonization of Greenland in 1721, the sale of European food to the Inuit was prohibited. It was not until 1860 that it became legal to sell coffee, tea, bread, and grain to the Inuit. As with many other indigenous peoples, there has been a shift from traditional foods to a "modern" diet since the mid-nineteenth century, with serious health consequences for the Inuit.

Using data from an 1855 survey, August and Marie Krogh estimated the food available per day to a traditional Inuit (table 10.1).

This diet, dominated by traditional foods, was high in both protein (47 percent energy) and fat (45 percent energy) but very low in carbohydrates (8 percent energy).[60] During the twentieth century, the contribution of traditional foods decreased in the Inuit diet. In a village population, traditional foods provided 54 percent of food energy in 1953 and only 41 percent in 1976 (in a nearby village). The contribution of traditional foods to the diet of town populations was lower than in villages, being 17–25 percent in 1953, and 9–13 percent in 2004-6.[61] The consumption of traditional foods also varied substantially among different segments of the population. A 2005–7 survey of dietary patterns found that only 8 percent of young men consumed significant amounts of "local food" compared to 45 percent of old men. Similarly, only 10 percent of young men consumed "seal, fish, and local meat" (caribou, musk ox, and wildfowl) compared to 49 percent of old men.[62]

It was not until the 1970s that the fatty acid composition of the traditional Inuit diet was determined. On their 1972 and 1976 expeditions, Bang and Dyerberg collected food from Inuit hunters, fishermen, and their wives for later fatty acid measurement and comparison to a normal Danish diet. Although the Danish and Inuit diets had approximately the same amount of fat (37–42 percent energy), they had very different fatty acid compositions. The omega balance of the Danish diet was 21 percent, compared to 51 percent for the 1972 Inuit diet,[63] and 72 percent for the 1976 Inuit diet (see note 61). Later, additional diet samples were obtained from town-dwelling Inuit. In these samples the omega balance was 35 percent in 2004 and 12 percent in 2006.[64] Over thirty years (1976 to 2006) there was a sixfold *decrease* in diet omega balance.

These changes in the food affected the Inuit's body composition. In 1976, the omega balance of plasma phospholipids was 61 percent

Table 10.1 Daily Food Available to a Traditional Inuit

Food source	Amount (in grams)
Meat (79% seal meat)	1,210
Fish (63% capelin)	1,100
Berries	55
Bread	27
Coffee and sugar	12
Eggs	6
Beans	6

Source: Estimated by August and Marie Krogh, based on an 1855 survey.

compared to 37 percent in 2004 and 25 percent in 2006 (see note 61). Once again, over thirty years (1976 to 2006) there was more than a twofold *decrease* in plasma omega balance.

These changes in diet and blood composition were associated with changes in Inuit health. Between 1901 and 1930, the most frequent cause of death in West Greenland was tuberculosis, followed by accidents and then pneumonia. There was no mention of ischemic heart disease.[64] Tuberculosis reached crisis levels in Greenland in the 1940s and 1950s, and following government controls, its incidence (per 1,000 persons) was dramatically reduced from about 23 in 1955 to about 1 in 1973.[65] Other health improvements over this period include dramatic reductions in death rate from acute infections[66] and a reduction in infant deaths (see note 65). However, several chronic diseases (obesity, ischemic heart disease, stroke, diabetes, and cancer) often described as "diseases of modernization," and previously relatively absent, are becoming common among the Inuit (see note 65). One of the most dramatic changes has been in mental health and its sad manifestation as suicide.

The annual suicide rate (per 100,000 persons) among Greenland Inuit between 1900 and 1930 was estimated to be 3, by 1960–64 it had risen to 14, and it averaged 101 in 1990–94, and 110 in 2010–11.[67] This represents a thirtyfold increase over the last century! The suicide rate was higher in towns (81 per 100,000) than villages (61 per 100,000) and was more than fivefold greater in young males than in old males. Between 2005 and 2010, among Greenland Inuit males, the annual incidence of suicidal thoughts was about 30 times the suicide rate.[68] These statistics describe a public health crisis.

I have concentrated on Greenland Inuit, but the same change from traditional to modern diets and similar public health changes (including increased suicide rate) have been recorded in other circumpolar Inuit populations, if sometimes with a different timeline (see note 67). Inuit from the Nunavik region of Canada (especially the young) consumed fewer traditional foods in 2004 than in 1992, and also consumed more alcohol and drugs, and the prevalence of suicidal ideation and suicide attempts increased.[69] Between 1982 and 1996, there was a fivefold increase in the suicide rate.[70] While it is common to include diet changes when examining causes of the increase in the chronic "diseases of modernization" (for example, obesity, heart disease, diabetes, cancer) it is rare for diet changes to be considered when examining changes in mental health (for example, anger, violence, depression, and suicide). I know of only one scientific paper that asked whether diet was an important factor in the mental health of circumpolar peoples.[71] In view of the numerous studies considered earlier in this chapter that show an increased omega balance is beneficial for mental health, it is a proposition well worth considering.

Psychosocial experiences, such as childhood abuse, early exposure to violence, and other factors are no doubt substantial contributors to psychological distress. However, although little considered, it is also plausible that the change from a traditional diet to a modern Western diet, with its consequent dramatic decrease in dietary omega balance, is also a contributor to the mental ill-health and suicide in modern Inuit populations. A health survey of the Nunavik Inuit in 1992 included both an assessment of psychological distress and a measurement of the fatty acid composition of plasma phospholipids. Participants with "psychological distress" had significantly lower plasma omega-3 levels than those without "psychological distress," although there was no difference in the plasma omega-6 levels. Further, plasma omega-3 levels were related to the degree of psychological distress. Individuals with the greatest degree of psychological distress had the lowest plasma omega-3.[72] A later Nunavik Inuit Health Survey (2004) measured the fatty acid composition of red blood cells and also found that individuals showing "serious psychological distress" had significantly lower omega-3 levels than those not showing distress and a greater risk of serious psychological distress in individuals with low red blood cell omega-3 levels.[73] The conclusion from these studies is that part of the dramatic changes in mental health of Inuit populations that has accompanied "modernization" can be explained by the change from the high omega balance traditional diet to the low omega balance modern diet.

CHAPTER 11

OF MICE AND MEN

Lessons from the Fat-1 mouse

Sometime in our past, our ancestors "lost" the enzymes to synthesize omega-6 as well as the enzymes to make omega-3 from omega-6; consequently, both are now essential requirements in our diet. As far as we know, this is true for all "higher" animals but it doesn't hold true for all animals. A simple nematode worm, about 1 millimeter long with the Latin name of *Caenorhabditis elegans*, still possesses the enzymes necessary to manufacture omega-3 and omega-6 fats. This worm was the first animal to have its genome sequenced and is a popular animal for much laboratory investigation. It eats bacteria, and because it can synthesize them, neither omega-3 nor omega-6 are "essential" components of its diet. Furthermore, it can convert omega-6 fats into omega-3 fats; the gene for this enzyme has been labeled the "Fat-1" gene.

In 2004, Jing Kang and colleagues from Harvard University reported that they had produced a transgenic mouse strain to which they had added the Fat-1 gene from *Caenorhabditis elegans*.[1] Individuals from this strain are called Fat-1 mice. To determine whether the gene was active, the researchers fed both "wild-type" and Fat-1 mice the same omega-3–deficient but omega-6–sufficient diet and measured the fatty acid composition of tissues and milk from both mice strains (figure 11.1). The extreme deficiency of omega-3 in the diet resulted in extremely low omega balance of fats in the tissues (2–20 percent) and milk (3 percent) from wild-type mice. The relative importance of membrane composition in the brain is evident by the fact that this tissue had the highest omega balance, retaining more

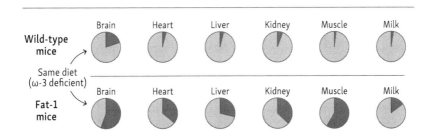

Figure 11.1 Comparison of the omega balance of fats extracted from selected tissues of wild-type mice and Fat-1 mice fed the same omega-3 deficient diet. See text for explanation and source of data.

of its omega-3 than the other tissues. In contrast, for the Fat-1 mice, the omega balance of tissues (29–59 percent) and milk (15 percent) were much higher, despite consuming a diet devoid of omega-3. Thus, unlike normal wild-type mice, Fat-1 mice do *not* have an essential requirement for omega-3 fats in their diet. Consequently, any differences between wild-type and Fat-1 mice fed identical diets (that are omega-6 adequate) will indicate activities that are influenced by omega balance. In this way, Fat-1 mice represent a separate experimental system that can either confirm or negate results obtained in other experiments where change in omega balance has been achieved by diet manipulation.

Fat-1 mice fed a high omega-6 diet do not develop obesity (or the fatty liver) as do wild-type mice.[2] Two separate studies have shown that when fed the same diet, Fat-1 mice have a higher glucose tolerance than wild-type mice.[3] These studies using the transgenic Fat-1 mouse support a role for omega balance of membrane fats being an important determinant for both obesity and Type 2 diabetes.

Compared to those of wild-type mice, the cells from Fat-1 mice show a reduced inflammatory response when challenged.[4] When wild-type mice and Fat-1 mice both had acute lung injury, the inflammatory response and the severity of the disease, as well as sickness behaviors, were reduced in the Fat-1 mice, which also recovered lung function more quickly than the wild-type mice.[5] Similarly, when acute liver inflammation was induced in both strains of mice by injection of a bacterial toxin, the inflammatory response and liver damage were less in the Fat-1 mice than in the wild-type mice.[6]

Allergic responses and autoimmune diseases are reduced in Fat-1 mice. Experimental induction of allergic airway inflammation produced a lower inflammatory response and a reduced bronchial hyper-responsiveness to the challenge in Fat-1 mice than in wild-type mice.[7] Similarly when allergic dermatitis (eczema) was induced in mice, both the inflammatory response and the damage to the skin were reduced in Fat-1 mice compared to the wild-type mice.[8] A mouse disease model used to investigate rheumatoid arthritis also shows a diminished inflammatory response and a lesser disease condition in Fat-1 mice compared to wild-type mice.[9] An experimental model of Type 1 diabetes, in which a microbial toxin initiates inflammatory responses that destroy the insulin-producing pancreatic cells, has been used for many years. A number of different groups of investigators have shown that, unlike wild-type mice, Fat-1 mice are resistant to this destructive process.[10] Multiple sclerosis is the autoimmune disease involving chronic inflammation and demyelination in the brain and spinal cord. After Fat-1 and wild-type mice were fed a chemical toxin for five weeks, they exhibited a similar degree of central nervous system demyelination; however, two weeks later the Fat-1 mice showed a greater degree of remyelination, suggesting that omega-3 are beneficial in the treatment of multiple sclerosis.[11]

The inflammatory response and the severity of colitis are much reduced in Fat-1 mice compared to wild-type mice.[12] In chronic obstructive pulmonary disease, inflammation can be induced by exposure to the fine particles associated with smoke and air pollution. Exposure to such fine particles has been shown to produce a reduced inflammatory response in Fat-1 mice compared to wild-type mice.[13] The development of new blood vessels in the retina (retinal neovascularization) is a particularly damaging aspect of macular degeneration, and Fat-1 mice show less retinal neovascularization than wild-type mice.[14]

A large number of studies have compared the development and growth of a variety of cancer cells in Fat-1 and wild-type mice. All have shown a reduced cancer and cancer activity in the Fat-1 mice. For example, fifteen days after the implantation of breast cancer cells into mice, tumors were still growing in wild-type mice but had completely disappeared in Fat-1 mice.[15] Others have similarly shown reduced growth of breast cancer in Fat-1 mice compared to wild-type mice.[16] Similar differences have also been noted for gastric cancers,[17] colon and colorectal cancers,[18] pancreatic cancer,[19] liver cancer,[20] skin cancer, and melanomas,[21] as well as prostate cancer.[22]

When fed a diet with negligible omega-3, Fat-1 mice have the same brain content of $22:6\omega$-3 content as normal mice fed a highly enriched omega-3 diet.[23] Japanese researchers examining early brain development found that mice fed a diet with a low omega balance (2 percent) had reduced neurogenesis, thinner brain cortex layers, and increased anxiety-related behaviors as adults. When this diet was fed to Fat-1 mice, there were no such deficiencies in brain development.[24] A different group of investigators similarly found that brain neurogenesis and learning were enhanced in the Fat-1 mice compared to the wild-type mice when both were fed an omega-3–deficient diet.[25] The injection of a bacterial toxin into normal laboratory mice can induce a neuro-inflammatory episode and result in impaired memory and diminished cognitive performance. When the same experiment was carried out in Fat-1 mice, pro-inflammatory mediators were lower, and the Fat-1 mice showed normal cognitive performance similar to noninjected wild-type mice.[26]

A number of different mice strains have been created as animal models for investigating Alzheimer's disease. Two independent studies, using different strains of Alzheimer's disease mice, have shown that when Fat-1 mice are interbred with these strains, the offspring that have the Fat-1 gene have a reduced neuro-pathology and cognitive deficits compared to the offspring without the Fat-1 gene.[27] Another study has shown that when both Fat-1 mice and wild-type mice are fed the same omega-3–deficient diet, the Fat-1 mice show a much greater rate of clearing amyloid-beta from the brain and that, compared to wild-type mice, Fat-1 mice also show much reduced neuronal damage when amyloid-beta is injected into their brain.[28]

We might also expect Fat-1 mice to not experience chronic pain with the same intensity as do wild-type mice. It is of course difficult to measure the pain experienced by other species. One protocol that has been used to investigate pain in mice consists of injecting a very small amount of dilute formalin solution under the skin on the sole of one of the hind feet of the mouse. Following this experience, the mice will experience pain and either lick, lift, or flinch the injected foot. By counting the combined number of licks, lifts, and flinches, it is possible to quantify the pain experienced by the mouse. When this protocol was carried out on normal wild-type mice, they exhibited a pain score of 50–60 (combined number of licks, lifts, and flinches of the injected foot) for the first 5 minutes after the injection, followed by a score of zero during the second 5-minute period. The pain score increases again after 10 minutes, peaking at about 20 minutes after the injection, and then slowly declines to zero by 60 minutes. It is assessed that the response during the first period corresponds to the "acute" pain, while the response during the second period is analogous to "chronic" pain, being associated with an inflammatory response. This response has also been described by examining changes in the structure and biochemistry of the pain neurons in the spinal cord that serve the injected foot and comparing them with the pain neurons that serve the non-injected foot. These changes include activation of macrophage cells that are an integral part of the spinal cord as well as activation of inflammatory processes in the pain neuron. When the same protocol was carried out on Fat-1 mice, they showed the same initial "acute" pain response as the wild-type mice, but the second "chronic" pain response was half that exhibited by the wild-type mice. Furthermore, activation of spinal macrophages and other inflammatory processes associated with chronic pain was much reduced in the Fat-1 mice compared to wild-type mice.[29] Considering that both types of mice are fed the same diet but differ in the composition of their cell membranes, these findings are an independent validation that the balance of omega-3 and omega-6 fatty acids in membranes is important in the perception of chronic pain.

The evidence from the Fat-1 mice is strong that an increase in the membrane content of omega-3 PUFA relative to omega-6 PUFA is very beneficial in lessening the occurrence and ill-health associated with various chronic disease conditions. It also strongly supports the notion that chronic inflammation is fundamental to much of the ill-health associated with these various diseases.

CHAPTER 12

THE OMEGA STORY AND SOLUTIONS

Food Composition, Labels, and Diet Choices

Change without Knowledge and Understanding

The omega story is a story of ignorance, a story of change in our food chain before knowledge of essential fats and our understanding of where they come from was realized. While the fats that humans first used were likely from animals, our extraction of oils from plants probably also has a long history. A fundamental aspect of the change in our modern food was the substitution of vegetable oils for animal fats, and this started more than a century ago. The use of "shortening" dates back to at least the eighteenth century, and "shortening" was originally synonymous with "lard." Similarly, margarine was originally made from beef tallow. Following the invention of hydrogenation, modern shortenings and margarines essentially contain only vegetable oils.[1]

Our early awareness of fat centered on storage fat (the "visible" fats of chapter 5), and although we knew that some fats were polyunsaturated (and had a different chemistry from that of other fats), we were ignorant of their nutritional importance. For the first decades of the twentieth century, much nutrition research centered on vitamins, and fat was generally perceived as important only as a carrier of "fat-soluble" vitamins or a source of energy. The discovery by George and Mildred Burr in 1929, that "fat" itself was essential in the diet of rats and their later identification, in the 1930s, that $18:2\omega$-6 was a specific essential fatty acid and that $18:3\omega$-3 was also essential, were initially met with skepticism. For the next few decades, only indirect evidence supported the proposal that these fatty acids were essential diet requirements for humans. Direct evidence for humans having an essential requirement of omega-6 came in the early 1970s, while for omega-3 it came in 1982.[2] The knowledge and understanding of the cellular importance of membrane fats (the "invisible" fats of chapter 5) and the 20- and 22-carbon fatty acids (made from the two 18-carbon polyunsaturated fats) grew slowly, with the modern understanding of "fluid mosaic" membranes dating from only 1972.[3]

However, despite this ignorance of omega-3 and omega-6 fats and their nutritional importance, significant changes in the modern food chain were already underway. From 1910 to 1960, the daily provision (per person) of polyunsaturated fats in the US food supply increased from 12g per person to 20g. This increase was due to a 716 percent increase in "vegetable oil" and a 685 percent increase in "margarine." Together, these two sources went from representing 9 percent of poly-unsaturated fats in 1910 to comprising 45 percent in 1960. Although, during this fifty-year period, there was little change in the supply of polyunsaturated fats from animal-based foods, the switch to in-creased "grain-feeding" of animals had also already begun. The omega balance of the US food supply went from about 40 percent in 1910 to about 18 percent in 1960 (see chapter 3).

Similar changes have continued over the half-century since 1960 in the United States and have also increasingly occurred in the food chain of other nations. In 1960, vegetable oils contributed more fat (per person per day) to the US food supply than all other plant sources, and their relative contribution has continued to increase since 1960. Other parts of the world (including Australia) have shown similar changes, but started from a lower level (see figure 4.1). The dramatic rise of vegetable oil in the modern food chain is closely linked to the rise of "ultraprocessed" foods. The increased consumption of vege-table oil has been the dominant influence on the reduced omega bal-ance of the modern food chain.

Although there have been smaller changes in consumption of fat from animal-sources, the changes that have occurred have also decreased the omega balance of our food. Changes include an increase in meat and dairy from grain-fed animals and the reduction of fat in dairy food. These changes have occurred with general ignorance that "leaves" are the primary source of omega-3 fats, while "seeds" are the dominant source of omega-6 fats, and that the omega balance of animal-sourced fats is determined by the balance of "leaves" and "seeds" in the animal's diet (see chapter 2). The omega balance of the US food supply further decreased from about 18 percent in 1960 to about 9 percent in 2010 (see chapter 4).

Consequences and Comorbidities

Coincident with changes in the food supply over the last half-century has been the unexpected and unexplained rise in the prevalence of many chronic diseases. These have been loosely called "modern epidemics," or sometimes the "diseases of modernity." The first was cardiovascular heart disease, which in the middle of the twentieth century was responsible for about half of the deaths of adult Americans. Although there has been a decreased mortality from cardiovascular disease in high-income countries over recent decades, it has been on the increase in developing countries.[4] Cardiovascular disease mortality rate (per 100,000 persons) in North America declined from 370 in 1950 to 171 in 2015,[5] and responsibility for this decline in death is largely due to advances in the medical response (heart transplants, bypass operations, imaging techniques, cardiac pacemakers, use of stents, pharmacological treatments) rather than a decrease in the disease prevalence.

The prevalence of several other chronic diseases and conditions has also increased in recent times: obesity, fatty liver disease, diabetes, asthma, allergy, autoimmune diseases, inflammatory bowel disease, neuro-degenerative diseases, depression, and other aspects of mental ill-health. Something is going on, but what is it? Two aspects emerged that are very significant. The first is that many of these diseases are co-morbid; it is common for individuals to have more than one chronic disease. The second is that it is increasingly apparent that many are also associated with chronic inflammation. Both findings suggest that there is something common to them all. This book suggests that the imbalance between omega-3 and omega-6 in the modern diet is responsible for many of these epidemics. This is *not* to suggest that the imbalance is necessarily the "cause" of the disease, but rather the imbalance is involved in the increased prevalence of the disease—that it amplifies the ill-health associated with the disease or condition. For example, the increased prevalence of allergies and asthma is due to a hyper-responsiveness to the irritation rather than an increased number of irritations.

There were two interesting but different responses to the first of these modern epidemics: the heart disease epidemic. The first was from Ancel Keys, a charismatic scientist, with little prior experience or knowledge of lipids, who proposed the "diet-heart" hypothesis. At a time when fats were primarily perceived as "fuel" and there was general ignorance that both omega-3 and omega-6 were essential requirements of the human diet, as well as little understanding of their importance in normal body function, Keys proposed that heart disease was due to too much saturated fat in the diet. With little evidential support, this proposal was adopted by the medical establishment and still dominates much nutritional advice today. The other response was from two Danish physicians, Hans Olaf Bang and Jorn Dyerberg, and their approach was a response to Keys's "diet-heart" hypothesis. They traveled to Greenland to investigate why Inuit, who consumed a diet dominated by saturated fat (seal and whale blubber) had minimal heart disease. Their discoveries resulted in the emergence of scientific interest in dietary omega-3 fats and their effects on various diseases. Their work partly lifted the veil of ignorance about these important fats (see chapter 7). The absence of other diseases in Greenland Inuit also stimulated other researchers. For example, the absence of diabetes in Greenland Inuit was the stimulus for Len Storlien to begin his research on the role of diet omega-3 in insulin resistance (see chapter 6).

The emergence of "ultraprocessed" foods in the modern diet has also stimulated research into their role in these chronic diseases. "Ultraprocessed" foods contribute increasingly larger amounts to total food energy in recent times in high-income countries such as the United States,[6] Canada,[7] the United Kingdom,[8] and Brazil,[9] and it is concerning that consumption of ultraprocessed food is *unevenly* distributed throughout the population. High ultraprocessed food consumption has been associated with greater all-cause mortality in the United States[10] and Spain (where it was also linked with obesity)[11] and in France,[12] where it was also associated with a higher risk of cardiovascular disease[13] and a higher incidence of cancer.[14] Most of these studies have not examined which specific aspects of ultraprocessed foods were responsible. Only the French study calculated the intake of omega-6 and omega-3 fats, and reported that high consumption of ultraprocessed food was associated with a significantly elevated consumption of omega-6 and a significantly reduced consumption of omega-3 fats.

Being observational, these studies are unable to prove cause-and-effect. A recent US randomized control trial examined a possible causal connection between ultraprocessed foods and obesity. In this experiment,[15] adults were fed either a diet of "ultraprocessed" food or a diet of "unprocessed" food for two weeks. All participants received both diets, the order of which was randomly determined. The diets were matched for calories, sugar, fiber, and macronutrients, and although they contained the same total fat content, they differed in their fatty acid composition, with the "ultraprocessed" diet having an omega balance of 7 percent compared to 16 percent for the "unprocessed" diet. Participants were instructed to "consume as much or as little as desired." When the two diet periods are compared, there was a minimal difference in energy expenditure but a significant difference in their food intake. Participants gained weight on the "ultraprocessed" diet and lost weight on the "unprocessed" diet. While it is not possible to determine why participants ate more of the "ultraprocessed" diet, its lower omega balance is compatible with mechanisms discussed in chapter 6.

Over the years I have been fortunate enough to visit many parts of the world; both highly developed and less developed countries. Because of my background, I have been doing a completely unquantitative and impressionistic assessment of the link between diet and obesity in these countries. My impression is that the more the people of a country or region get their food as "produce" from markets, the less the prevalence of obesity.

Omega Balance, not Minimum Requirements

Omega balance is a simple concept. It is the percentage of total polyunsaturated fat that is omega-3. The remaining percentage is omega-6. Although it might appear to some as a ratio, it is not, and, as explained in chapter 2, it has distinct mathematical advantages over a ratio.

Conventional nutrition advice, especially when considering nutrients that are "essential," is to recommend a "minimum requirement" of the specific nutrient. This approach considers individual nutrients in isolation, and while it might be adequate when considering intake of vitamins and amino acids, it is inadequate for the omega-6 and omega-3 fats. These essential nutrients exert their effects primarily through their abundance in cell membranes and they *compete* for their incorporation into cell membranes. Consequently, because of this competition, it is their abundance *relative* to each other that is an important influence on their effects. Omega balance is a measure of their relative abundance. In this way, separate minimum dietary requirements are inadequate for the essential fats.

In the 1930s, when it was discovered that rats did *not* synthesize either 18:2ω-6 or 18:3ω-3 and that they were thus *both* essential dietary requirements, it was early appreciated that these omega-6 and omega-3 fats competed. It was identified that 18:3ω-3 "competitively inhibited" the effectiveness of 18:2ω-6 in preventing the symptoms of essential fatty acid deficiency (see note 2). My own awareness of this competition was sparked by a finding from our 12-diet rat experiment (see chapter 5). While 20:4ω-6 (absent in all 12 diets) was the most abundant polyunsaturated fat in membranes, and displayed the greatest diet-induced variation, the best predictor of 20:4ω-6 content was *not* dietary omega-6 content but instead was diet omega balance.[16] Furthermore, this was also the case when we reanalyzed the results of early experiments on rats, by Ralph Holman, using very low-fat diets.[17] This supported the finding that some enzymes responsible for membrane remodeling are highly selective for polyunsaturated fats but do *not* discriminate between omega-6 and omega-3 fats.[18] The incorporation of omega-3 and omega-6 fats in membranes will thus depend on the omega balance in the region of the responsible enzymes.

An important aspect of omega balance is that it emphasizes the "whole-of-diet" intake of omega-3 and omega-6, whereas the "minimum requirement" approach supports a "dietary supplement" provision of omega-3. The omega balance approach essentially says that a minimum requirement of omega-3 cannot be specified unless the intake of omega-6 is already known.

Unfortunately, the "minimum requirement" approach has influenced the design of many experimental trials intended to test the influence of omega-3 in humans. Such trials have often used fish-oil supplements as the experimental treatment, and many have used only very small doses of omega-3 relative to a background diet often dominated by omega-6. The net effect is that such treatments sometimes achieve only trivial changes in "whole-of-diet" omega balance and consequently often report no statistically significant effect of the experimental treatment. Hopefully, a change to the omega balance concept will result in more realistic design of trials examining the influence of omega-3 on human health.

The Rise of Trans Fats

In recent years, the presence of "trans" fats in modern foods and their possible ill-health effects have become a concern in several jurisdictions. In 2003, the US Food and Drug Administration (FDA) required content of trans fats to be listed on foods. Foods with less than 0.5g per serving can be labeled as having 0g per serving. In 2015, the FDA moved to eliminate industrial trans fats from the US food supply, giving manufacturers a deadline of three years. The rise of trans fats is very closely connected to the dramatic rise of vegetable oils in the modern food chain.

When vegetable oils were substituted for animal fats in foods, a disadvantage was that a "liquid" oil replaced a "solid" fat. Hydrogenation of liquid oils, patented in 1902, overcame this problem.[19] Hydrogenation involves using both high temperature and a metal catalyst in the presence of hydrogen to add hydrogen atoms to the previously "unsaturated" carbon atoms. *Complete* hydrogenation is the alchemy of converting an unsaturated fatty acid (a liquid) to a saturated fatty acid (solid), and the process of hydrogenation was envisioned to allow vegetable oils to replace animal fats in food, at the same time increasing chemical stability and giving the food a longer shelf-life. However, food companies discovered that *incomplete* hydrogenation (or "partial hydrogenation") enabled better control of the characteristics of the ultimate food product, but a problem of partial hydrogenation was the production of "trans" unsaturated fatty acids (commonly known as "trans fats").

I'm sure chapter 5 was complicated enough for the average reader, and I purposefully did not mention that double-bonds come in two types; "*cis*" and "*trans*" double-bonds. In most naturally occurring unsaturated fatty acids (certainly all that I have mentioned thus far), the double bonds are of the *cis* variety. Partial hydrogenation of vegetable oils converts many of the normal *cis*-double bonds to *trans*-double bonds and this change affects the behavior of the fat. A *trans*-unsaturated fat behaves more like a saturated fat than a *cis*-unsaturated fat, and *trans* fats cannot be legally labelled as "unsaturated" but are classified in the same category as saturated fats. The process of partial hydrogenation likely marks the beginning of "ultraprocessing" in the modern food chain.

Trans fats can be divided into two groups: industrial and natural. We humans have been consuming naturally-produced trans fats for several thousand years, because microbes in the gut of ruminants (cattle, goats, sheep) also produce trans fats.[20] Consequently, in milk and meat from ruminants, natural trans fats constitute about 3 percent of total fat. In frying fats, shortenings, and margarines, industrial trans fats can constitute up to 35 percent of total fat depending on the degree of partial hydrogenation of the vegetable oil.[21]

Estimated daily intake of trans fat (per person) are about 6g in the United States, [22] about 3g in Europe,[23] and about 0.2g in Japan.[24]Concerns were raised when observational studies[25] and experimental diet manipulation[26] found that increased consumption of trans fat was associated with elevated inflammation markers and increased risk of coronary heart disease.[27] A meta-analysis of observational studies[28] found that intake of "industrial" trans fats was associated with increased CHD-mortality, but that intake of "ruminant" trans fats had no significant effect on CHD-mortality. Intake of industrial trans fats is a correlate of vegetable oil intake, and thus, diets high in industrial trans fats will have a low omega balance. Trans fats may not be as "bad" as they are often portrayed. For example, trans fats can protect endogenous lipids from oxidation in both LDL particles and bilayer membranes.[29] Some of the ruminant trans fats (specifically conjugated linoleic acids) likely have beneficial effects on some disease conditions.[30] It is also little appreciated that because omega-3 fats are more reactive to hydrogenation than omega-6 fats, partial hydrogenation also has the effect of decreasing the omega balance. For example, in an experiment comparing consumption of a high saturated fat diet, a low trans fat diet, and a high trans fat diet, the omega balance of the three diets were respectively 15, 13, and 9 percent.[31] Personally, I think the alarm about trans fats may been overstated and that what is being analyzed is a "correlate" rather than a "cause." Their removal from the human food chain may not have the desired effects on prevalence of chronic disease, especially, if it does not decrease the consumption of vegetable oils in the modern human diet.

A Long Life?

If an increase in the omega balance of food results in a decreased mortality from many modern diseases, then it should also be associated with a longer life. Is there any evidence?

A recent study analyzed the mortality rates of a cohort of offspring from the Framingham Heart study. Low levels of red blood cell omega-3 fats were associated with early death in this cohort, and this association was almost identical to the degree that smoking status resulted in early death.[32] High red blood cell omega-3 was associated with a longer life. The similarity between the influence of smoking and a low red blood cell omega-3 level on longevity suggests that a low diet omega balance should be of public health concern.

Centenarians have red blood cells with a high omega balance compared to non-centenarians.[33] However, such an observation is not evidence that the connection is causal. Because lifespan is partly inherited (a large study of Danish twins suggests inheritance is about one-quarter responsible for determination of lifespan),[34] Italian researchers measured and compared the fatty acid composition of red blood cells of the offspring of nonagenarians (90+ year old citizens) and matched controls from the Cilento area of southern Italy. The offspring were all healthy and had an average age of 68 years. The control group were from the same region and matched for age, gender, smoking behavior, diet, and absence of known medical conditions. The omega balance of the nonagenarian offspring was 17 percent, compared to 8 percent for the matched controls.[35] While not definitive, this result is supportive that a higher omega balance is associated with a longer life.

A Happy Life?

A close colleague was concerned when he learned that I intended to include "happiness" as one of the effects of an increased food omega balance. After I pointed out that there was evidence that an increased omega balance of the diet was associated with less chronic pain, less anxiety, less aggression, less depression, and less suicide, he was sat-isfied that it was reasonable to assume that an increased diet omega balance was likely associated with an increase in "happiness."

That "chronic pain" has increased in recent times is manifest by a sixfold global increase, between 1995 and 2015, in the combined use of the top five opioid analgesics.[36] By far, their greatest use was in North America, but other regions have also experienced dramatic increases. While the "opioid crisis" is related to the addictive nature of these analgesics (despite the advertising of some as being nonad-dictive), and their marketing and overprescription for pain relief, it is little appreciated that the low omega balance of the modern US diet is also likely a contributor to the crisis by increasing the prevalence of chronic pain. The great benefit when such a realization becomes more widespread is that it suggests appropriate dietary change will result in significant improvement in well-being of both individuals and affected communities.

Although dietary omega-3 are considered important for good brain development, rarely is diet omega balance mentioned with re-spect to mental health issues. This is disappointing, as it is relatively easily assessed, and more importantly, dietary imbalances can be relatively easily remedied. The "mind-body" dualism acts to mini-mize consideration that the brain is part of the body and that the building blocks, essential for its normal function, are an important consideration for its optimal function. Individuals can often be very resistant to considering that diet might be an important influence on mental health. Yet they have no problems considering drugs as pow-erful ways of influencing thinking, perception, and mental health. There is no doubt that psychosocial factors are very significant con-tributors to mental ill-health, and these are often treated by various forms of psychotherapy and counselling. Much of this psychological treatment is effectively "learning" new ways to think, "learning" how to more beneficially interpret situations and personal interactions as well as "learning" how to handle emotions. There is now consid-erable evidence that omega-3 in the diet improves "learning." I can see no reason why an increase in diet omega balance would not result in both better mental health and greater benefits from such mental health treatments. I await the day that a low diet omega balance appears as a "risk factor" for poor mental health.

When I heard that, once again, the "World Happiness Report 2021" ranked Finland as the "happiest" country in the world, I decided to see whether there was any statistical relationship between the "happiness" of nations and their food supply. The Happiness Report started in 2012 and uses the Gallup World Poll, in which individuals from many nations indicate their "happiness" on a scale of 0 to 10, and scores for each country are then averaged. In figure 12.1, I have plotted the average happiness score (2017–2019) for the twenty happiest nations against the percent of the 2018 total fat supply that comes from vegetable oils.[37] Statistically, there is a highly significant relationship. The greater the contribution of vegetable oils to the total fat supply of the nation (which is likely indicative of a low omega balance of the national diet), the lower the average self-assessed "happiness score" for the nation. Although I have only plotted the data for the twenty happiest nations, there is also a highly significant statistical relationship when data for all 143 nations are compared. The relationship is provocative and surprised even me!

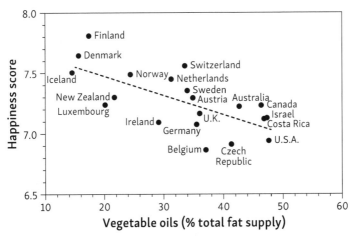

Figure 12.1 Correlation between self-assessed "happiness" (2017–2019) and contribution of "vegetable oils" to 2018 provision of fat in the food supply of the world's twenty "happiest" countries. See text for details and sources.

Food Labels and Databases

Occasionally, I have been asked by colleagues and friends: "How much omega-3 should I take?" My answer is a question: "How much omega-6 do you eat? I can't advise you about your omega-3 intake unless I know your omega-6 intake." Their response is often: "I have no idea of my omega-6 intake. How would I find out?"

Current food labels would be of *no* help. With respect to "fat," they generally list only "saturated fat," "monounsaturated fat," and "polyunsaturated fat," with no indication of either "omega-3 polyunsaturated fat" or "omega-6 polyunsaturated fat." Yet the information is available. In order to determine the fatty acid composition of anything, the procedure is to extract the fat, convert the total fat to a mixture of fatty acids, then separate and quantify the individual fatty acids from the mixture. The final step is to add up all the "saturated," "monounsaturated," and "polyunsaturated" fatty acids. Thus, in order to know the "polyunsaturated" fat content of anything, the quantity of both all omega-3 and all omega-6 fats have been combined. Considering it has now been known for decades that omega-3 and omega-6 are separate essential fats that cannot be interconverted and have very different effects, there is really *no* excuse for their respective amounts not to be identified on food labels, especially given that these amounts have actually been measured.

To be told the "total polyunsaturated" fatty acid content of a food, but not its omega-6 nor omega-3 content, is a bit like being given a mood-altering drug, being told it contains both "uppers" and "downers," and told the combined amount but not the individual amounts of either "uppers" or "downers." Not good! It's time for food labels to change.

Food databases have the same deficiency. In chapter 2, I used both the USDA "FoodData Central"[38] and the FSANZ "Australian Food Composition"[39] online databases to calculate the omega balance of a variety of foods. Both databases list the content of individual fatty acids in foods and generally identify individual polyunsaturated fatty acids as either omega-3 or omega-6. However, although both present the value of "total polyunsaturated fats," neither give values for "total omega-3" or for "total omega-6"—in my view a significant deficiency, easily remedied. Of course, I would like to see both food labels and online databases provide the omega balance of the various foods either as a numerical value or as a pie chart (as presented in chapter 2).

Dietary Guidelines

Dietary advice has been provided to Americans for a considerable time, but initially did not include any advice about fat. A 1940 book titled *The American and His Food* did not mention dietary fat.[40] It was the post–World War II drive in the United States to understand heart disease that gave rise to advice about dietary fat. The suggestion by Ancel Keys that saturated fat was responsible resulted in the American Heart Association issuing a report in 1961 with the explicit advice of "Reduce intake of total fat, saturated fat, and cholesterol. Increase intake of polyunsaturated fat." In 1977, a select committee of the US Senate issued "Dietary Goals for the United States," giving more specific goals that included: (1) increase carbohydrate consumption to 55–60 percent of energy intake; (2) reduce total fat consumption to 30 percent of energy intake; (3) reduce saturated fat intake to about 10 percent of energy intake; and (4) polyunsaturated fat consumption should be 10 percent of energy intake (see note 40). None of these reports differentiated between omega-3 and omega-6 fats.

The US Department of Agriculture also issued dietary guidelines and in 1990 was given the responsibility to issue them every five years. The latest version is the *Dietary Guidelines for Americans, 2020-2025*.[41] They are little changed since 1977. Although guidelines regarding total fat intake are gone, the advice to keep saturated fat below 10 percent of energy intake and to consume more polyunsaturated oils remains. The obsession with saturated fat is perplexing. As Nina Teicholz points out in her 2014 book *The Big Fat Surprise: Why Butter, Meat, and Cheese Belong in a Healthy Diet*,[42] it has no strong scientific basis yet has become dietary dogma. There is no separate consideration of omega-6 and omega-3, and the words themselves appear only once in the *Dietary Guidelines* (on page 60). It is worrying that a healthy diet for adults recommends "oils" to be 12 percent of energy, as they are a good source of "essential fatty acids," yet there is *no* consideration of the difference between omega-3 and omega-6 fats. The level of scientific ignorance regarding the essential fats in this document is truly alarming.

Many other countries base their dietary advice on the US guidelines and thus have similar recommendations. The most recent Australian Dietary Guidelines also suggest limiting saturated fat intake and include suggestions to consume reduced-fat dairy and replacing products with saturated fat, such as butter and cream, with polyunsaturated oils.[43] Unsaturated fats are featured because they are not saturated fats, but once again there is no differentiation between omega-3 and omega-6 fats. In the document, there is a single mention of omega-3 fatty acids (that fish are a source) but no mention of omega-6 fatty acids. In a section titled "Not all fats are equal," the first sentence finishes with "some oils contain unsaturated fats (polyunsaturated and monounsaturated) that are essential for health." The implication that monounsaturated fats are essential fatty acids is worrying in an important document presumably written by professional nutritionists. Similarly, the most recent UK dietary guidelines suggest reducing saturated fat intake, using low-fat dairy or dairy alternatives (such as soya drinks), and replacing butter with vegetable oil spreads.[44] It states that unsaturated fats are healthier fats but contains no acknowledgment that there are omega-3 and omega-6 fats (although it does say fish are healthy).

Although there is no advice about separate consumption of omega-3 and omega-6 fats in these national dietary guidelines, this is not the case with the premier scientific society concerning lipid research. In 2004, ISSFAL (International Society for the Study of Fatty Acids and Lipids) issued a series of recommendations for dietary intake of the essential fats by healthy adults. They made no comment about consumption of the *nonessential* saturated and monounsaturated fats but instead proposed that adequate intake of 18:2ω-6 is 2 percent of energy, and a healthy intake of 18:3ω-3 is 0.7 percent of energy as well as recommending a minimum intake of 500mg/d of 20:5ω-3 and 22:6ω-6. These ISSFAL recommendations for daily intake correspond to a diet omega balance of about 30 percent.[45]

The recommended intakes contrast markedly with the average *actual* daily intakes by the US population (from a 1999–2000 survey), which correspond to a diet omega balance of 9 percent.[46] Similarly, a dietary survey of the Australian population revealed the average daily intake in 1995 corresponded to a diet omega balance of 11 percent.[47] Both the United States and Australia (and likely many other developed high-income countries) have omega-6 intakes much *higher* and omega-3 intakes *lower* than the recommended levels.

Some Final Comments

It should be obvious that I find the "nutritionist" community sadly deficient with respect to their relative lack of concern and attention to the balance of omega-3 and omega-6 fats in the modern diet. Much of the information that we, the general public, receive about nutrition and disease these days comes from epidemiological studies, and despite such studies raising connections between particular diet components and disease, they generally show little interest in examining potential mechanisms linking the two. A realistic and feasible mechanism should be essential before proposing that a particular aspect of a diet is associated with a particular disease or condition. I have emphasized a concern for explanatory mechanisms, and examination of the role of the two types of essential fats in cell membranes as potential mechanisms will, I'm sure, bring many seemingly unconnected observations into a more holistic understanding of the chronic diseases that unfortunately affect too many of us.

Unfortunately, the public's awareness of the beneficial effects of omega-3 fats is dominated by "fish oil" capsules. The phrase "found in fish oils," so often repeated after mention of omega-3 has limited the understanding of omega-3 fats and resulted in them being perceived as some sort of supplement rather than an essential part of our diet. Omega-3 fats are found in so many other components of our diet. Although not perfect, the "seeds" versus "leaves" perspective can make food more understandable. A "whole-of-diet" approach is also an important component in understanding the importance of these two types of fats. After I became aware of omega-3 fats in the 1980s, I started taking fish-oil capsules daily, but after I became more aware of the distribution of both omega-3 and omega-6 in my food, I stopped taking these daily supplements and nowadays use a whole-of-diet approach.

My approach is to minimize my omega-6 intake and to maximize my omega-3 intake, as much as possible. The most important aspect of food and eating is that it should be enjoyable, and although I use small amounts of vegetable oils occasionally (for their particular taste), I avoid them as much as possible and have gone back to largely cooking in butter. I have a few rules that I use, and all will be obvious from the reading of this book. They are based around the concept of trying to keep as high an omega balance as possible. When choosing food in an eating establishment, I consider the whole meal and try to figure out what the entire meal is made from and how it is prepared.

My personal rules are:
- Eat lots of green-leaf vegetables.
- Avoid deep-fried foods.
- Always choose grass-fed over grain-fed produce.
- Choose dairy from grass-fed cattle and always full-fat, never reduced-fat.
- Use butter for cooking instead of vegetable oils.
- Choose fish, seafood, and lamb, rather than chicken or pork.
- When buying canned fish (tuna, salmon, sardines), never choose "in oil."
- Choose beans (high omega balance) rather than peas.
- Bread, most commonly, is "soy and linseed."

- Minimize snacks (potato chips, corn chips) and cakes.
- Minimize ultraprocessed foods.

As I mentioned in the preface, I hope that this book influences what we feed others. I'm sure that more attention to the diets provided by all our institutions, to ensure they have a good omega balance, will likely have beneficial effects for everyone. Most importantly, I hope that this book influences what we feed to our children. Special concern is the effects that excessive omega-6 fats in food has on (1) the proliferation of fat cells in young children and the future development of obesity, as well as (2) the debilitating effects of mental health issues such as anxiety, aggression, and depression. The fact that many of the modern chronic diseases are being increasingly diagnosed in our children deserves special attention, and a diet with a good omega balance will hopefully ensure that this alarming problem lessens in the future.

This book started with a parent's nightmare. It is appropriate that it ends with the advice commonly given by many parents to their children:

"Don't forget to eat your greens!"

OMEGA BALANCE AND COVID-19

I completed my writing just before the start of the COVID-19 pandemic, and thus it was not considered. Yet the story I have outlined also has implications for the severity of COVID-19 experienced by many. COVID-19 is a contagious disease caused by the SARS-CoV-2 virus that especially (but not solely) affects the lungs. Following the first phase of virus replication (resulting in virus-mediated tissue damage), there is a secondary phase involving the immune system that sometimes results in an "inflammatory storm." Autopsies of deceased COVID-19 patients show little active viral infection but substantial activated immune cells, which suggests that death results from the excessive inflammatory response and not viral-induced tissue damage.[1] The "inflammatory storm" involves excessive release of both lipid and non-lipid inflammation mediators.[2] Lipid inflammation mediators include the "eicosanoids" made from 20:4ω-6 in membranes, which is influenced by diet omega balance, and, as chapter 7 describes, the non-lipid mediators also include many whose production is influenced by diet omega balance. This "inflammatory storm" is associated with excessive fluid accumulation in lungs, and diminished tissue repair, resulting in respiratory distress often requiring mechanical ventilation and supplemental oxygen to minimize chance of death.

While "age" is a dominant risk factor for death from COVID-19 (as it is for many diseases), so are a series of co-morbid chronic diseases. They include obesity, diabetes, and cardiovascular disease (including hypertension) as well as asthma, chronic obstructive lung disease

(COPD), and some autoimmune diseases.[3] These chronic diseases are discussed in the second half of this book as being influenced by diet omega balance.

One of the successful treatments for hospitalized patients with severe COVID-19 has been the use of synthetic glucocorticoids (especially dexamethasone).[4] The anti-inflammatory action of the glucocorticoids involves inhibition of the enzyme responsible for removing 20:4ω-6 from membrane lipids and thus these glucocorticoids inhibit the production of inflammatory mediators from this omega-6 fatty acid (see chapter 7).

Because death from COVID-19 is due largely to the hyper-inflammatory response and a low diet omega balance is associated with elevated inflammation, then the obvious question is: "Does a diet with a low omega balance affect mortality due to COVID-19 infection?"

A number of recent studies shed light on the answer to this question. One study of 74 severe COVID-19 patients found those with lowest blood omega-3 index had the greatest risk of death.[5] Another prospective study of the blood of 24,727 individuals in the UK Biobank found that a high ω-6/ω-3 ratio (a low omega balance) was associated with both greater susceptibility to COVID-19 and greater severity of the disease once infected.[6] As well, a pilot study of a hundred hospitalized COVID-19 patients suggested that high blood omega-3 levels are associated with a reduced mortality.[7]

It has also been assessed whether intervention to improve a patient's omega balance is beneficial. A randomized clinical trial of 128 critically ill COVID-19 patients found that the one-month survival was 21 percent in the intervention group (given 1g fish oil daily) compared to 3 percent in the non-intervention group.[8] Similarly, fish diets have found to be associated with a lower probability of moderate-to-severe COVID-19.[9]

Of course, death from COVID-19 in any particular nation will be affected by many parameters, most notably the quality of its health care system and the degree of vaccination. To test if the national diet may also be an influence, in early March 2022, I collected three sets of data for thirty-six nations defined by the United Nations as "developed economies" and thus likely to have good health care systems.[10] The data sets were: (1) national percent fatality rate due to COVID-19 up to March 2022, (2) national vaccination rates as of late February 2022, and (3) national percent of total fat supply provided by vegetable oils in 2018 (latest available data).[11] The average fatality rate for these 36 nations was 0.87 percent of total COVID cases, and values ranged from 0.03 to 3.26 percent. Almost half of the variation could be statistically explained by vaccination rates (which ranged from 29.6 to 91.3 percent). The contribution of vegetable oils to total fat in the national food supply (which I have used as an indicator of the omega balance of the national food chain) could statistically explain nearly 10 percent in the variation in percent fatality due to COVID-19. Of these 36 nations, the 18 with the lowest vegetable oil contribution to fat in their diet (average 25 percent) had an average fatality of 0.70 percent compared to 1.05 percent for the 18 nations with the highest vegetable oil contribution (average 41 percent). In other words, those countries with high food omega balance (as assessed by low vegetable oil contribution in total fat) tend to have lower death due to COVID-19 than those with low food omega balance. This was not due to differences in vaccination status, as for both groups the average vaccination rates were 70 percent.

Acknowledgments

My journey from zoophysiology to this book has been influenced by many fruitful scientific collaborations, too many to individually thank here (but they know who they are). The late Len Storlien was especially significant in the emergence of my interest in omega-3 fats in the late 1980s. I began writing this book in 2009, and I thank Mary Brand and Karina Kelly for reading and commenting on the drafts of early chapters. After a break, it was completed in 2019 (just before the coronavirus pandemic), and I thank Len Storlien, Martin Denny, Paul Else, Bill Buttemer and Leife Hulbert for feedback on the full version of the manuscript. During its writing, the efforts of Alexandra Elbakyan were helpful in obtaining much information. The help of Dotti Le Sage in early versions of some figures is appreciated and my sincere thanks also go to Joe Rusko, my editor at Johns Hopkins University Press. I also thank my agent Cathy Baker for being Cathy Baker, and for encouraging the completion of what I hope is a significant contribution to the future good health and wellness of my fellow humans on this planet.

APPENDIX 1

Omega Balance and Polyunsaturated Fat (PUFA) Content of Selected Foods

Food	Omega balance (ω-3 % PUFA)	PUFA content (g/100g food)	Source	ID #	
Vegetable oils					
safflower oil	0	74.6	USDA	171026	*
palm kernel oil	0	1.6	USDA	171422	*
peanut (groundnut) oil	0	32.0	USDA	110386	*
cottonseed oil	0	51.9	USDA	110359	*
sunflower oil	0	65.7	USDA	1103867	*
grapeseed oil	0	58.7	FSANZ	F006167	
almond oil	0	17.4	USDA	1103856	
hazelnut oil	0	10.2	USDA	171427	
poppyseed oil	0	62.4	USDA	171423	
macadamia oil	0	1.2	FSANZ	F006169	
sesame oil	1	41.7	USDA	1103865	
coconut oil	1	1.7	USDA	1103857	*
argan oil	1	35.0	Ref. 1		
corn oil	2	54.7	USDA	1103858	*
palm oil	2	9.3	USDA	171015	*
oat oil	4	40.9	USDA	173576	
ricebran oil	5	35.0	USDA	171013	*
olive oil	7	10.5	USDA	1103861	*
avocado oil	7	13.5	USDA	173573	
soybean oil (partially hydrogenated)	7	37.6	USDA	171012	
soybean oil	12	57.7	USDA	1103866	*
walnut oil	16	63.3	USDA	1103868	
hempseed oil	23	74.7	Ref. 2		
mustard oil	28	21.2	USDA	172337	
canola oil	32	28.1	USDA	1103863	*
flaxseed (linseed) oil	79	67.9	USDA	1103860	

Food	Omega balance (ω-3 % PUFA)	PUFA content (g/100g food)	Source	ID #	
Grains and cereal-based food					
corn chips	2	16.4	USDA	167537	*
corn	3	2.2	USDA	170288	*
rice	4	0.2	USDA	168883	*
wheat	4	0.8	USDA	169720	*
muesli	5	0.9	USDA	169075	*
millet	6	2.1	USDA	169702	*
corn flakes	6	0.3	USDA	174648	*
pumpernickel bread	7	1.2	USDA	174918	*
rye bread	8	0.8	USDA	172684	*
white bread	10	1.6	USDA	174924	*
multigrain bread	11	1.9	USDA	168013	*
rye crispbread	14	0.6	USDA	172739	*
Nuts, seeds, and soybean products					
almonds (dry roasted)	0	13.0	USDA	170158	*
brazil nuts (dry)	0	24.4	USDA	170569	*
hazelnuts (dry roasted)	1	8.5	USDA	170583	*
pine nuts (dry)	1	34.1	USDA	170591	*
pistachio (dry roasted)	2	13.3	USDA	170185	*
cashews (dry roasted)	2	7.8	USDA	170571	*
potato chips (cooked in soybean oil)	3	9.2	USDA	170248	
margarine (soybean oil)	7	20.9	USDA	171018	*
chestnuts (roasted)	11	0.9	USDA	170190	
soy lecithin (emulsifier)	11	45.3	USDA	171426	*
soyflour (full fat)	12	11.7	USDA	174273	*
soymilk (lite)	12	0.4	USDA	1097543	*
soymilk (plain)	14	1.2	USDA	1750337	*
miso (soybean paste)	14	2.9	USDA	172442	*
walnuts	19	44.2	USDA	170594	
hemp seed (hulled)	24	38.1	USDA	170148	
chia seed	79	28.7	USDA	1100612	

Food	Omega balance (ω-3 % PUFA)	PUFA content (g/100g food)	Source	ID #	
Peas and beans					
chickpeas (raw)	4	2.7	USDA	173756	*
mung beans (raw)	7	0.4	USDA	174256	*
broadbeans (fava beans, raw)	7	0.6	USDA	175205	*
split peas, green (raw)	16	1.0	USDA	172428	*
green peas (raw)	19	0.2	USDA	170419	*
lentils (raw)	21	0.5	USDA	172420	*
lima beans (raw)	31	0.3	USDA	174252	*
baked beans (canned)	45	0.2	USDA	168128	*
black beans (raw)	46	0.6	USDA	173734	*
white (cannellini) beans (raw)	46	0.4	USDA	175202	*
green beans (raw)	61	0.1	USDA	169961	*
red kidney beans (raw)	61	0.6	USDA	173744	*
Leaf vegetables					
cabbage (raw)	53	0.1	USDA	169335	*
broccoli (raw)	56	0.1	USDA	170379	*
Chinese cabbage (pak choi, raw)	57	0.1	USDA	170390	*
brussels sprouts (raw)	65	0.2	USDA	170383	*
watercress	66	0.04	USDA	170068	*
lettuce, red-leaf (raw)	70	0.1	USDA	168431	*
lettuce, cos/romaine (raw)	71	0.2	USDA	169247	*
lettuce, green-leaf (raw)	71	0.1	USDA	169249	*
dandelion (wild, raw)	72	0.2	Ref. 3		*
spinach (raw)	84	0.2	USDA	168462	*
spinach (cooked)	84	0.1	USDA	170531	
peppermint (raw)	86	0.5	USDA	173474	*
purslane (wild, raw)	91	0.2	Ref. 3		*
peppers (green, sweet, raw)	13	0.1	USDA	170427	
Pork, beef, and lamb					
pork spare ribs	2	4.0	USDA	167853	
pork, cured bacon, raw	5	5.8	USDA	168277	*

Food	Omega balance (ω-3 % PUFA)	PUFA content (g/100g food)	Source	ID #	
pork, cured bacon, pan-fried	5	6.1	USDA	168322	
pork, ground, 16% fat	6	2.1	USDA	168372	*
pork, trimmed retail cuts	6	1.6	USDA	167888	
pork, ground, 4% fat	7	0.7	USDA	169190	
pork, loin	7	1.3	USDA	167818	*
pork, leg (ham)	7	2.0	USDA	168222	*
pork, ground (Aus)	10	1.4	FSANZ	F007057	
beef, chuck, stew (all grades)	2	0.3	USDA	171206	
beef, chuck, stew (choice)	2	0.3	USDA	170810	
beef, roast, lean only	7	0.2	USDA	746761	*
beef, porterhouse steak	7	0.3	USDA	746762	*
beef, ground (30% fat)	9	0.7	USDA	168652	*
beef, ground (3% fat)	11	0.2	USDA	173111	
beef, porterhouse steak (Aus)	24	0.5	FSANZ	F000825	
beef, ground (low fat) (Aus)	28	0.2	FSANZ	F000666	
beef, ground (high fat) (Aus)	31	0.3	FSANZ	F000655	*
beef, imported (New Zealand)	42	0.2	USDA	173086	
lamb, shoulder, 1/4"fat	22	1.7	USDA	172496	
lamb, foreshank, 1/4"fat	23	1.1	USDA	172481	
lamb, trimmed retail cuts	23	1.7	USDA	172479	*
lamb, ground	23	1.9	USDA	174370	*
lamb, rib, 1/4" fat	23	2.7	USDA	174321	*
lamb, ground, 15% fat (Aus)	29	1.1	USDA	172608	*
Other meats					
buffalo, ground	11	0.7	USDA	174421	
camel, rump	18	0.4	FSANZ	F002206	
rabbit, wild	20	1.1	USDA	174347	
rabbit, farmed, composite cuts	20	1.1	USDA	172521	*
buffalo, top round steak	20	0.1	USDA	167649	*
crocodile, back leg	21	0.6	FSANZ	F003299	*
venison (deer), ground	26	0.4	USDA	172602	*

Food	Omega balance (ω-3 % PUFA)	PUFA content (g/100g food)	Source	ID #	
kangaroo, rump	29	0.2	FSANZ	F004790	*
horse	45	0.7	USDA	175086	*
Offal					
pork, kidney	4	0.3	USDA	168270	
pork, heart	7	1.1	USDA	168267	
pork, liver	9	0.9	USDA	167862	
pork, brain	55	1.4	USDA	168264	
beef, kidney	1	0.5	USDA	169449	*
beef, heart	2	0.5	USDA	174723	*
beef, liver	2	0.5	USDA	169451	*
beef, kidney (New Zealand)	32	0.6	USDA	174727	
beef, heart (New Zealand)	28	0.6	USDA	174723	*
beef, liver (New Zealand)	40	0.9	USDA	174729	*
beef, brain	77	1.6	USDA	168622	*
lamb, liver	9	0.8	USDA	172531	
lamb, liver (New Zealand)	62	0.9	USDA	172615	
lamb, kidney	35	0.6	USDA	174354	
lamb, heart	42	0.6	USDA	172527	
lamb, brain	70	0.9	USDA	172525	
Animal fats and dairy					
lard	9	11.2	USDA	171401	*
cream, light (coffee cream)	10	0.8	USDA	170857	
butter (unsalted)	10	3.0	USDA	173430	*
cheese, Parmesan	11	1.2	USDA	325036	*
sour cream	11	0.8	USDA	171257	
cheese, cheddar	12	1.2	USDA	328637	*
milk, low-fat (1%)	13	0.03	USDA	746772	*
milk, full-fat (3.25%)	14	0.1	USDA	746782	*
cheese, ricotta	14	0.4	USDA	746766	
beef tallow	15	4.0	USDA	171400	*
milk, full-fat (3.5%) (Aus)	25	0.1	FSANZ	F005634	*

Food	Omega balance (ω-3 % PUFA)	PUFA content (g/100g food)	Source	ID #	
yogurt, natural, regular (Aus)	25	0.1	FSANZ	F009694	
sour cream (Aus)	26	0.8	FSANZ	F003269	
beef dripping (tallow) (Aus)	28	2.5	FSANZ	F003627	
cheese, ricotta (Aus)	29	0.3	FSANZ	F002488	
ghee (clarified butter) (Aus)	32	1.8	FSANZ	F004205	
butter (unsalted) (Aus)	32	1.5	FSANZ	F001971	*
milk, low-fat (1%) (Aus)	33	0.03	FSANZ	F005614	*
cream, thickened, regular (Aus)	49	1.4	FSANZ	F003270	
cheese, Parmesan (Aus)	52	1.0	FSANZ	F002479	*
cheese, cheddar (Aus)	55	1.3	FSANZ	F002414	*
Poultry and eggs					
chicken liver	1	1.3	USDA	171060	*
egg, chicken (whole)	1	1.8	USDA	748967	*
egg, quail (whole)	3	1.3	USDA	172191	*
emu, ground	4	0.6	USDA	172832	
egg, turkey (whole)	5	1.7	USDA	172192	*
chicken, drumstick	5	2.0	USDA	172373	*
turkey, whole (meat and skin)	5	1.5	USDA	171081	*
turkey, ground	6	2.2	USDA	171505	
chicken, whole (meat and skin)	6	3.2	USDA	171447	*
chicken breast	6	2.0	USDA	171474	*
chicken, ground	6	1.5	USDA	171116	
quail breast	6	0.8	USDA	172829	
egg, duck (whole)	8	1.2	USDA	172189	*
duck, domesticated	8	5.1	USDA	172408	*
duck, wild	8	2.0	USDA	174468	
chicken, roasting, meat only	10	0.7	USDA	173636	
emu, rump steak	11	0.3	USDA	174479	*
quail, meat and skin	15	3.0	USDA	172418	*
Seafood					
catfish, farmed	13	1.1	USDA	175165	

Food	Omega balance (ω-3 % PUFA)	PUFA content (g/100g food)	Source	ID #	
tuna, canned in oil, drained	16	3.0	USDA	175157	*
sardines, canned in oil, drained	31	5.1	USDA	175139	*
shrimp	43	0.2	USDA	175179	
tilapia	47	0.4	USDA	175176	
salmon, chinook, smoked	53	1.0	USDA	173687	
trout, rainbow, farmed	59	1.5	USDA	173717	*
catfish, wild	63	0.9	USDA	174186	
trout rainbow, wild	71	1.2	USDA	175154	*
salmon, Atlantic, farmed	67	3.9	USDA	175167	*
salmon, Atlantic, wild	83	2.5	USDA	173686	*
lobster, spiny	71	0.6	USDA	174211	
sardines, in tomato sauce	80	2.1	USDA	175140	*
shark, mixed species	84	1.2	USDA	173697	
snapper, mixed species	85	0.5	USDA	173698	*
mussels, blue	85	0.6	USDA	174216	
oysters, eastern, wild	86	0.5	USDA	171978	
oysters, eastern, farmed	89	0.6	USDA	175172	
scallops, mixed species	87	0.1	USDA	174220	*
tuna, skipjack	87	0.3	USDA	175156	
tuna, canned in water, drained	90	1.1	USDA	175158	*
salmon, chinook	90	2.8	USDA	173688	
oyster, Pacific	92	0.9	USDA	174219	
caviar, black and red	92	7.4	USDA	174188	*
tuna, bluefin	93	1.4	USDA	173706	
squid (calamari) mixed species	96	0.5	USDA	174223	*

Whole meals

Food	Omega balance (ω-3 % PUFA)	PUFA content (g/100g food)	Source		
sweet & sour pork	2	5.1	Ref. 4		
fish & chips	4	7.9	Ref. 4		
KFC® 2-piece feed	6	1.6	Ref. 4		
saté beef & rice	8	0.8	Ref. 4		
vegetarian pizza	10	1.6	Ref. 4		

Food	Omega balance (ω-3 % PUFA)	PUFA content (g/100g food)	Source	ID #
supreme pizza	11	2.6	Ref. 4	
spaghetti bolognaise	11	0.6	Ref. 4	
Whopper® & fries	11	3.1	Ref. 4	
chicken & vegetables	12	0.7	Ref. 4	
Subway® turkey & salad	13	1.1	Ref. 4	
lasagna	13	1.1	Ref. 4	
chicken curry & rice	13	0.5	Ref. 4	
Filet-o-Fish® & fries	13	3.1	Ref. 4	
pork & vegetables	14	2.2	Ref. 4	
Big Mac® & fries	14	2.4	Ref. 4	
hamburger (with fixings)	14	2.2	Ref. 4	
beef kebab	26	0.9	Ref. 4	
lamb & vegetables	30	1.0	Ref. 4	
bean burrito	30	1.2	Ref. 4	
steak & vegetables	31	0.2	Ref. 4	
salad (with dressing)	41	0.4	Ref. 4	
salad (no dressing)	45	0.4	Ref. 4	
salmon & salad	80	2.8	Ref. 4	

The omega balance of foods with * in last column is illustrated in figures 2.1 and 2.2

Sources: USDA: US Department of Agriculture, Agricultural Research Service, FoodData Central, https://fdc.nal.usda.gov/index.html; FSANZ: Food Standards, Australia-New Zealand, https://www.foodstandards.gov.au/science/monitoringnutrients/afcd/Pages/default.aspx.

Ref. 1: Rueda A et al. (2014). Characterization of fatty acid profile of argan oil and other edible vegetable oils by gas chromatography and discriminant analysis. *J. Chem.* vol. 2014, Article ID 843908, https://doi.org/10.1155/2014/843908.

Ref. 2: Kiralan M et al. (2010). Fatty acid composition of hempseed oils from different locations in Turkey. *Span. J. Agric. Res.* 8:385–390, https://doi.org/10.5424/sjar/2010082-1220.

Ref. 3: Liu L et al. (2002). Fatty acid profiles of leaves of nine edible wild plants: an Australian study. *J. Food Lipids* 9:65–71, https://doi.org/10.1111/j.1745–4522.2002.tb00209.x.

Ref. 4: Turner N et al. (2011). The ω-3 and ω-6 fats in meals: A proposal for a simple new label. *Nutrition* 27:719–726, https://doi.org/10.1016/j.nut.2010.07.019.

List of Common Fatty Acids

Number identifier	Common name (abbreviation)
Saturated	
14:0	myristic acid
16:0	palmitic acid
18:0	stearic acid
20:0	arachidic acid
22:0	behenic acid
Monounsaturated	
14:1	myristoleic acid
16:1	palmitoleic acid
18:1	oleic acid (OA)
Omega-6 polyunsaturated	
18:2ω-6	linoleic acid (LA)
18:3ω-6	γ-linolenic acid (GLA)
20:3ω-6	dihomo-γ-linolenic acid. (DGLA)
20:4ω-6	arachidonic acid (AA)
22:5ω-6	osbond acid
Omega-3 polyunsaturated	
18:3ω-3	α-linolenic acid (ALA)
18:4ω-3	stearidonic acid (SDA)
20:5ω-3	eicosapentaenoic acid (EPA)
22:5ω-3	docosapentaenoic acid (DPA)
22:6ω-3	docosahexaenoic acid (DHA)

Notes

Chapter 1. Essentials of Nutrition

1. Allport S (2006) *The Queen of Fats: Why Omega-3s Were Removed from the Western Diet and What We Can Do to Replace Them.* Berkeley: University of California Press.

2. Holman RT et al. (1982) A case of human linolenic acid deficiency involving neurological abnormalities. *Am. J. Clin. Nutr.* 35:617–623, https://doi.org/10.1093/ajcn/35.3.617.

3. Holman found little omega-3 and omega-6 in the blood samples of the two patients intravenously fed the fat-free solutions; however, he observed very high levels of monounsaturated fats and also a large amount of an unusual omega-9 PUFA (mead acid) which is not normally found in animals with adequate diet supply of essential fats. Its presence is now used as an indication of essential fat deficiency.

4. Holman RT (1988) George O. Burr and the discovery of essential fatty acids. *J. Nutr.* 118:535–540, https://doi.org/10.1093/jn/118.5.535.

5. Burr GO, Burr MM (1929) A new deficiency disease produced by the rigid exclusion of fat from the diet. *J. Biol. Chem.* 82:345–367, https://doi.org/10.1111/j.1753-4887.1973.tb06008.x.

6. Burr GO, Burr MM (1930) The nature and role of fatty acids essential in nutrition. *J. Biol. Chem.* 86:587–621, https://doi.org/10.1016/S0021-9258(20)78929-5.

7. Holman 1988, 537.

8. William Brown; see Holman 1988.

9. Arild Hansen; see Holman 1998. The slow discovery of the importance of w3 essential fatty acids in human health. *J. Nutr.* 128:427S–433S, https://doi.org/10.1093/jn/128.2.427S.

10. Castell JD et al. (1972) Essential fatty acids in the diet of rainbow trout (*Salmo gairdneri*): growth, feed conversion and some gross deficiency symptoms. *J Nutr.* 102:77–86, https://doi.org/10.1093/jn/102.1.93.

11. An enzyme is a specific protein molecule made by a cell to catalyse a specific biochemical reaction. They may either catalyse reactions inside the cell or be secreted from the cell to catalyse reactions outside the cell. They can be free in solution or attached to cell membranes. Enzymes have a shape specific for the catalytic task they perform. An enzyme protein is specified by a gene, which is a part of the DNA chain with a specific sequence of nucleic acid bases that in turn determines the specific sequence of amino acids in the protein which in turn determines the shape of that protein.

12. Values are from USDA FoodData Central, https://fdc.nal.usda.gov/index.html, FDC ID 169097 (oranges), 167746 (lemons), 170194 (thymus), and 169454 (spleen).

13. Organic molecules are those that contain, in their structure, at least one carbon atom bonded to a hydrogen atom.
14. Hulbert AJ et al. (2014) Polyunsaturated fats, membrane lipids and animal longevity. *J. Comp. Physiol. B* 184:149–166, https://doi.org/10.1007/s00360 -013-0786-8.
15. Collins FD et al. (1969) Linoleic deficiency in man. *Circulation* 40 (issue 4, supp. 3): III 5; Collins FD et al (1971). Plasma lipids in human linoleic deficiency. *Nutr. Metab.* 13:150–167, https://doi.org/10.1159/000175332.
16. Fienes RNT-W et al. (1973) Essential fatty acid studies in primates. Linolenic acid requirements of Capuchins. *J. Med. Primatology* 2:155–169, https://doi .org/10.1159/000460319.
17. Rivers JPW et al. (1975) Inability of cats to desaturate essential fatty acids. *Nature* 258:171–173, https://doi.org/10.1038/258171a0.

Chapter 2. Omega Balance of Foods
1. Poincelot RP (1976) Lipid and fatty acid composition of chloroplast envelope membranes from species with differing net photosynthesis. *Plant Physiol.* 58:595–598, https://doi.org/10.1104/pp.58.4.595.
2. Taubes G (2008) *Good Calories, Bad Calories: Challenging the Conventional Wisdom on Diet, Weight Control, and Disease.* New York: Anchor Books; Teicholz N (2014) *The Big Fat Surprise: A Nutritional Investigation.* New York: Simon & Schuster.
3. US Department of Agriculture, FoodData Central database (https://fdc.nal .usda.gov/index.html). Data for each food from this website is identified by its FDC ID number. The other source is "Food Standards Australia and New Zealand" (https://www.foodstandards.gov.au/science/monitoringnutrients /afcd/Pages/foodsearch.aspx). Data from this website is identified as FSANZ followed by its 'Public Food Key' number. (see appendix 1).
4. FAOSTAT database: Food and Agricultural Organisation of the United Nations. Food Balance Sheets 2018 data (http://www.fao.org/faostat/en/#data/FBS). Using the production quantity, imports, exports, variation in stock, amounts used for feed, for seed, amount processed, as well as losses and other uses, the amount used for food supply is calculated. Knowing population size, the "per capita food supply" of a wide range of food items is calculated for each year. Using the fat contents for each of the food items, the daily per capita supply of fat for each food category is calculated. This database takes into account the "non-food" uses of the specific food. For example, significant amounts of various oilseeds are grown for industrial uses, such as bio-fuel production, but these are excluded in the calculated provision of fat from vegetable oils (or oilseeds) in the food supply.
5. Sources of data for figure 2.1 and other plant-based foods mentioned in the text are provided in appendix 1.
6. FAOSTAT database: Food and Agricultural Organisation of United Nations. Food Balance Sheets 2018 data (http://www.fao.org/faostat/en/#data/FBS).

7. Combined values for cereals, pulses, treenut, and oilcrops.

8. Clapham WM et al (2005) Fatty acid composition of traditional and novel forages. *J. Agric. Food Chem.* 53:10068–10073, https://doi.org/10.1021/jf0517039.

9. Data for figure 2.2 and other animal-based foods mentioned in the text are provided in appendix 1.

10. Dawczynski C et al (2007) Amino acids, fatty acids, and dietary fibre in edible seaweed products. *Food Chem.* 103:891–899, https://doi.org/10.1016 /j.foodchem.2006.09.041; Takagi T et al (1985) Fatty acid composition of twelve algae from Japanese waters. *J. Japan Oil Chem.* 34:12–16, https://doi .org/10.5650/jos1956.34.1008

11. Reynolds JE et al (2006) Human health implications of omega-3 and omega-6 fatty acids in blubber of the bowhead whale (*Balaena mysticetus*). *Arctic* 59:155–164, https://www.jstor.org/stable/40512790.

12. Egeland GM et al (2009) Back to the future: using traditional food and knowledge to promote a healthy future among Inuit. In *Indigenous Peoples' Food Systems* (pp 10–22) Centre for Indigenous Peoples' Nutrition and Environment. Rome: FAO.

13. Proust F et al (2016) Fatty acid composition of birds and game hunted by the Eastern James Bay Cree people of Quebec. *Int. J. Circumpolar Health* 75:30583, https://doi.org/10.3402/ijch.v75.30583.

14. Gladyshev MI et al (2016) Comparison of fatty acid compositions in birds feeding in aquatic and terrestrial ecosystems. *Contemporary Problems of Ecology* 9:503–513, https://doi.org/10.1134/S1995425516040065.

15. Wood JD et al (2008) Fat deposition, fatty acid composition and meat quality: A review. *Meat Science* 78:343–358 (table 14), https://doi.org/10.1016/j.meatsci .2007.07.019.

16. Benbrook CM et al (2018) Enhancing the fatty acid profile of milk through forage-based rations, with nutrition modeling of diet outcomes. *Food Sci Nutr.* 6:681–700 (table 3), https://doi.org/10.1002/fsn3.610.

17. Fisher AV et al (2000) Fatty acid composition and eating quality of lamb types derived from four diverse breed × production systems. *Meat Science* 55:141–147 (table 3), https://doi.org/10.1016/s0309-1740(99)00136-9.

18. Fonteles NLO et al (2018) Fatty acid composition of polar and neutral meat lipids of goats browsing in native pasture of Brazilian Semiarid. *Meat Science* 139:149–156 (table 5), https://doi.org/10.1016/j.meatsci.2018.01.021.

19. Parunovic N et al (2012) Fatty acid profile and cholesterol content of *m. longissimus* of free-range and conventionally reared Mangalitsa pigs. *S. Afr. J. Anim. Sci.* 42:101–113 (table 3), http://www.scielo.org.za/scielo.php?script=sci _arttext&pid=S0375-15892012000200002.

20. Forrester-Anderson IT et al (2006) Fatty acid content of pasture-reared fryer rabbit meat. *J Food Comp. & Anal.* 19:715–719 (table 4), https://doi.org /10.1016/j.jfca.2006.02.011.

21. Strazdiòa V et al (2013) Nutrition value of wild animal meat. *Proc. Latvian Acad. Sci. B* 67:373–377 (table 2), https://doi.org/10.2478/prolas-2013-0074.

22. Bernard L et al (2009) Effect of plant oils in the diet on performance and milk fatty acid composition in goats fed diets based on grass hay or maize silage. *Brit. J. Nutr.* 101:213–224 (table 3), https://doi.org/10.1017/S0007114508006533.

23. Turner N et al (2011) Omega-3 and omega-6 fats in meals: a proposal for a simple new label. *Nutrition* 27:719–726, https://doi.org/10.1016/j.nut.2010.07.019.

Chapter 3. Earlier Diets

1. Data are from Stevens CE & Hume ID (1995) *Comparative Physiology of the Vertebrate Digestive System*, 2nd ed. Cambridge: Cambridge University Press; Kararli TT (1995) Comparison of gastrointestinal anatomy, physiology, and biochemistry of humans and commonly used laboratory animals. *Biopharm. & Drug Disposition* 16:351–380, https://doi.org/10.1002/bdd.2510160502; Dressman JB (1986) Comparison of canine and human gastrointestinal physiology. *Pharm. Res.* 3:123–131, https://doi.org/10.1023/A:1016353705970.

2. Milton K (2003) The critical role played by animal source foods in human (*Homo*) evolution. *J. Nutr.* 133:3886S–3892S, https://doi.org/10.1093/jn/133.11.3886S.

3. Hatch MD (2002) C4 photosynthesis: discovery and resolution. *Photosynthesis Res.* 73:251–256, https://doi.org/10.1023/A:1020471718805.

4. Schwarcz HP & Schoeniinger MJ (1991) Stable isotope analysis in human nutritional ecology *Year of Physical Anthropology* 34:283–321, https://doi.org/10.1002/ajpa.1330340613.

5. Hedges REM, Reynard LM (2007) Nitrogen isotopes and the trophic level of humans in archaeology. *J. Archaeol. Sci.* 34:1240–1251, https://doi.org/10.1016/j.jas.2006.10.015.

6. Balter M (2014) The killing ground. *Science* 344:1080–1083, https://www.jstor.org/stable/i24742038.

7. Richards MP (2002) A brief review of the archaeological evidence for Palaeolithic and Neolithic subsistence. *Eur. J. Clin. Nutr.* 56:1270–1278, https://doi.org/10.1038/sj.ejcn.1601646.

8. Richards MP et al. (2008) Isotopic dietary analysis of a Neanderthal and associated fauna from the Jonzac (Charente-Maritime), France. *J. Human Evol.* 55:179–185, https://doi.org/10.1016/j.jhevol.2008.02.007.

9. Richards MP Schmitz RW (2008) Isotope evidence for the diet of the Neanderthal type specimen. *Antiquity* 82:553–559, https://doi.org/10.1017/S0003598X00097210.

10. Wißing C et al (2016) Isotopic evidence for dietary ecology of late Neandertals in North-Western Europe. *Quaternary Internat.* 411:327–345, https://doi.org/10.1016/j.quaint.2015.09.091.

11. Richards MP, Trinkhaus E (2009) Isotopic evidence for the diets of European Neanderthals and early modern humans. *Proc Nat. Acad. Sci. USA* 106:16034–16039, https://doi.org/10.1073/pnas.0903821106.

12. Hu Y et al (2009) Stable isotope dietary analysis of the Tianyuan 1 early modern

human. *Proc Nat. Acad. Sci. USA* 106:10971–10974, https://doi.org/10.1073/pnas
.09048261.

13. Richards MP et al (2005) Isotope evidence for the intensive use of marine
foods by Late Upper Palaeolithic humans. *J. Human Evol.* 49:390–394, https://
doi.org/10.1016/j.jhevol.2005.05.002.

14. Cordain L et al (2002) Fatty acid analysis of wild ruminant tissues: evolutionary implications for reducing diet-related chronic disease. *Eur. J. Clin. Nutr.*
56:181–191, https://doi.org/10.1038/sj.ejcn.1601307.

15. Cordain L et al (2000) Plant-animal subsistence ratios and macronutrient
energy estimations in worldwide hunter-gather diets. *Am J. Clin. Nutr.*
71:682–692, https://doi.org/10.1093/ajcn/71.3.682.

16. I have described the first category as "gathered plant food" rather than
"gathering of wild plants and small land fauna" as in the original atlas. This
will overestimate the "plant-based" contribution and underestimate "animal-
sourced" foods.

17. Cordain L et al (2002) The paradoxical nature of hunter-gatherer diets: meat-
based, yet non-atherogenic. *Eur. J. Clin. Nutr.* 56 (suppl 1): S42–S52, https://
doi.org/10.1038/sj.ejcn.1601353.

18. Cordain L (2002) The nutritional characteristics of a contemporary diet based
upon paleolithic food groups. *J. Am. Nutraceutical Assoc.* 5:15–24, https://www
.researchgate.net/publication/237630815_The_Nutritional_Characteristics
_of_a_Contemporary_Diet_Based_Upon_Paleolithic_Food_Groups.

19. In Cordain's paper, the saturated fat, monounsaturated and polyunsaturated
fat contents (table 3) do not add up. I have used the values of 14.2g for omega-6
and 9.6g for omega-3 fat content.

20. Wikipedia, s.v. List of domesticated plants, https://en.wikipedia.org/wiki/List
_of_domesticated_plants

21. Larson G et al (2012) Rethinking dog domestication by integrating genetics,
archaeology, and biogeography. *Proc Nat. Acad. Sci. USA* 109:8878–8883,
https://doi.org/10.1073/pnas.1203005109.

22. Guixe EG et al (2006) Paleodiets of humans and fauna at the Spanish Meso-
lithic site of El Collado. *Current Anthropol.* 47:549–556, https://doi.org/10.1086
/504170.

23. Richards MP et al (2003) Sharp shift in diet at onset of Neolithic. *Nature*
425:366, https://doi.org/10.1038/425366a.

24. Jay M, Richards MP (2006) Diet in the Iron Age cemetery population at Wet-
wang Slack, East Yorkshire, UK: carbon and nitrogen stable isotope evidence.
J. Archaeol. Sci. 33:653–662, https://doi.org/10.1016/j.jas.2005.09.020.

25. Richards MP et al (2006) Stable isotope palaeodietary study of humans and
fauna from the multi-period (Iron Age, Viking and Late Medieval) site of
Newark Bay, Orkney. *J. Archaeol. Sci.* 33:122–131, https://doi.org/10.1016
/j.jas.2005.07.003.

26. Muldner G, Richards MP (2007) Stable isotope evidence for 1500 years of

human diet at the city of York, UK. *Amer. J. Phys. Anthropol.* 133:682–697, https://doi.org/10.1002/ajpa.20561.

27. Muldner G, Richards MP (2008) Fast or feast: reconstructing diet in later medieval England by stable isotope analysis. *J. Archaeol. Sci.* 35:2960–2965, https://doi.org/10.1016/j.jas.2004.05.007.

28. Choy K, Richards MP (2009) Stable isotope evidence of human diet at the Nukdo shell midden site, South Korea. *J. Archaeol. Sci.* 36:1312–1318, https://doi.org/10.1016/j.jas.2009.01.004.

29. Hu Y et al. (2008) Stable isotope analysis of humans from Xiaojingshan site: implications for understanding the origin of millet agriculture in China. *J. Archaeol. Sci.* 35:2960–2965, https://doi.org/10.1016/j.jas.2008.06.002.

30. Dickson JH et al. (2004) Kwaday Dan Ts'inchi, the first ancient body of a man from a North American glacier: Reconstructing his last days by intestinal and biomolecular analyses. *Holocene* 14:481–486, https://doi.org/10.1191/0959683604hl742rp; Richards MP et al (2007) Radiocarbon dating and dietary stable isotope analysis of Kwaday Dan Ts'inchi. *American Antiquity* 72:719–733, https://doi.org/10.2307/25470442.

31. Macko SA et al. (1999) Documenting the diet in ancient human populations through stable isotope analysis of hair. *Phil. Trans. R. Soc Lond. B* 354:65–76, https://doi.org/10.1098/rstb.1999.0360; Dickson JH (2000) The omnivorous Tyrolean Iceman: colon contents (meat, cereals, pollen, moss and whipworm) and stable isotope analyses. *Phil. Trans. R. Soc. Lond. B* 355:1843–1849, https://doi.org/10.1098/rstb.2000.0739; Maixner et al. (2018) The Iceman's last meal consisted of fat, wild meat, and cereals. *Current Biology* 28:1–8, https://doi.org/10.1016/j.cub.2018.05.067

32. Wilson AS, et al. (2007) Stable isotope and DNA evidence for ritual sequences in Inca child sacrifice. *Proc Nat. Acad. Sci. USA* 104:16456–16461, https://doi.org/10.1073/pnas.0704276104.

33. Wu X et al. (2012) Early pottery at 20,000 years ago in Xianrendong Cave, China. *Science* 336:1696–1700, https://doi.org/10.1126/science.1218643.

34. Evershed RP et al. (2008) Experimental evidence for the processing of marine animal products and other commodities containing polyunsaturated fatty acids in pottery vessels. *Archaeometry* 50:101–113, https://doi.org/10.1111/j.1475-4754.2007.00368.x .

35. Evershed RP et al. (1999) Lipids as carriers of anthropogenic signals from prehistory. *Phil. Trans. R. Soc. Lond. B* 354:19–31, https://doi.org/10.1098/rstb.1999.0357.

36. Dudd S, Evershed RP (1998) Direct demonstration of milk as an element of archaeological economies. *Science* 282:1478–1481, https://doi.org/10.1126/science.282.5393.1478.

37. Evershed RP et al. (2008) Earliest date for milk use in the Near East and south-eastern Europe linked to cattle herding. *Nature* 455:528–531, https://www.academia.edu/564299/Earliest_Date_for_Milk_Use_in_the_Near_East_and_Southeastern_Europe_Linked_to_Cattle_Herding.

38. Copley MS et al .(2003) Direct chemical evidence for widespread dairying in prehistoric Britain. *Proc Nat. Acad. Sci. USA* 100:1524–1529, https://doi.org /10.1073/pnas.0335955100.

39. Outram AK et al. (2009) The earliest horse harnessing and milking. *Science* 323:1332–1335, https://doi.org/10.1126/science.1168594.

40. Milk Composition—Species Table' accessed from *Milk Composition and Synthesis Resource Library* on July 6, 2018, http://ansci.illinois.edu/static/ansc438 /Milkcompsynth/milkcomp_table.html.

41. Vesa TH et al (2000) Lactose Intolerance. *J. Am. Coll. Nutr.* 19:165S–175S, doi: 10.1080/07315724.2000.10718086; Deng Y et al (2015) Lactose Intolerance in Adults: Biological Mechanism and Dietary Management. *Nutrients* 7:8020–8035, https://doi.org/10.3390/nu7095380.

42. Ranciaro A et al. (2014) Genetic origins of lactase persistence and spread of pastoralism in Africa. *Am. J. Human Gen.* 94:496–510, https://doi.org/10.1016 /j.ajhg.2014.02.009.

43. Curry A (2013) The milk revolution. *Nature* 500:20–22, https://doi.org/10.1038 /500020a.

44. Salque M et al. (2013) Earliest evidence for cheese making in the sixth millennium BC in northern Europe. *Nature* 493:522–525, https://doi.org/10.1038 /nature11698.

45. Nestel P (1986) A society in transition: developmental and seasonal influences on the nutrition of Maasai women and children. In: *Food and Nutrition Bulletin 8*. The United Nations University Press, https://hdl.handle.net/10568/50112.

46. Food and Agricultural Organisation of United Nations (2001) Pastoralism in the new millennium. FAO Animal Production and Health Paper 150. http:// www.fao.org/docrep/005/Y2647E/y2647e00.htm#toc.

47. US Dept. Agriculture, Food and Nutrition Service, Nutrient Content of the US Food Supply Reports. https://www.fns.usda.gov/resource/nutrient-content -us-food-supply-reports spreadsheets downloaded: (1) Food calories and macronutrients per capita per day, (2) Polyunsaturated fatty acids contributed from major food groups, and (3) Fatty acids per capita per day.

Chapter 4. The Omega Story

1. FAOSTAT "Food Balance Sheets" website, http://www.fao.org/faostat/en /#data/FBS.

2. World Bank "Commodity Market Outlook" January 2013, p. 13, http:// pubdocs.worldbank.org/en/450001461935833268/CMO-2013-January.pdf.

3. Monteiro CA et al. (2019) Ultra-processed foods, diet quality, and health using the NOVA classification system. Rome: Food and Agriculture Organisation.

4. Wikipedia, s.v. "ultra-processed food," https://en.wikipedia.org/wiki/Ultra -processed_food.

5. Shurtleff W, Aoyagi A (2004) *History of Soybeans and Soyfoods, 1100 B.C. to the 1980s.* https://www.soyinfocenter.com/HSS/shortening1.php.

6. Baker P et al. (2020) Ultra-processed foods and the nutrition transition: Global,

regional and national trends, food systems transformations and political economy drivers. *Obesity Rev.* 21: e13126, https://doi.org/10.1111/obr.13126.

7. US Department of Agriculture, Food and Nutrition Service, Nutrient Content of the US Food Supply Reports, https://www.fns.usda.gov/resource/nutrient-content-us-food-supply-reports; spreadsheets downloaded: (1) Food calories and macronutrients per capita per day, (2) Polyunsaturated fatty acids contributed from major food groups, and (3) Fatty acids per capita per day.

8. Archer E et al. (2018) The failure to measure dietary intake engendered a fictional discourse on diet-disease relations. *Front. Nutr.* 5:105, https://doi.org/10.3389/fnut.2018.00105.

9. Katan MB et al. (1994) Effects of fats and fatty acids on blood lipids in humans: an overview. *Am. J. Clin. Nutr.* 60(suppl):1017S–1022S, https://doi.org/10.1093/ajcn/60.6.1017S.

10. Jonnalagadda SS et al. (1995) Fatty acid consumption pattern of Americans: 1987–1988 USDA Nationwide Food Consumption Survey. *Nutr. Res.* 15:1767–1781, https://doi.org/10.1016/0271-5317(95)02046-2.

11. Ervin RB et al (2004) Dietary intake of fats and fatty acids for the United States population: 1999–2000. *National Center for Health Statistics CDC*, vol. 348. Hyattsville, MD.

12. What We Eat in America, NHANES 2017–2018 https://www.ars.usda.gov/ARSUserFiles/80400530/pdf/1718/tables_1-56_2017-2018.pdf.

13. Van Rossum CTM et al. (2011) Dutch National Food Consumption Survey 2007–2010: Diet of children and adults aged 7 to 69 years. Bilthoven: National Institute for Public Health and the Environment.

14. Pietinen P et al. (2010) FINDIET 2007 Survey: energy and nutrient intakes. *Publ. Health Nutr.* 13:920–924, https://doi.org/10.1017/S1368980010001102.

15. Iwasaki M et al. (2011) Dietary ratio of n-6 to n-3 polyunsaturated fatty acids and periodontal disease in community-based older Japanese: A 3-year follow-up study. *Prost. Leuk. and Essent. Fatty Acids* 85:107–112, https://doi.org/10.1016/j.plefa.2011.04.002.

16. Murakami K et al (2008) Total n-3 polyunsaturated fatty acid intake is inversely associated with serum C-reactive protein in young Japanese women. *Nutr. Res.* 28:309–314, https://doi.org/10.1016/j.nutres.2008.03.008.

17. Meyer BJ et al. (2003) Dietary intakes and food sources of omega-6 and omega-3 polyunsaturated fatty acids. *Lipids* 38:391–398, https://doi.org/10.1007/s11745-003-1074-0.

18. Meyer BJ (2016) Australians are not meeting the recommended intakes for omega-3 long chain polyunsaturated fatty acids: results of an analysis from the 2011–2012 National Nutrition and Physical Activity Survey. *Nutrients* 8:111, https://doi.org/10.3390/nu8030111.

19. Pot GK et al. (2012) National Diet and Nutrition Survey: fat and fatty acid intakes from the first year of the rolling programme and comparison with previous surveys. *Br. J. Nutr.* 107:405–415, https://doi.org/10.1017/S0007114511002911.

20. Baek Y et al. (2015) Dietary intake of fats and fatty acids in the Korean population: Korea National Health and Nutrition Examination Survey, 2013.
Nutr. Res. Prac. 9:650–657, https://doi.org/10.4162/nrp.2015.9.6.650.

21. Ramírez-Silva I et al. (2011) Fatty acids intake in the Mexican population.
Results of the National Nutrition Survey 2006. *Nutr. Metab.* 8:33, https://doi
.org/10.1186/1743-7075-8-33.

22. Variation in omega-3 and omega-6 intake between individuals may be associated with differences in total PUFA intake or variation in omega balance between individuals or both. It is not possible to differentiate between these
conditions unless the omega-3 intake and omega-6 intake are measured and
compared for each individual.

23. Sheppard KW, Cheatham CL (2018) Omega-6/omega-3 fatty acid intake of
children and older adults in the U.S.: dietary intake in comparison to current
dietary recommendations and the Healthy Eating Index. *Lipids in Health and
Disease* 17:43, https://doi.org/10.1186/s12944-018-0693-9.

24. The basic assumption is that ratio values belong to a "normal" distribution.
If this is the case, 68% of values lie between the mean ± 1 S.D., and 96% of
values lie between the mean ± 2 S.D. Once the respective ratio values were
determined, they were individually converted to omega balance values. The
assumption that ratio values follow a "normal distribution" is likely untrue,
but I have used it to illustrate the potential variation in individual diet omega
balance values within a population.

25. Mann NJ et al. (2006) Fatty acid composition of habitual omnivore and vege-
tarian diets. *Lipids* 41:637–646, https://doi.org/10.1007/s11745-006-5014-9.

26. Knoll N et al. (2011) High content of long-chain n-3 polyunsaturated fatty
acids in red blood cells of Kenyan Maasai despite low dietary intake. *Lipids
in Health and Disease* 10:141, https://doi.org/10.1186/1476-511X-10-141.

27. Egeland GM et al (2009) Back to the future: using traditional food and knowledge to promote a healthy future among Inuit. In *Indigenous Peoples Food Systems*, pp. 10–22. Rome: Food and Agriculture Organisation, Centre for
Indigenous Peoples' Nutrition and Environment.

28. Deutch B et al. (2007) Traditional and modern Greenlandic food—Dietary
composition, nutrients and contaminants. *Science of the Total Environment*
384:106–119, https://doi.org/10.1016/j.scitotenv.2007.05.042.

29. Nichols PD et al. (2014) Readily available sources of long-chain omega-3 oils:
Is farmed Australian seafood a better source of the good oil than wild-caught
seafood? *Nutrients* 6:1063–1079, https://doi.org/10.3390/nu6031063.

30. US Department of Agriculture, Food and Nutrition Service, Nutrient Content
of the US Food Supply Reports, https://www.fns.usda.gov/resource/nutrient
-content-us-food-supply-reports; spreadsheet downloaded: *Protein contributed
from major food groups*. Because both full-fat whole milk and low-fat milks
have the same protein content, "protein" can be used as a measure of supply
of the two types of milk.

Chapter 5. The Importance of Cell Membranes

1. Energy content (kJ/g) of fat is 39.6; carbohydrate is 17.5, and protein is 18.6. The human body stores less than 1 day's energy requirements as carbohydrate; during a fast, this is used first, with initial weight loss being predominantly loss of associated water.
2. There are hundreds of membrane fats. They are described by their head-group and the combination of the fatty acids. Membrane fats include phospholipids, sphingolipids, and glycolipids (consult biochemistry textbooks for more details).
3. "Bacteria" is used to describe our prokaryotic ancestors, which include a huge variety of Archea and Bacteria. Comments about "bacteria" generally refer to the intestinal bacteria *Escherischia coli* and not to all bacteria.
4. Alvarez HM, Steinbuchel A (2002) Triacylglycerols in prokaryotic organisms. *Appl. Microbiol. Biotechnol.* 60:367–376, https://doi.org/10.1007/s00253-002-1135-0.
5. The "membrane fat" is "phosphatidic acid" from which both triglycerides and other phospholipids can be made. See Nelson DL, Cox MM (2005) *Lehninger Principles of Biochemistry*, 4th ed., p. 805, New York: Freeman.
6. The forces that hold nonpolar regions of molecules together are called hydrophobic interactions and are also important in determining the orientation of proteins in bilayer membranes. See Nelson and Cox 2005, chapter 2, for more information.
7. A lipoprotein is an assembly of lipids (fats) and proteins. The inside of the assembly is hydrophobic, while the surface of the lipoprotein particle is hydrophilic and is where the phospholipids and proteins are located. Blood lipoproteins are classified by their relative density (VLDL = very low-density lipoprotein; LDL = low density lipoprotein; HDL = high density lipoprotein).
8. See Nelson and Cox 2005, 369–389, for more information.
9. The "temperature'" of a system is a measure of movement of molecules in the system. The "goldilocks" level of movement required for life is manifest as the temperature that animals regulate their body temperature (such as mammals and birds) is generally in the 35–40 °C range.
10. Frye LD, Edidin M (1970) The rapid intermixing of cell surface antigens after formation of mouse-human heterokaryons. *J. Cell Sci.* 7:319–335, https://doi.org/10.1242/jcs.7.2.319.
11. Singer SJ, Nicolson GL (1972) The fluid mosaic model of the structure of cell membranes. *Science* 175:720–731, https://doi.org/10.1016/B978-0-12-207250-5.50008-7.
12. See Nelson and Cox 2005, 794.
13. In mammals, 22:6ω-3 and 22:5ω-6 are made by an unusual microsomal-peroxisomal process, see Sprecher H, Chen Q (1999) Polyunsaturated fatty acid biosynthesis: a microsomal-peroxisomal process. *Prost. Leukot. Essent. Fatty Acids* 60:317–321, https://doi.org/10.1016/s0952-3278(99)80006-4;

and Hulbert et al. (2014) Polyunsaturated fats, membrane lipids and animal longevity. *J. Comp. Physiol. B* 184:149–166, https://doi.org/10.1007/s00360 -013-0786-8 Simple animals such as *C. elegans* are unable to make 22:6ω-3. Some marine bacteria have evolved the ability to synthesize 22:6ω-3 by the anaerobic polyketide synthase pathway, see Wang et al. (2021) Docosahexaenoic acid production by *Schizochytrium* sp: review and prospect. *Food Biotech.* 35:111–135, https://doi.org/10.1080/08905436.2021.1908900. Some 22:6ω-3 in marine food passes up the food chain from this source.

14. Lutz PL (2002) *The Rise of Experimental Biology.* Totowa, NJ: Humana Press.
15. See Hulbert AJ (2014) A sceptics view: "Kleiber's Law" or the "3/4 Rule" is neither a law nor a rule but rather is an empirical approximation. *Systems* 2:186–202, https://doi.org/10.3390/systems2020186.
16. Hulbert, A.J. (2007) Chapter 22: Energy metabolism, pp 591–602. In *Lecture Notes: Human Physiology* 5th ed. (ed. O. Petersen), Oxford: Blackwell.
17. Wikipedia, s.v. Candle, https://en.wikipedia.org/wiki/Candle.
18. Endosymbiosis is the leading proposal for the origin of eukaryotic cells of animals and plants. According to this theory, mitochondria and chloroplasts are descended from former free-living bacteria.
19. As well as ATP formation, transmembrane ion gradients are also used as energy source to perform work and are sometimes used to transport other molecules (such as glucose) against a concentration gradient.
20. Rolfe DFS, Brown GC (1997) Cellular energy utilization and molecular origin of standard metabolic rate in mammals. *Physiol. Rev.* 77:731–758, https://doi.org/10.1152/physrev.1997.77.3.731.
21. Couture P, Hulbert AJ (1995) On the relationship between body mass, tissue metabolic rate and sodium pump activity in mammalian liver and kidney. *Am. J. Physiol.* 268:R641–R650, https://doi.org/10.1152/ajpregu.1995.268.3.R641.
22. Ho D et al. (2011) Heart rate and electrocardiography monitoring in mice. *Curr. Protocol. Mouse Biol.* 1:123–139, https://doi.org/10.1002/9780470942390 .mo100159.
23. Gudbjarnason S et al. (1978) Modification of cardiac phospholipids and catecholamine stress tolerance, pp. 297–310 in: deDuve C, Hayaishi O (eds.) *Tocopherol, Oxygen and Biomembranes.* Amsterdam: Elsevier.
24. Couture P, Hulbert AJ (1995) Membrane fatty acid composition is related to body mass of mammals. *J. Membrane Biol.* 148:27–39, https://doi.org/10.1007 /BF00234153; Hulbert AJ et al. (2002) The acyl composition of mammalian phospholipids: an allometric analysis. *Comp. Biochem. Physiol. B* 132:515–527, https://doi.org/10.1016/s1096-4959(02)00066-0.
25. Hulbert AJ et al. (2002) Acyl composition of muscle membranes varies with body size in birds. *J. Exp. Biol.* 205:3561–3569, https://doi.org/10.1242/jeb .205.22.3561; Brand MD et al. (2003) Proton conductance and fatty acyl composition of liver mitochondria correlates with body mass in birds. *Biochem. J.* 376:741–748, https://doi.org/10.1042/BJ20030984; Else PL et al. (2004)

Respiration rate of hepatocytes varies with body size in birds. *J. Exp. Biol.* 207:2305–2311, https://doi.org/10.1242/jeb.01017.

26. Else PL, Hulbert AJ (1981) A comparison of the "mammal machine" and the "reptile machine": energy production. *Am. J. Physiol.* 240:R3–R9, https://doi.org/10.1152/ajpregu.1981.241.5.R350; Else PL, Hulbert AJ (1985b) An allometric comparison of the mitochondria of mammalian and reptilian tissues: the implications for the evolution of endothermy. *J. Comp. Physiol. B.* 156:3–11, https://doi.org/10.1007/BF00692920.

27. Hulbert AJ, Else PL (1981) A comparison of the "mammal machine" and the "reptile machine": energy use and thyroid activity. *Am. J. Physiol.* 241:R350–R356, https://doi.org/10.1152/ajpregu.1981.241.5.R350; Else PL, Hulbert AJ (1987) The evolution of mammalian endothermic metabolism: "leaky membranes" as a source of heat. *Am. J. Physiol.* 253:R1–R7, https://doi.org/10.1152/ajpregu.1987.253.1.R1.

28. Hulbert AJ, Else PL (1990) The cellular basis of endothermic metabolism: a role for "leaky" membranes? *News in Physiological Sciences* 5:25–28, https://doi.org/10.1152/physiologyonline.1990.5.1.25.

29. Else PL et al. (1996) Molecular activity of sodium pumps in endotherms and ectotherms. *Am. J. Physiol.* 271:R1287–R1294, https://journals.physiology.org/doi/pdf/10.1152/ajpregu.1996.271.5.R1287.

30. Hulbert AJ, Else PL (1989) The evolution of mammalian endothermic metabolism: mitochondrial activity and changes in cellular composition. *Am. J. Physiol.* 256:R63–R69, https://doi.org/10.1152/ajpregu.1989.256.1.R63.

31. Else PL, Wu BJ (1999) What role for membranes in determining the higher sodium pump molecular activity of mammals compared to ectotherms. *J. Comp. Physiol. B* 169:296–302, https://doi.org/10.1007/s003600050224.

32. Wu BJ et al. (2004) Membrane lipids and sodium pumps of cattle and crocodiles: an experimental test of the membrane pacemaker theory of metabolism. *Am. J. Physiol.* 287:R633–R641, https://doi.org/10.1152/ajpregu.00549.2003.

33. Wu BJ et al. (2001) Molecular activity of Na^+,K^+-ATPase from different sources is related to packing of membrane lipids. *J. Exp. Biol.* 204:4271–4280, https://doi.org/10.1242/jeb.204.24.4271.

34. Brand MD et al. (1991) Evolution of energy metabolism: proton permeability of the inner membrane of liver mitochondria is greater in a mammal than in a reptile. *Biochem. J.* 275:81–86, https://doi.org/10.1042/bj2750081.

35. Brand MD et al. (1994) Liposomes from mammalian liver mitochondria are more polyunsaturated and leakier to protons than those from reptiles. *Comp. Biochem. Physiol.* 108B:181–188, https://doi.org/10.1016/0305-0491(94)90064-7.

36. While there is freedom of rotation around carbon-carbon single bonds, carbon-carbon double bonds are shorter and do not allow free rotation around the bond. See Nelson and Cox 2005, p. 13.

37. The six double bonds in 22:6ω-3 reduces chain flexibility, but this also means the chain undergoes rapid transitions between vastly different shapes. See

Feller SE et al. (2002) Polyunsaturated fatty acids in lipid bilayers: intrinsic and environmental contributions to their unique physical properties. *J. Am. Chem. Soc.* 124:318–326, https://doi.org/10.1021/ja0118340.

38. Wikipedia, s.v. Stearic acid, https://en.wikipedia.org/wiki/Stearic_acid, Wikipedia, s.v. List of unsaturated fatty acids, https://en.wikipedia.org/wiki/List_of_unsaturated_fatty_acids

39. For discussion see: Hulbert AJ (2021) The under-appreciated fats of life: the two types of polyunsaturated fats. *J. Exp. Biol.* 224: jeb232538, https://doi.org/10.1242/jeb.232538.

40. Ishinaga et al. (1979) Distribution of phospholipid molecular species in outer and cytoplasmic membranes of Escherichia coli. *J. Biochem.* 86:161–165, PMID: 383707; Rock Co et al. (1996) Lipid metabolism in prokaryotes, pp. 35–74, in *Biochemistry of Lipids, Lipoproteins and Membranes* (ed. DE Vance and JE Vance) New York: Elsevier.

41. Sinensky M (1974) Homeoviscous adaptation–a homeostatic process that regulates viscosity of membrane lipids in *Escherichia coli. Proc. Natl. Acad. Sci. USA* 71:522–525, https://doi.org/10.1073/pnas.71.2.522.

42. Hazel JR (1972) The effect of temperature acclimation upon succinic dehydrogenase activity activity from the epiaxial muscle of the common goldfish (Carassius auratus L.)–Lipid reactivation of the soluble enzyme. *Comp. Biochem. Physiol.* B 43:863–882, https://doi.org/10.1016/0305-0491(72)90230-1.

43. Raynard RS, Cossins AR (1991) Homeoviscous adaptation and thermal compensation of sodium pump of trout erythrocytes. *Am J. Physiol.* 260:R916–R924, https://doi.org/10.1152/ajpregu.1991.260.5.R916.

44. Schmid PC et al. (1995) Generation and remodeling of phospholipid molecular species in rat hepatocytes. *Arch. Biochem. Biophys.* 319:168–176, https://doi.org/10.1006/abbi.1995.1279.

45. "Phospholipase" enzymes remove fatty acid chains from specific membrane fats, "acyltransferase" enzymes selectively add specific fatty acids to membrane fats, "transacylase" enzymes catalyze the transfer of acyl chains between different lipids.

46. Yamashita A et al. (1997) Acyltransferases and transacylases involved in fatty acid remodelling of phospholipids and metabolism of bioactive lipids in mammalian cells. *J. Biochem.* 122:1–16, https://doi.org/10.1093/oxfordjournals.jbchem.a021715; Fryst H et al. (1996) Formation of vesicles by the action of acyl-CoA:1-acyllysophosphatidylcholine acyltransferase from rat liver microsomes: optimal solubilization conditions and analysis of lipid composition and enzyme activity. *Biochem.* 35:2644–2650, https://doi.org/10.1021/bi952268m.

47. Giron-Calle J et al. (1997) Effects of oxidative stress on glycerolipid acyl turnover in rat hepatocytes. *Lipids* 32:917–923, https://doi.org/10.1007/s11745-997-0118-9

48. Lands WE et al. (1982) Selective incorporation of polyunsaturated fatty acids

into phosphatidylcholine by rat liver microsomes. *J. Biol. Chem.* 257: 14968–14972, https://doi.org/10.1016/S0021-9258(18)33378-7.

49. Hulbert AJ et al. (2005) Dietary fats and membrane function: implications for metabolism and disease. *Biol. Rev.* 80:155–169, https://doi.org/10.1017/s146 4793104006578.

50. The 2018 world food supply (http://www.fao.org/faostat/en/#data/FBS) provided 12,255 kJ energy and 86.2 g fat per person per day. Assuming 39.6 kJ per g fat, the fat supply is equivalent to about 28 percent of food energy.

51. Ervin RB et al. (2004) Dietary intake of fats and fatty acids for the United States population: 1999–2000. *National Center for Health Statistics CDC*, vol. 348. Hyattsville, Maryland.

52. Abbott SK et al. (2010) Membrane fatty acid composition of rat skeletal muscle is most responsive to the balance of dietary n-3 and n-6 polyunsaturated fatty acids. *Brit. J. Nutr.* 103:522–529, https://doi.org/10.1017/S0007114509992133; Abbott SK et al. (2012) Fatty acid composition of membrane bilayers: importance of diet polyunsaturated fat balance. *Biochim. Biophys. Acta–Biomembranes* 1818:1309–1317, https://doi.org/10.1016/j.bbamem.2012.01.011.

53. Allport S (2006) *The Queen of Fats: Why Omega-3s Were Removed from the Western Diet and What We Can Do to Replace Them.* Berkeley: University of California Press.

54. Allport S. (2010). One person's response to a high omega-6 diet, https://www.aocs.org/stay-informed/read-inform/featured-articles/one-persons-response-to-a-high-omega-6-diet-november-2010 .

55. Omega balance was calculated from results kindly provided by Susan Allport. Analyses were performed in the Bibus laboratory at the University of Minnesota.

56. Mitchell DC et al. (2003) Enhancement of G protein–coupled signaling by DHA phospholipids. *Lipids* 38:437–443, https://doi.org/10.1007/s11745-003-1081-1.

57. Arshavsky VY et al. (2002) G proteins and phototransduction. *Annu. Rev. Physiol.* 64:153–87, https://doi.org/10.1146/annurev.physiol.64.082701.102229.

58. Arshavsky VY, Burns ME (2014) Current understanding of signal amplification in phototransduction. *Cellular Logistics*, 4:2, e29390, https://doi.org/10.4161/cl.29390.

59. Jastrzebska B et al. (2011) Role of membrane integrity on G protein-coupled receptors: rhodopsin stability and function. *Prog Lipid Res.* 50:267–277, https://doi.org/10.1016/j.plipres.2011.03.002.

60. Wikipedia, s.v. G Protein, https://en.wikipedia.org/wiki/G_protein.

61. Niu S-L et al. (2004) Reduced G protein-coupled signaling efficiency in retinal rod outer segments in response to *n*-3 fatty acid deficiency. *J. Biol. Chem.* 279:31098–31104, https://doi.org/10.1074/jbc.M404376200.

62. Centers for Disease Control and Prevention (2012). Second National Report on Biochemical Indicators of Diet and Nutrition in the U.S. Population, https://www.cdc.gov/nutritionreport/pdf/Nutrition_Book_complete508_final.pdf

63. Cho HP et al. (1999) Cloning, expression, and fatty acid regulation of the human delta-5 desaturase. *J. Biol. Chem.* 274:37335–37339, https://doi.org/10.1074/jbc.274.52.37335; Rapoport SI et al. (2010) Quantitative contributions of diet and liver synthesis to docosahexaenoic acid homeostasis. *Prost. Leukot. Essent. Fatty Acids* 82:273–276, https://doi.org/10.1016/j.plefa.2010.02.015.

64. Rapoport SI et al. (2007) Brain metabolism of nutritionally essential polyunsaturated fatty acids depends on both the diet and the liver. *Prost. Leukot. Essent. Fatty Acids* 77:251–261, https://doi.org/10.1016/j.plefa.2007.10.023

65. See figure 2 in Hulbert AJ et al. (2014) Polyunsaturated fats, membrane lipids and animal longevity. *J. Comp. Physiol. B* 184:149–166, https://doi.org/10.1007/s00360-013-0786-8.

66. R^2 values for relationship between two variables can vary from 0 (which says there is no relationship) to 1.0 (which says one variable can fully predict the other variable). The respective R^2 values for relationships between membrane 20:4ω-6 content of tissues and (1) diet omega-6 content and (2) diet omega balance were respectively; 0.38 and 0.89 for brain; 0.18 and 0.87 for heart, 0.39 and 0.94 for skeletal muscle; 0.54 and 0.89 for liver, 0.31 and 0.95 for red blood cells. Also see figure 3 in Hulbert (2021) The under-appreciated fats of life: the two types of polyunsaturated fats. *J. Exp Biol.* 224:jeb232538, https://doi.org/10.1242/jeb.232538.

67. Mohrhauer H, Holman RT (1963) Effect of linolenic acid upon the metabolism of linoleic acid. *J. Nutr.* 81:67–74, https://doi.org/10.1093/jn/84.1.15; Mohrhauer H, Holman RT (1963) Alteration of the fatty acid composition of brain lipids by varying levels of dietary essential fatty acids. *J. Neurochem.* 10:523–530, https://doi.org/10.1111/j.1471-4159.1963.tb09855.x. Analysis of the data in these papers, gives the respective R^2 values for relationships between membrane 20:4ω-6 content and (1) diet omega-6 content and (2) diet omega balance of respectively; 0.39 and 0.89 for brain, 0.40 and 0.77 for heart and 0.49 and 0.90 for liver.

Chapter 6. Obesity and Diabetes

1. Ng M et al. (2014) Global, regional, and national prevalence of overweight and obesity in children and adults during 1980–2013: a systematic analysis for the Global Burden of Disease Study 2013. *Lancet* 384:715–828, https://doi.org/10.1016/S0140-6736(14)60460-8; NCD Risk Factor Collaboration (2016) Trends in adult body-mass index in 200 countries from 1975 to 2014: a pooled analysis of 1698 population-based measurement studies with 19·2 million participants. *Lancet* 387:1377–96, https://doi.org/10.1016/S0140-6736(16)30054-X; Chooi YC et al (2019) The epidemiology of obesity. *Metab Clin. & Exp.* 92:6–10, https://doi.org/10.1016/j.metabol.2018.09.005.

2. Hulbert AJ (2007) Energy metabolism. Chapter 22, pp 591–602 in: *Lecture Notes: Human Physiology 5th Edition* (ed. O. Petersen). Oxford: Blackwell.

3. Wikipedia, s.v. Leptin, https://en.wikipedia.org/wiki/Leptin.

4. DeLany JP et al (2013) High energy expenditure masks low physical activity in obesity. *Int. J. Obes.* 37:1006–1011, https://doi.org/10.1038/ijo.2012.172.

5. Hill RS, Davies PSW (2001) The validity of self-reported energy intake as determined using the doubly labelled water technique. *Brit. J. Nutr.* 85:415–430, https://doi.org/10.1079/bjn2000281.

6. Fothergill E et al (2016) Persistent metabolic adaptation 6 years after "The Biggest Loser" competition. *Obesity* 24:1612–1619, https://doi.org/10.1002/oby.21538.

7. Hall KD (2013) Diet versus exercise in "The Biggest Loser" weight loss competition. *Obesity* 21:957–959, https://doi.org/10.1002/oby.20065.

8. Luke A, Cooper RS (2013) Physical activity does not influence obesity risk: time to clarify the public health message. *Int. J. Epidemiol.* 42:1831–1836, https://doi.org/10.1093/ije/dyt159.

9. La Berge AF (2008) How the ideology of low fat conquered America. *J. History Med. & Allied Sci.* 63:139–177, https://doi.org/10.1093/jhmas/jrn001.

10. Yudkin J (1957) Diet and coronary thrombosis. Hypothesis and fact. *The Lancet.* 270:155–162, https://doi.org/10.1016/s0140-6736(57)90614-1.; Yudkin J (1972) *Pure, White and Deadly: The Problem of Sugar.* London: Davis-Poynter.

11. Taubes G. (2007) *Good Calories, Bad Calories.* New York: Anchor Books.

12. Teicholz N. (2014) *The Big Fat Surprise.* New York: Simon & Schuster.

13. Lai M et al (2014) You are what you eat, or are you? The challenges of translating high-fat-fed rodents to human obesity and diabetes. *Nutrition & Diabetes* 4: e135, https://doi.org/10.1038/nutd.2014.30.

14. Teklad custom research diets. Diet induced obesity, https://www.envigo.com/products-services/teklad/laboratory-animal-diets/custom-research/diet-induced-obesity/

15. Abbott, Sarah K., (2011) The influence of dietary fatty acid profile on membrane fatty acid composition in the rat and its metabolic implications, Ph.D. thesis, University of Wollongong. http://ro.uow.edu.au/theses/3260 : Search of 2008 Medline database for "high fat diet induced obesity" and "rats and mice" provided 81 papers that averaged 51 percent energy as fat.

16. Montgomery MK et al (2013) Mouse strain-dependent variation in obesity and glucose homeostasis in response to high-fat feeding. *Diabetologia* 56:1129–1139, https://doi.org/10.1007/s00125-013-2846-8.

17. Ikemoto S et al (1996) High-fat diet-induced hyperglycemia and obesity in mice: differential effects of dietary oils. *Metabolism* 45:1539–1546, https://doi.org/10.1016/s0026-0495(96)90185-7.

18. Couet C et al (1997) Effect of dietary fish oil on body fat mass and basal fat oxidation in healthy adults. *Int. J. Obesity* 21:637–643, https://doi.org/10.1038/sj.ijo.0800451.

19. Kabir M et al (2007) Treatment for 2 mo with n-3 polyunsaturated fatty acids reduces adiposity and some atherogenic factors but does not improve insulin sensitivity in women with type 2 diabetes: a randomized controlled study. *Am J Clin Nutr* 86:1670–1679, https://doi.org/10.1093/ajcn/86.5.1670.

20. Thorsdottir I et al (2007) Randomized trial of weight-loss-diets for young

adults varying in fish and fish oil content. *Int. J. Obesity* (2007) 31:1560–1566, https://doi.org/10.1038/sj.ijo.0803643.

21. Munro IA, Garg ML (2013) Prior supplementation with long chain omega-3 polyunsaturated fatty acids promotes weight loss in obese adults: a double-blinded randomised controlled trial. *Food Funct.* 4:650–658, https://doi.org /10.1039/c3fo60038f.

22. Mohammadi-Sartang M et al (2017) The effect of flaxseed supplementation on body weight and body composition: a systematic review and meta-analysis of 45 randomized placebo-controlled trials. *Obesity Reviews* 18:1096–1107, https://doi.org/10.1111/obr.12550.

23. Storlien LH et al (1996) Skeletal muscle membrane lipids and insulin resistance. *Lipids* 31:S261–S265, https://doi.org/10.1007/BF02637087. The relationship published was between BMI and the muscle omega-6:omega-3 ratio (see figure 1). I converted the ratio values to omega balance. The combined populations were (1) 52 Pima Indians (average BMI = 33), (2) 27 Caucasian Australians (average BMI = 27), (3) 13 Caucasian Australians (average BMI = 23).

24. The data for "obese" individuals are unpublished results of Hulbert AJ, Mitchell TW, Else PL and Shikora S. The experimental protocol was approved by both the University of Wollongong Human Research Ethics Committee (Australia) and the New England Medical Center Hospital Ethics Committee (United States). All subjects were non-smoking Caucasians undergoing elective obesity surgery at NEMCH/Tufts University Boston USA and gave informed written consent. The non-obese values are taken as non-obese healthy adult controls from the following scientific literature (after each reference the following code identifies what data was used for: M = Membrane fats, S = Storage fats, mu = skeletal muscle, ad = adipose tissue, pl = plasma) sources are: Burke PA et al (2001) *J. Par. & Ent. Nutr* 25:188–193. (M:mu,ad,pl); Di Marino L et al (2000) *Metabolism* 49:1164–1166. (M:mu); Rodriguez Y, Christophe AB (2004) *Ann Nutr. Metab.* 48:335–342. (M:pl); Phinney SD et al (1990) *Am J Clin. Nutr.* 51:385–392. (M:pl, S:pl); Zeleniuch-Jacquotte A et al (2000) *Eur J Clin Nutr* 54:367–372. (M:pl); Field CJ et al (1985) *Amer. J. Clin. Nutr.* 42:1206–1220. (S:ad); Andersson A et al (1998) *Am J Physiol.* 274:E432-E438. (M:mu); Andersson A et al (2002) *Am J Clin Nutr* 76:1222–1229. (M:mu,pl); Cunnane SC et al (1993) *Nutrition* 9:423–429. (S:ad,pl); Ullrich NFE et al (2001). *J Invest Med* 49:273–275. (S:ad); Skeaff CM et al (2006) *J Nutr* 136:565–569. (S:pl); Li D, Sinclair A et al (1999) *Am J Clin Nutr* 69:872–882. (S:pl); Sekine K (1995) *Int Med* 34:139–143. (S: ad); Hodson L et al (2008) *Prog Lipid Res* 47:348–380. (S:ad,pl).

25. Elizondo A et al (2007) Polyunsaturated fatty acid pattern in liver and erythrocyte phospholipids from obese patients. *Obesity* 15:24–31, https://doi.org /10.1038/oby.2007.518.

26. Sansone A et al (2016) Hexadecenoic fatty acid isomers in human blood lipids and their relevance for the interpretation of lipidomic profiles. *PLoS ONE* 11: e0152378, https://doi.org/10.1371/journal.pone.0152378.

27. Cazzola R et al (2004) Decreased membrane fluidity and altered susceptibility to peroxidation and lipid composition in overweight and obese female erythrocytes. *J. Lipid Res.* 45:1846–1851, https://doi.org/10.1194/jlr.M300509-JLR200; Karlsson M et al (2006) Serum phospholipid fatty acids, adipose tissue, and metabolic markers in obese adolescents. *Obesity* 14:1931–1939, https://doi.org/10.1038/oby.2006.225.
28. Négrel R et al (1989) Prostacyclin as a potent effector of adipose cell differentiation. *Biochem J.* 257:399–405, https://doi.org/10.1042/bj2570399.; Gaillard D et al (1989) Requirement and role of arachidonic acid in the differentiation of pre-adipose cells. *Biochem J.* 257:389–397, https://doi.org/10.1042/bj2570389.; Ailhaud G (2008) Omega-6 fatty acids and excessive adipose tissue development. *World Rev Nutr Diet.* 98:51–61, https://doi.org/10.1159/000152921.
29. Spalding KL et al (2008) Dynamics of fat cell turnover in humans. *Nature* 453:783–787, https://doi.org/10.1038/nature06902.
30. Freedman DS et al (2001) Relationship of childhood obesity to coronary heart disease risk factors in adulthood: The Bogalusa Heart Study. *Pediatrics* 108:712–718, https://doi.org/10.1542/peds.108.3.712
31. Barquissau V et al (2017) Control of adipogenesis by oxylipins, GPCRs and PPARs. *Biochimie* 136:3–11, https://doi.org/10.1016/j.biochi.2016.12.012.
32. Okuno M et al (1997) Perilla oil prevents the excessive growth of visceral adipose tissue in rats by down-regulating adipocyte differentiation. *J. Nutr.* 127:1752–1757, https://doi.org/10.1093/jn/127.9.1752.
33. Donahue SMA et al (2011) Prenatal fatty acid status and child adiposity at age 3 y: results from a US pregnancy cohort. *Am. J. Clin. Nutr.* 93:780–788, https://doi.org/10.3945/ajcn.110.005801.
34. Savva SC et al (2004) Association of adipose tissue arachidonic acid content with BMI and overweight status in children from Cyprus and Crete. *Brit. J. Nutr.* 91:643–649, https://doi.org/10.1079/BJN20031084.
35. Jensen CL et al (1997) Effect of dietary linoleic/alpha-linolenic acid ratio on growth and visual function of term infants. *J. Pediatr.* 131:200–209, https://doi.org/10.1016/s0022-3476(97)70154-9.
36. Dayton S et al (1996) Composition of lipids in human serum and adipose tissue during prolonged feeding of a diet high in unsaturated fat. *J. Lipid Res.* 7:103–111, https://doi.org/10.1016/S0022-2275(20)39591-2.
37. Hui-Lin Li (1974) An archaeological and historical account of cannabis in China. *Econ. Bot.* 28:437–448, https://doi.org/10.1007/BF02862859.
38. Abel EL (1975) Cannabis: effects on hunger and thirst. *Behav. Biol.* 15:255–281, https://doi.org/10.1016/s0091-6773(75)91684-3.
39. Gaoni Y, Mechoulam R (1964) Isolation, structure, and partial synthesis of an active constituent of hashish. *J. Am. Chem. Soc.* 86:1646–1647, https://doi.org/10.1021/ja01062a046.
40. Devane WA et al (1988) Determination and characterization of a cannabinoid receptor in rat brain. *Mol. Pharmacol.* 34:605–613

41. Munro S et al (1993) Molecular characterization of a peripheral receptor for cannabinoids. *Nature* 365:61–65, https://doi.org/10.1038/365061a0.

42. Devane W et al (1992) Isolation and structure of a brain constituent that binds to the cannabinoid receptor. *Science* 258:1946–1949, https://doi.org/10.1126/science.1470919.

43. Mechoulam R et al (1995) Identification of an endogenous 2-monoglyceride, present in canine gut, that binds to cannabinoid receptors. *Biochem. Pharmacol.* 50:83–90, https://doi.org/10.1016/0006-2952(95)00109-d.

44. Horn H et al (2018) Endocannabinoids in body weight control. *Pharmaceuticals* 11:55–103, https://doi.org/10.3390/ph11020055.

45. Fride E (2004) The endocannabinoid-CB1 receptor system in pre- and post-natal life. *Eur. J. Pharmacol.* 500:289–297, https://doi.org/10.1016/j.ejphar.2004.07.033.

46. Di Marzo V, Matias I (2005) Endocannabinoid control of food intake and energy balance. *Nature Neuroscience* 8:585–589, https://doi.org/10.1038/nn1457.

47. Mazier W et al (2015) The endocannabinoid system: pivotal orchestrator of obesity and metabolic disease. *Trends Endocrinol. & Metab.* 26:524–537, https://doi.org/10.1016/j.tem.2015.07.007.

48. Hillard CJ (2018) Circulating endocannabinoids: from whence do they come and where are they going? *Neuropsychopharmacol.* 43:155–172, https://doi.org/10.1038/npp.2017.130.

49. Engeli S et al (2005) Activation of the peripheral endocannabinoid system in human obesity. *Diabetes* 54:2838–2843, https://doi.org/10.2337/diabetes.54.10.2838.

50. Di Marzo V et al (2009) Role of insulin as a negative regulator of plasma endocannabinoid levels in obese and nonobese subjects. *Eur. J. Endocrinol.* 161:715–722, https://doi.org/10.1530/EJE-09-0643; Little TJ et al (2018) Plasma endocannabinoid levels in lean, overweight and obese humans: relationships with intestinal permeability markers, inflammation and incretin secretion. *Amer. J. Physiol. Endocrinol. Metab.* 315:E489–E495, https://doi.org/10.1152/ajpendo.00355.2017.

51. Bluher M et al (2006) Dysregulation of the peripheral and adipose tissue endocannabinoid system in human abdominal obesity. *Diabetes* 55:3053–3060, https://doi.org/10.2337/db06-0812; Cote M et al (2007) Circulating endocannabinoid levels, abdominal adiposity and related cardiometabolic risk factors in obese men. *Int. J. Obesity* 31:692–699, https://doi.org/10.1038/sj.ijo.0803539; Abdulnour J et al (2014) Circulating endocannabinoids in insulin sensitive vs. insulin resistant obese postmenopausal women. A MONET group study. *Obesity* 22:211–216, https://doi.org/10.1002/oby.20498; Fernandez-Aranda F et al (2014) Moderate-vigorous physical activity across body mass index in females: moderating effect of endocannabinoids and temperament. *PLoS ONE* 9(8): e104534, https://doi.org/10.1371/journal.pone.0104534; Pastor A et al (2016) A lower olfactory capacity is related to higher circulating concentrations of endocannabinoid 2-arachidonoylglycerol and higher body

mass index in women. *PLoS ONE* 11(2): e0148734, https://doi.org/10.1371/journal.pone.0148734.

52. Ravinet Trillou C et al (2004) CB1 cannabinoid receptor knockout in mice leads to leanness, resistance to diet-induced obesity and enhanced leptin sensitivity. *Int. J. Obesity* 28:640–648, https://doi.org/10.1038/sj.ijo.0802583

53. Hildebrandt AL et al (2003) Antiobesity effects of chronic cannabinoid CB1 receptor antagonist treatment in diet-induced obese mice. *Eur. J. Pharmacol.* 462:125–132, https://doi.org/10.1016/s0014-2999(03)01343-8.

54. Di Marzo V, Després J-P (2009) CB1 antagonists for obesity—what lessons have we learned from rimonabant? *Nat. Rev. Endocrinol.* 5:633–638, https://doi.org/10.1038/nrendo.2009.197.

55. Watanabe S et al (2003) n-3 Polyunsaturated fatty acid (PUFA) deficiency elevates and n-3 PUFA enrichment reduces brain 2-arachidonoylglycerol level in mice. *Prost. Leukot. Essen. Fatty Acids* 69:51–59, https://doi.org/10.1016/s0952-3278(03)00056-5; Wood JT et al (2010) Dietary docosahexaenoic acid supplementation alters select physiological endocannabinoid-system metabolites in brain and plasma. *J. Lipid Res.* 51:1416–1423, https://doi.org/10.1194/jlr.M002436.; Artmann A et al (2008) Influence of dietary fatty acids on endocannabinoid and N-acylethanolamine levels in rat brain, liver and small intestine. *Biochim. Biophys. Acta* 1781:200–212, https://doi.org/10.1016/j.bbalip.2008.01.006; Batetta B et al (2009) Endocannabinoids may mediate the ability of (n-3) fatty acids to reduce ectopic fat and inflammatory mediators in obese Zucker rats. *J. Nutr.* 139:1495–1501, https://doi.org/10.3945/jn.109.104844.

56. Alvheim AR et al (2012) Dietary linoleic acid elevates endogenous 2-AG and anandamide and induces obesity. *Obesity* 20:1984–1994, https://doi.org/10.1038/oby.2012.38.

57. Banni S et al (2011) Krill oil significantly decreases 2-arachidonoylglycerol plasma levels in obese subjects. *Nutr. & Metab.* 8:7 , https://doi.org/10.1186/1743-7075-8-7.

58. Berge K et al (2013) Chronic treatment with krill powder reduces plasma triglyceride and anandamide levels in mildly obese men. *Lipids in Health and Disease* 12:78, https://doi.org/10.1186/1476-511X-12-78.

59. Mele M et al (2011) Enrichment of Pecorino cheese with conjugated linoleic acid by feeding dairy ewes with extruded linseed: Effect on fatty acid and triglycerides composition and on oxidative stability. *Int. Dairy J.* 21:365–372, https://doi.org/10.1016/j.idairyj.2010.12.015; Pintus S et al (2013) Sheep cheese naturally enriched in α-linolenic, conjugated linoleic and vaccenic acids improves the lipid profile and reduces anandamide in the plasma of hypercholesterolaemic subjects. *Brit. J. Nutr.* 109:1453–1462, https://doi.org/10.1017/S0007114512003224.

60. ACC is "acetyl-CoA-carboxylase" and commits the 2-carbon acetyl unit (as acetyl-CoA) to lipogenesis; FAS is "fatty acid synthase" and through several

cycles combines 2-carbon units to make 16:0 as the final product; SCD is "stearoyl-CoA-desaturase" and converts 16:0 to 16:1, enabling lipogenesis to continue by removing "product inhibition."

61. Hellerstein MK (1999) De novo lipogenesis in humans: metabolic and regulatory aspects. *Eur. J. Clin. Nutr.* 53:Suppl 1:S53–S65, https://doi.org/10.1038/sj.ejcn.1600744.

62. Guo ZK et al (2000) De novo lipogenesis in adipose tissue of lean and obese women: application of deuterated water and isotope ratio mass spectrometry. *Int. J. Obesity* 24:932–937, https://doi.org/10.1038/sj.ijo.0801256.

63. Kim H-J et al (1999) Fish oil feeding decreases mature sterol regulatory element-binding protein 1 (SREBP-1) by down-regulation of SREBP-1c mRNA in mouse liver. A possible mechanism for down-regulation of lipogenic enzyme mRNAs. *J. Biol. Chem.* 274:25892–25898, https://doi.org/10.1074/jbc.274.36.25892.

64. "Message levels" refers to the messenger-RNA for the respective enzymes. Compared to the liver m-RNA levels for ACC, FAS and SCD in mice fed the high-carbohydrate diet those for mice fed the omega-6 diet were respectively reduced by 47%, 0% and 67%, compared to respective reductions of 91%, 41% and 95% in mice fed the omega-3 diet.

65. Himsworth HP (1936) Diabetes Mellitus: Its differentiation into insulin-sensitive and insulin-insensitive types. *The Lancet* 227:127–130, https://doi.org/10.1093/ije/dyt203.

66. Reaven GM (1988) Role of insulin resistance in human disease. *Diabetes* 37:1595–1607, https://doi.org/10.2337/diab.37.12.1595.

67. Storlien LH et al (1986) Fat feeding causes widespread in vivo insulin resistance, decreased energy expenditure, and obesity in rats. *Am. J. Physiol.* 251:E576–E583, https://doi.org/10.1152/ajpendo.1986.251.5.E576.

68. Storlien LH et al (1987) Fish oil prevents insulin resistance induced by high-fat feeding in rats. *Science* 237:885–888, https://doi.org/10.1126/science.3303333.

69. Storlien LH et al (1991) Influence of dietary fat composition on development of insulin resistance in rats. Relationship to muscle triglyceride and ω-3 fatty acids in muscle phospholipid. *Diabetes* 40:280–89, https://doi.org/10.2337/diab.40.2.280.

70. Ghafoorunissa, IA, Natarajan S (2005) Substituting dietary linoleic acid with α-linolenic acid improves insulin sensitivity in sucrose fed rats. *Biochim. Biophys. Acta* 1733:67–75, https://doi.org/10.1016/j.bbalip.2004.12.003.

71. Borkman M et al (1993) The relationship between insulin sensitivity and the fatty acid composition of phospholipids of skeletal muscle. *N. Engl. J. Med.* 328:238–244, https://doi.org/10.1056/NEJM199301283280404.

72. Pan DA et al (1995) Skeletal muscle membrane lipid composition is related to adiposity and insulin action. *J. Clin. Invest.* 96:2802–2808, https://doi.org/10.1172/JCI118350

73. Schulz LO, Chaudhari LS (2015) High-risk populations: the Pimas of Arizona and Mexico. *Curr. Obes. Rep.* 4:92–98, https://doi.org/10.1007/s13679-014 -0132-9.

74. Storlien LH et al (1996) Skeletal muscle membrane lipids and insulin resistance. *Lipids* 31:S261–S265, https://doi.org/10.2522/ptj.20080018.

75. Baur LA et al (1998) The fatty acid composition of skeletal muscle membrane phospholipid: Its relationship with the type of feeding and plasma glucose levels in young children. *Metabolism* 47:106–112, https://doi.org/10.1016 /s0026-0495(98)90202-5.

76. Patel PS et al (2009) The association between type of dietary fish and seafood intake and the risk of incident type 2 diabetes: The EPIC-Norfolk cohort study. *Diabetes Care* 32:1857–1863, https://doi.org/10.2337/dc09-0116.

77. Kabir M et al (2007) Treatment for 2 mo with n-3 polyunsaturated fatty acids reduces adiposity and some atherogenic factors but does not improve insulin sensitivity in women with type 2 diabetes: a randomized controlled study. *Am. J. Clin. Nutr.* 86:1670–1679, https://doi.org/10.1093/ajcn/86.5.1670.

78. Mostad IL et al (2006) Effects of n-3 fatty acids in subjects with type 2 diabetes: reduction of insulin sensitivity and time-dependent alteration from carbohydrate to fat oxidation. *Am. J. Clin. Nutr.* 84:540–550, https://doi.org /10.1093/ajcn/84.3.540.

79. Rhee Y, Brunt A (2011) Flaxseed supplementation improved insulin resistance in obese glucose intolerant people: a randomized crossover design. *Nutr. J.* 10:44–51, https://doi.org/10.1186/1475-2891-10-44.

80. Carter P et al (2010) Fruit and vegetable intake and incidence of type 2 diabetes mellitus: systematic review and meta-analysis. *BMJ* 341: 543 (c4229), https://doi.org/10.1136/bmj.c4229.

81. Barnard RJ et al (1998) Diet-induced insulin resistance precedes other aspects of the metabolic syndrome. *J. Appl. Physiol.* 84:1311–1315, https://doi.org/10 .1152/jappl.1998.84.4.1311 (personal communication that diet fat was lard).

82. Cohen JC et al (2011) Human fatty liver disease: old questions and new insights. *Science* 332:1519–1523, https://doi.org/10.1126/science.1204265; Leslie M (2015) The liver's weighty problem. *Science* 349:18–20, https://doi.org/10.1126/science .349.6243.18

83. Alwayn IPJ et al (2005) Omega-3 fatty acids improve hepatic steatosis in a murine model: potential implications for the marginal steatotic liver donor. *Transplant.* 79:606 –608, https://doi.org/10.1097/01.tp.0000150023.86487 .44; El-Badry AM et al (2007) Omega 3 – omega 6: What is right for the liver? *J. Hepat.* 47:718–725, https://doi.org/10.1016/j.jhep.2007.08.005.

84. Pan DA et al (1997) Skeletal muscle triglyceride levels are inversely related to insulin action. *Diabetes* 46:983–988, https://doi.org/10.2337/diab.46.6.983.

85. Agha M, Agha R (2017) The rising prevalence of obesity: part A: impact on public health. *Int. J. Surg. Oncol.* 2:e17, https://doi.org/10.1097/IJ9 .0000000000000017.

Chapter 7. Cardiovascular Disease and Inflammation

1. Finegold JA et al. (2013) Mortality from ischaemic heart disease by country, region, and age: Statistics from World Health Organisation and United Nations. *Int. J. Cardiol.* 168:934–945, https://doi.org/10.1016/j.ijcard.2012.10.046.

2. Mahmood SS et al. (2013) The Framingham Heart Study and the epidemiology of cardiovascular disease: a historical perspective. *The Lancet* 383:999–1008, https://doi.org/10.1016/S0140-6736(13)61752-3

3. Keys A (1953) Atherosclerosis: a problem in newer public health. *J. Mt. Sinai Hosp. NY* 20:118–139.

4. Keys A (1970) Coronary heart disease in seven countries. *Circulation* 41:186–195, https://doi.org/10.1016/s0899-9007(96)00410-8.

5. Dietary goals for the United States, prepared by the staff of the Select Committee on Nutrition and Human Needs, United States Senate. US GPO, 1977. available at: https://thescienceofnutrition.files.wordpress.com/2014/03/dietary-goals-for-the-united-states.pdf/.

6. U S Department of Agriculture and US Department of Health and Human Services. Dietary Guidelines for Americans, 2020–2025. 9th ed. (December 2020). available at: https://www.dietaryguidelines.gov.

7. National Health and Medical Research Council (2013) Australian Dietary Guidelines Summary. Canberra: National Health and Medical Research Council. Available at www.nhmrc.gov.au/guidelines-publications/n55a.

8. Taubes G. (2007) *Good Calories, Bad Calories*. New York/:Anchor Books, Teicholz N. (2014) *The Big Fat Surprise*. New York: Simon & Schuster.

9. Siri-Tarino PW et al. (2010) Meta-analysis of prospective cohort studies evaluating the association of saturated fat with cardiovascular disease. *Am. J. Clin. Nutr.* 91:535–46, https://doi.org/10.3945/ajcn.2009.27725.

10. Astrup A et al. (2020) Saturated fats and health: a reassessment and proposal for food-based recommendations: JACC State-of-the-Art review. *J. Am. Coll. Cardiol.* 76:844–857, https://doi.org/10.1016/j.jacc.2020.05.077; Ho FK et al. (2020) Associations of fat and carbohydrate intake with cardiovascular disease and mortality: prospective cohort study of UK Biobank participants. *BMJ* 368:m688, https://doi.org/10.1016/S0140-6736(17)32252-3.

11. For information about Bang and Dyerberg's trip to Greenland I am indebted to Susan Allport (2006) *The Queen of Fats*. Berkeley: University of California Press.

12. Bang HO et al. (1971) Plasma lipid and lipoprotein pattern in Greenlandic West-coast Eskimos. *The Lancet* 1:1143–1146, https://doi.org.10.1016/s0140-6736(71)91658-8.

13. Bang HO et al. (1976) The composition of food consumed by Greenland Eskimos. *Acta Med. Scand.* 200:69–73, https://doi.org/10.1111/j.0954-6820.1976.tb08198.x.

14. Dyerberg J et al. (1975) Fatty acid composition of the plasma lipids in Greenland Eskimos. *Am. J. Clin. Nutr.* 28:958–966, https://doi.org/10.1093/ajcn/28.9.958.

15. Page IH et al. (1961) Dietary fat and its relation to heart attacks and strokes. Report by the central committee for medical and community program of the American Heart Association. *Circulation.* 23:133–136.

16. Woodhill JM et al. (1978) Low fat, low cholesterol diet in secondary prevention of coronary heart disease. *Adv. Exp. Med. Biol.* 109:317–30, https://doi.org /10.1007/978-1-4684-0967-3_18.

17. Ramsden CE et al. (2013) Use of dietary linoleic acid for secondary prevention of coronary heart disease and death: evaluation of recovered data from the Sydney Diet Heart Study and updated meta-analysis. *BMJ* 346:e8707, https:// doi.org/10.1136/bmj.e8707.

18. Frantz Jr. ID et al. (1989) Test of effect of lipid lowering by diet on cardiovascular risk. The Minnesota Coronary Survey. *Arteriosclerosis* 9:129–139, https:// doi.org/10.1161/01.atv.9.1.129.

19. Begley S (2016). Records found in dusty basement undermine decades of dietary advice, STAT, April 12, 2016, https://www.statnews.com/2016/04/12 /unearthed-data-challenge-dietary-advice/

20. Ramsden CE et al. (2016) Re-evaluation of the traditional diet-heart hypothesis: analysis of recovered data from Minnesota Coronary Experiment (1968–73) *BMJ* 353:i1246, https://doi.org/10.1136/bmj.i1246.

21. Marchioli R, and GISSI-Prevenzione Investigators (1999) Dietary supplementation with n-3 polyunsaturated fatty acids and vitamin E after myocardial infarction: results of the GISSI-Prevenzione trial. *Lancet* 354:447–55, https:// doi.org/10.1016/S0140-6736(99)07072-5.

22. Lavie CJ et al. (2009) Omega-3 polyunsaturated fatty acids and cardiovascular diseases. *J. Am. Coll. Cardiol.* 54:585–94, https://doi.org/10.1016/j.jacc.2009 .02.084.

23. Abdelhamid AS et al. (2018) Omega-3 fatty acids for the primary and secondary prevention of cardiovascular disease. *Cochrane Database of Systematic Reviews* Issue 7. Art. No.: CD003177, https://doi.org/10.1002/14651858.CD003177.

24. Ervin RB et al. (2004) Dietary intake of fats and fatty acids for the United States population: 1999–2000. *National Center for Health Statistics CDC*, vol. 348. Hyattsville, Maryland, https://www.cdc.gov/nchs/data/ad/ad348.pdf.

25. Wikipedia, s.v. French paradox, https://en.wikipedia.org/wiki/French_paradox.

26. Allender S et al. (2008) European cardiovascular disease statistics. 2008 edition. see *Table 1.4 Age-standardized death rates from CHD, adults aged 0 to 64, by sex, 1972 to 2005, Europe,* and *Table 5.5 Percentage of total energy from saturated fat, Europe, 1998* https://www.researchgate.net/publication/234653504

27. Renaud S, de Lorgeril M (1992) Wine, alcohol, platelets, and the French paradox for coronary heart disease. *Lancet.* 339:1523–1526, https://doi.org/10.1016 /0140-6736(92)91277-f.

28. Dehghan M, et al. (2018) Association of dairy intake with cardiovascular disease and mortality in 21 countries from five continents (PURE): a prospective cohort study. *Lancet* 392:2288–2297, https://doi.org/10.1016/S0140-6736 (18)31812-9.

29. Yam D et al. (1996) Diet and disease–the Israeli paradox: possible dangers of a high omega-6 polyunsaturated fatty acid diet. *Israel J Med. Sci.* 32:1134–1143.

30. FAOSTAT database: http://www.fao.org/faostat/en/#data/FBS.

31. World Health Organization, SDR(0–64), Ischaemic heart disease, per 100 000 https://gateway.euro.who.int/en/indicators/hfamdb_429-sdr-0-64-ischaemic -heart-disease-per-100-000/visualizations/#id=30295.

32. Siegel-Itzkovich J (2016). Since 1998, Israeli death rate from heart disease has dropped by 50%. Jerusalem Post, March 8, 2016, https://www.jpost.com /Business-and-Innovation/Health-and-Science/Since-1998-Israeli-death -rate-from-heart-disease-has-dropped-by-50-percent-447176.

33. Levitan I et al. (2010) Oxidized LDL: diversity, patterns of recognition, and pathophysiology. *Antioxid. & Redox Signal.* 13:39–75, https://doi.org/10.1089 /ars.2009.2733

34. The fatty acid composition of cholesterol esters, phospholipids, triglycerides from human plasma was averaged from: Skeaff CM et al. (2006) Dietary-induced changes in fatty acid composition of human plasma, platelet, and erythrocyte lipids follow a similar time course. *J.Nutr.* 136:565–569, https:// doi.org/10.1093/jn/136.3.565; and King IB et al. (2006) Effect of a low-fat diet on fatty acid composition in red cells, plasma phospholipids, and choles-terol esters: investigation of a biomarker of total fat intake. *Am. J. Clin. Nutr.* 83:227–236, https://doi.org/10.1093/ajcn/83.2.227.

35. Libby P (2012) Inflammation in atherosclerosis. *Arterioscler Thromb Vasc Biol.* 32:2045–2051, https://doi.org/10.1161/ATVBAHA.108.179705

36. Malek AM et al. (1999) Hemodynamic shear stress and its role in atherosclero-sis. *JAMA.* 282:2035–2042, https://doi.org/10.1001/jama.282.21.2035.

37. Haraszthy VI et al. (2000) Identification of periodontal pathogens in athero-matous plaques. *J Periodontol* 71:1554–1560, https://doi.org/10.1902/jop .2000.71.10.1554.

38. Steinberg D et al. (1989) Beyond cholesterol. modifications of low-density lipoprotein that increase its atherogenicity. *N. Engl. J. Med.* 320:915–924, https://doi.org/10.1056/NEJM198904063201407.

39. Brunzell JD et al. (2008) Lipoprotein management in patients with cardio-metabolic risk. Consensus conference report from the American Diabetes Association and the American College of Cardiology Foundation. *J. Am. Coll. Cardiol.* 51:1512–1524, https://doi.org/10.1016/j.jacc.2008.02.034.

40. Funk CD (2001) Prostaglandins and leukotrienes: advances in eicosanoid biol-ogy. *Science* 294:1871–1875, https://doi.org/10.1126/science.294.5548.1871.

41. Dennis EA, Norris PC (2015) Eicosanoid storm in infection and inflammation. *Nat, Rev. Immunol.* 15:511–523, https://doi.org/10.1038/nri3859.

42. Breyer RM et al. (2001) Prostanoid receptors: subtypes and signalling. *Annu. Rev. Pharmacol. Toxicol.* 41:661–90, https://doi.org/10.1146/annurev.pharmtox.41.1.661.

43. Nakanishi M, Rosenberg DW (2013) Multifaceted roles of PGE2 in inflamma-tion and cancer. *Semin Immunopathol.* 35:123–137, https://doi.org/10.1007 /s00281-012-0342-8

44. Pepys MH, Hirschfield GM (2003) C-reactive protein: a critical update. *J. Clin. Invest.* 111:1805–1812, https://doi.org/10.1172/JCI18921.

45. Oxidative damage generally involves the addition of oxygen atoms to the polyunsaturated fatty acid chain which will result in the chain being less "fat-loving" and the membrane fat molecule will "float" higher in the membrane bilayer, in turn resulting in the headgroup of the oxidatively damaged membrane fat being more accessible to the C-reactive protein and consequently removed from the membrane.

46. Chang M-Y et al. (2002) C-reactive protein binds to both oxidized LDL and apoptotic cells through recognition of a common ligand: phosphorylcholine of oxidized phospholipids. *Proc. Nat. Acad. Sci. USA* 99:13043–13048, https://doi.org/10.1073/pnas.192399699.

47. Wikipedia, s.v. History of aspirin, https://en.wikipedia.org/wiki/History_of_aspirin

48. Abbott SK et al. (2010) Membrane fatty acid composition of rat skeletal muscle is most responsive to the balance of dietary n-3 and n-6 polyunsaturated fatty acids. *Brit. J. Nutr.* 103:522–529, https://doi.org/10.1017/S0007114509992133; Abbott SK et al. (2012) Fatty acid composition of membrane bilayers: importance of diet polyunsaturated fat balance. *Biochim. Biophys. Acta –Biomembranes* 1818:1309–1317, https://doi.org/10.1016/j.bbamem.2012.01.011; Hulbert AJ (2021) The under-appreciated fats of life: the two types of polyunsaturated fats. *J. Exp. Biol.* 224:jeb232538, https://doi.org/10.1242/jeb.232538.

49. Peterson LD et al. (1998) Eicosapentaenoic and docosahexaenoic acids alter rat spleen leukocyte fatty acid composition and prostaglandin E2 production but have different effects on lymphocyte functions and cell-mediated immunity. *Lipids* 33:171–180, http://doi.org/10.1007/s11745-998-0193-y; and see Innes JK, Calder PC (2018) Omega-6 fatty acids and inflammation. *Prost. Leuk. Essent. Fatty Acids* 132:41–48, http://doi.org/10.1016/j.plefa.2018.03.004.

50. Farzaneh-Far R et al. (2009) Inverse association of erythrocyte n-3 fatty acid levels with inflammatory biomarkers in patients with stable coronary artery disease: the heart and soul study. *Atherosclerosis* 205:538–543, https://doi.org/10.1016/j.atherosclerosis.2008.12.013.

51. Micallef MA et al. (2009) An inverse relationship between plasma n-3 fatty acids and c-reactive protein in healthy individuals. *Eur. J. Clin. Nutr.* 63:1154–1156, https://doi.org/10.1038/ejcn.2009.20.

52. Kalogeropoulos N et al. (2010) Unsaturated fatty acids are inversely associated and n-6/n-3 ratios are positively related to inflammation and coagulation markers in plasma of apparently healthy adults. *Clin. Chim. Acta* 411:584–591, https://doi.org/10.1016/j.cca.2010.01.023.

53. Ferrucci L et al. (2006) Relationship of plasma polyunsaturated fatty acids to circulating inflammatory markers. *J. Clin. Endocrinol. Metab.* 91:439–446, https://doi.org/10.1210/jc.2005-1303.

54. Reinders I et al. (2012) Association of serum n-3 polyunsaturated fatty acids with C-reactive protein in men. *Eur. J. Clin. Nutr.* 66:736–741, https://doi.org/10.1038/ejcn.2011.195.

55. Niu K et al. (2006) Dietary long-chain n-3 fatty acids of marine origin and serum C-reactive protein concentrations are associated in a population with a diet rich in marine products. *Am. J. Clin. Nutr.* 84:223–229, https://doi.org/10.1093/ajcn/84.1.223.

56. Ma Y-J et al. (2016) Perioperative ω-3 polyunsaturated fatty acid nutritional support in gastrointestinal cancer surgical patients: a systematic evaluation. *Nutr. & Cancer* 68:568–576, https://doi.org/10.1080/01635581.2016.1158291.

57. Muhammad K et al. (2011) Treatment with ω-3 fatty acids reduces serum C-reactive protein concentration. *Clin. Lipidology* 6:723–729, https://doi.org/10.2217/clp.11.54.

58. Li Y-H et al. (2015) Efficacy of poly-unsaturated fatty acid therapy on patients with nonalcoholic steatohepatitis. *World J. Gastroenterol.* 21:7008–7013, https://doi.org/10.3748/wjg.v21.i22.7008.

59. Paschos GK et al. (2004) Background diet influences the anti-inflammatory effect of α-linolenic acid in dyslipidaemic subjects. *Brit. J. Nutr.* 92:649–655, https://doi.org/10.1079/bjn20041230.

60. Zhao G et al. (2004) Dietary α-linolenic acid reduces inflammatory and lipid cardiovascular risk factors in hypercholesterolemic men and women. *J. Nutr.* 134:2991–2997, https://doi.org/10.1093/jn/134.11.2991.

61. Serhan CN et al. (2015) Lipid mediators in the resolution of inflammation. *Cold Spring Harb. Perspect. Biol.* 7:a016311, https://doi.org/10.1101/cshperspect.a016311.

62. Endres S et al. (1989) The effect of dietary supplementation with n-3 polyunsaturated fatty acids on the synthesis of interleukin-1 and tumor necrosis factor by mononuclear cells. *N. Engl. J. Med.* 320:265–271, https://doi.org/10.1056/NEJM198902023200501; Endres S et al. (1993) Dietary supplementation with n-3 fatty acids suppresses interleukin-2 production and mononuclear cell proliferation. *J. Leukocyte Biol.* 54:599–603, https://doi.org/10.1002/jlb.54.6.599.

63. Pahwa R et al. (2020) Chronic inflammation. NCBI Bookshelf. National Institutes of Health. StatPearls Publishing; https://www.ncbi.nlm.nih.gov/books/NBK493173/

64. Couzin-Frankel J (2010) Inflammation bares a dark side. *Science* 330:1621, https://doi.org/10.1126/science.330.6011.1621.

Chapter 8. Allergies, Auto-immune Diseases, and Cancer

1. Kromann N, Green A (1980) Epidemiological studies in the Upernavik District, Greenland. Incidence of some chronic diseases 1950–1974. *Acta Med. Scand.* 208:401–406, https://pubmed.ncbi.nlm.nih.gov/7457208/.

2. Wikipedia, s.v. Asthma, https://en.wikipedia.org/wiki/Asthma#cite_note-Ana2010-19.

3. Debeuf N, Lambrecht BN (2018) Eicosanoid control over antigen presenting cells in asthma. *Front. Immunol.* 9:2006, https://doi.org/10.3389/fimmu.2018 .02006.

4. Leynaert B et al. (2012) Gender differences in prevalence, diagnosis and incidence of allergic and non-allergic asthma: a population-based cohort. *Thorax* 67:625–631, https://doi.org/10.1136/thoraxjnl-2011-201249.

5. Eder W et al. (2006) The asthma epidemic. *N. Engl. J. Med.* 355:2226–2235, https://doi.org/10.1056/NEJMra054308.

6. ISAAC Steering Committee (1998) Worldwide variation in prevalence of symptoms of asthma, allergic rhinoconjunctivitis, and atopic eczema. *Lancet* 351:1225–32, https://www.thelancet.com/pdfs/journals/lancet/PIIS0140 -6736(97)07302-9.pdf.

7. Burns JS et al. (2007) Low dietary nutrient intakes and respiratory health in adolescents. *Chest* 132:238–245, https://doi.org/10.1378/chest.07-0038; Li J et al. (2013) Intakes of long-chain omega-3 (n-3) PUFAs and fish in relation to incidence of asthma among American young adults: the CARDIA study. *Am. J. Clin. Nutr.* 97:173–178, https://doi.org/10.3945/ajcn.112.041145.

8. Woods RK et al. (2003) Food and nutrient intakes and asthma risk in young adults. *Am. J. Clin. Nutr.* 78:414–421, https://doi.org/10.1093/ajcn/78.3.414.

9. Hodge L et al. (1996) Consumption of oily fish and childhood asthma risk. *Med. J. Aust.* 164:137–140, https://doi.org/10.5694/j.1326-5377.1996.tb122010.x.

10. Kim JL et al. (2005) Current asthma and respiratory symptoms among pupils in relation to dietary factors and allergens in the school environment. *Indoor Air* 15:170–182, https://doi.org/10.1111/j.1600-0668.2005.00334.x.

11. Barros R et al. (2011) Dietary intake of α-linolenic acid and low ratio of n-6:n-3 PUFA are associated with decreased exhaled NO and improved asthma control. *Brit. J. Nutr.* 106:441–450, https://doi.org/10.1017/S0007114511000328.

12. McKeever TM et al. (2008) The relation between dietary intake of individual fatty acids, FEV1 and respiratory disease in Dutch adults. *Thorax* 63:208–214, https://doi.org/10.1136/thx.2007.090399.

13. Thien FCK et al. (2011) Dietary marine fatty acids (fish oil) for asthma in adults and children (Review). *Evid.-Based Child Health* 6:984–1012, https://doi.org /10.1002/14651858.CD001283.

14. Tecklenburg-Lund S et al. (2010) Randomized controlled trial of fish oil and montelukast and their combination on airway inflammation and hyperpnea-induced bronchoconstriction. *PLoS ONE* 5:e13487, https://doi.org/10.1371 /journal.pone.0013487.

15. Olsen SF et al. (2008) Fish oil intake compared with olive oil intake in late pregnancy and asthma in the offspring: 16 y of registry-based follow-up from a randomized controlled trial. *Am. J. Clin. Nutr.* 88:167–175, https://doi.org /10.1093/ajcn/88.1.167.

16. Furuhjelm C et al. (2009) Fish oil supplementation in pregnancy and lactation may decrease the risk of infant allergy. *Acta Pædiatrica* 98:1461–1467, https://

doi.org/10.1111/j.1651-2227.2009.01355.x; Warstedt K et al. (2016) High levels of omega-3 fatty acids in milk from omega-3 fatty acid-supplemented mothers are related to less immunoglobulin E-associated disease in infancy. *Acta Pædiatrica* 105:1337–1347, https://doi.org/10.1111/apa.13395; Furuhjelm C et al. (2011) Allergic disease in infants up to 2 years of age in relation to plasma omega-3 fatty acids and maternal fish oil supplementation in pregnancy and lactation. *Pediatr. Allergy Immunol.* 22:505–514, https://doi.org/10.1111/j.1399-3038.2010.01096.x.

17. Palmer DJ et al. (2013) Randomized controlled trial of fish oil supplementation in pregnancy on childhood allergies. *Allergy* 68:1370–1376, https://doi.org/10.1111/all.12233.

18. Branum AM, Lukacs SL (2009) Food allergy among children in the United States. *Pediat.* 124:1–7, https://doi.org/10.1542/peds.2009-1210.

19. Loh W, Tang MLK (2018) The epidemiology of food allergy in the global context. *Int. J. Environ. Res. Public Health* 15:2043, https://doi.org/10.3390/ijerph15092043.

20. Tang MLK, Mullins RJ (2017) Food allergy: is prevalence increasing? *Int. Med. J.* 47:256–261, https://doi.org/10.1111/imj.13362.

21. Prescott SL (2011) *The Allergy Epidemic: A Mystery of Modern Life.* Perth: University of Western Australia Publishing.

22. Hayter SM, Cook MC (2012) Updated assessment of the prevalence, spectrum and case definition of autoimmune disease. *Autoimmun. Rev.* 11:754–765, https://doi.org/10.1016/j.autrev.2012.02.001.

23. Araújo VMA et al. (2015) Relationship between periodontitis and rheumatoid arthritis: review of the literature. *Mediators of Inflammation* 2015, Article 259074, https://doi.org/10.1016/j.autrev.2012.02.001.

24. Buch M, Emery P (2002) The aetiology and pathogenesis of rheumatoid arthritis. *Hospital Pharmacist* 9:5–10, https://doi.org/10.1016/j.autrev.2012.02.001.

25. Rudan I et al. (2015) Prevalence of rheumatoid arthritis in low- and middle-income countries: a systematic review and analysis. *J. Global Health* 5:010409, https://doi.org/10.7189/jogh.05.010409.

26. Peschken CA, Esdaile JM (1999) Rheumatic diseases in North America's indigenous peoples. *Semin Arthritis Rheum* 28:368–391, https://doi.org/10.1016/s0049-0172(99)80003-1.

27. Jacobson DL et al. (1997) Epidemiology and estimated population burden of selected autoimmune diseases in the United States. *Clin. Immunol. & Immunopathol.* 84:223–243, https://doi.org/10.1006/clin.1997.4412.

28. Safiri S et al. (2019) Global, regional and national burden of rheumatoid arthritis 1990–2017: a systematic analysis of the Global Burden of Disease study 2017. *Ann. Rheum. Dis.* 78:1463–1471, https://doi.org/10.1136/annrheumdis-2019-215920.

29. Shapiro JA et al. (1996) Diet and rheumatoid arthritis in women: a possible protective effect of fish consumption. *Epidemiol.* 7:256–263, https://doi.org/10

.1097/00001648-199605000-00007; Rosell M et al. (2009) Dietary fish and fish oil and the risk of rheumatoid arthritis. *Epidemiol.* 20:896–90, https://doi .org/10.1097/EDE.0b013e3181b5f0ce1; Johansson K et al. (2018) Mediterranean diet and risk of rheumatoid arthritis: a population-based case-control study. *Arthrit. Res. & Therapy* 20:175, https://doi.org/10.1186/s13075-018-1680-2.

30. Tedeschi SK et al. (2018) Relationship between fish consumption and disease activity in rheumatoid arthritis. *Arthrit. Care & Res.* 70:327–332, https://doi .org/10.1002/acr.23295.

31. Sparks JA et al. (2019) Association of fish intake and smoking with risk of rheumatoid arthritis and age of onset: a prospective cohort study. *BMC Musculoskeletal Disorders* 20:2, https://doi.org/10.1186/s12891-018-2381-3; Di Giuseppe D et al. (2014) Fish consumption and risk of rheumatoid arthritis: a dose-response meta-analysis. *Arthrit. Res. & Therap.* 16:446, https://doi.org/10.1186 /s13075-014-0446-8; Nguyen Y, Salliot C, Mariette X, Boutron-Ruault MC, Seror R. (2022)Fish Consumption and Risk of Rheumatoid Arthritis: Findings from the E3N Cohort Study. Nutrients. 2022;14(4):861, https://doi.org/10.3390 /nu14040861.

32. He J et al.. (2016) Dietary intake and risk of rheumatoid arthritis—a cross section multicenter study. *Clin Rheumatol* 35:2901–2908, https://doi.org /10.1007/s10067-016-3383-x.

33. Tedeschi SK et al. (2017) Diet and rheumatoid arthritis symptoms: survey results from a rheumatoid arthritis registry. *Arthritis Care & Res.* 69:1920–1925, https://doi.org/10.1002/acr.23225.

34. Gioxari A et al. (2018) Intake of ω-3 polyunsaturated fatty acids in patients with rheumatoid arthritis: A systematic review and meta-analysis. *Nutrition* 45:114–124, https://doi.org/10.1016/j.nut.2017.06.023.

35. Hayter SM, Cook MC (2012) Updated assessment of the prevalence, spectrum and case definition of autoimmune disease. *Autoimmun. Rev.* 11:754–765, https://doi.org/10.1016/j.autrev.2012.02.001.

36. Tuomilehto J (2013) The emerging global epidemic of Type 1 diabetes. *Curr. Diab. Rep.* 13:795–804, https://doi.org/10.1007/s11892-013-0433-5.

37. Norris JM et al. (2007) Omega-3 polyunsaturated fatty acid intake and islet autoimmunity in children at increased risk for Type 1 diabetes. *JAMA.* 298:1420–1428, https://doi.org/10.1001/jama.298.12.1420.

38. Stene LC et al. (2003) Use of cod liver oil during the first year of life is associated with lower risk of childhood-onset type 1 diabetes: a large, population-based, case-control study. *Am. J. Clin. Nutr.* 78:1128–1134, https://doi.org /10.1093/ajcn/78.6.1128.

39. Lewis EJH et al. (2017) Effect of omega-3 supplementation on neuropathy in type 1 diabetes. a 12-month pilot trial. *Neurology* 88:1–8, https://doi.org/10.1212 /WNL.0000000000004033.

40. Frohman EM et al. (2006) Multiple sclerosis—the plaque and its pathogenesis. *N. Engl. J. Med.* 354:942–55, https://doi.org/10.1056/NEJMra052130.

41. Dobson R, Giovannoni G (2019) Multiple sclerosis—a review. *Eur. J. Neurol.* 26:27–40, https://doi.org/10.1111/ene.13819.

42. Kingwell E et al. (2008) High incidence and increasing prevalence of multiple sclerosis in British Columbia, Canada: findings from over two decades (1991–2010). *J. Neurol.* 262:2352–2363, https://doi.org/10.1007/s00415-015 -7842-0; Alonso A, Hernán MA (2008) Temporal trends in the incidence of multiple sclerosis. a systematic review. *Neurology* 71:129–135, https://doi.org /10.1212/01.wnl.0000316802.35974.34; Koch-Henriksen N, Sørensen PS (2010) The changing demographic pattern of multiple sclerosis epidemiology. *Lancet Neurol* 9:520–32, https://doi.org/10.1016/S1474-4422(10)70064-8; Trojano M et al.. (2012) Geographical variations in sex ratio trends over time in multiple sclerosis. *PLoS ONE* 7:e48078, https://doi.org/10.1371/journal .pone.0048078.

43. Bjørnevik K et al. (2017) Polyunsaturated fatty acids and the risk of multiple sclerosis. *Multiple Sclerosis J.* 23:1830–1838, https://doi.org/10.1177 /1352458517691150.

44. Bjørnevik K et al. (2019) α-Linolenic acid is associated with MRI activity in a prospective cohort of multiple sclerosis patients. *Multiple Sclerosis J.* 25:987–993, https://doi.org/10.1177/1352458518779925.

45. Cortese M et al. (2015) Timing of use of cod liver oil, a vitamin D source, and multiple sclerosis risk: the EnvIMS study. *Multiple Sclerosis J.* 21:1856–1864, https://doi.org/10.1177/1352458515578770.

46. Kampman MT et al. (2007) Outdoor activities and diet in childhood and adolescence relate to MS risk above the Arctic Circle. *J. Neurol.* 254:471–477, https://doi.org/10.1007/s00415-006-0395-5.

47. Bäärnhielm M et al. (2014) Fatty fish intake is associated with decreased occurrence of multiple sclerosis. *Multiple Sclerosis J.* 20:726–732, https://doi .org/10.1177/1352458513509508.

48. Ghadirian P et al. (1998) Nutritional factors in the aetiology of multiple sclero-sis: a case-control study in Montreal, Canada. *Int. J. Epidemiol.* 27:845–852, https://doi.org/10.1093/ije/27.5.845.

49. Hoare S et al. (2016) Higher intake of omega-3 polyunsaturated fatty acids is associated with a decreased risk of a first clinical diagnosis of central nervous system demyelination: results from the Ausimmune Study. *Multiple Sclerosis J.* 22:884–892, https://doi.org/10.1177/1352458515604380.

50. Bates D et al. (1989) A double-blind controlled trial of long chain n-3 polyun-saturated fatty acids in the treatment of multiple sclerosis. *J. Neurol. Neuro-surg. Psychiat.* 52:18–22, https://doi.org/10.1136/jnnp.52.1.18.

51. Torkildsen O et al. (2012) Omega-3 fatty acid treatment in multiple sclerosis (OFAMS Study). a randomized, double-blind, placebo-controlled trial. *Arch. Neurol.* 69:1044–1051, https://doi.org/10.1001/archneurol.2012.283.

52. Ramirez-Ramirez V et al. (2013) Efficacy of fish oil on serum of TNFα, IL-1β, and IL-6 oxidative stress markers in multiple sclerosis treated with interferon

Beta-1b. *Oxid. Med. Cell Longevity* 2018:709493, https://doi.org/10.1155/2013/709493; Kouchaki E et al. (2018) High-dose ω-3 fatty acid plus vitamin D3 supplementation affects clinical symptoms and metabolic status of patients with multiple sclerosis: a randomized controlled clinical trial. *J. Nutr.* 148:1–7, https://doi.org/10.1093/jn/nxy116; Nordvik I et al. (2000) Effect of dietary advice and n-3 supplementation in newly diagnosed MS patients. *Acta Neurol. Scand.* 102:143–149, https://doi.org/10.1034/j.1600-0404.2000.102003143.x; Weinstock-Guttman B et al. (2005) Low fat dietary intervention with ω-3fatty acid supplementation in multiple sclerosis patients. *Prost., Leukot. Essent. Fatty Acids* 73:397–404, https://doi.org/10.1016/j.plefa.2005.05.024.

53. Lani Prideaux L et al. (2011) Serological antibodies in inflammatory bowel disease: a systematic review. *Inflamm Bowel Dis.* 18:1340–1355, https://doi.org/10.1002/ibd.21903; Mitsuyama K et al. (2016) Antibody markers in the diagnosis of inflammatory bowel disease. *World J. Gastroenterol.* 22:1304–1310, https://doi.org/10.3748/wjg.v22.i3.1304.

54. Stenson WF (1990) Role of eicosanoids as mediators of inflammation in inflammatory bowel disease. *Scand. J. Gastroenterol.* 25:13–18, https://doi.org/10.3109/00365529009091903.

55. Kaplan GG, Ng SC (2017) Understanding and preventing the global increase of inflammatory bowel disease. *Gastroenterology* 152:313–321, https://doi.org/10.1053/j.gastro.2016.10.020

56. Shoda R et al. (1996) Epidemiologic analysis of Crohn disease in Japan: increased dietary intake of n-6 polyunsaturated fatty acids and animal protein relates to the increased incidence of Crohn disease in Japan. *Am. J. Clin. Nutr.* 63:741–745, https://doi.org/10.1093/ajcn/63.5.741.

57. Ananthakrishnan AN et al. (2014) Long-term intake of dietary fat and risk of ulcerative colitis and Crohn's disease. *Gut* 63:776–784, https://doi.org/10.1136/gutjnl-2013-305304

58. John S et al. (2010) Dietary n-3 polyunsaturated fatty acids and the aetiology of ulcerative colitis: a UK prospective cohort study. *Eur. J. Gastroenter. & Hepatol.* 22:602–606, https://doi.org/10.1097/MEG.0b013e3283352d05.

59. Amre DK et al. (2007) Imbalances in dietary consumption of fatty acids, vegetables, and fruits are associated with risk for Crohn's disease in children. *Am. J. Gastroenterol.* 102:2016–2025, https://doi.org/10.1111/j.1572-0241.2007.01411.x.

60. IBD in EPIC Study Investigators (2009) Linoleic acid, a dietary n-6 polyunsaturated fatty acid, and the aetiology of ulcerative colitis: a nested case–control study within a European prospective cohort study. *Gut* 58:1606–1611, https://doi.org/10.1136/gut.2008.169078.

61. Opstelten JL et al. (2016) Dairy products, dietary calcium, and risk of inflammatory bowel disease: results from a European prospective cohort investigation. *Inflamm Bowel Dis.* 22:1403–1411, https://doi.org/10.1097/MIB.0000000000000798.

62. Lev-Tzion R et al. (2014) Omega 3 fatty acids (fish oil) for maintenance of

remission in Crohn's disease. Cochrane Database of Systematic Reviews, Issue 2 Art. No. CD006320, https://doi.org/10.1002/14651858.CD006320.pub4.

63. Uchiyama K et al. (2010) N-3 polyunsaturated fatty acid diet therapy for patients with inflammatory bowel disease. *Inflamm. Bowel Dis.* 16:1696–1707, https://doi.org/10.1002/ibd.21251.

64. Pinto-Plata VM et al. (2006) C-reactive protein in patients with COPD, control smokers and non-smokers. *Thorax* 61:23–28, https://doi.org/10.1136/thx.2005 .042200.

65. Adeloye D et al. (2015) Global and regional estimates of COPD prevalence: Systematic review and meta-analysis. *J. Global Health* 5:020415, doi: 10.7189 /jogh.05-020415.

66. Shahar E et al. (1994) Dietary n-3 polyunsaturated fatty acids and smoking-related chronic obstructive pulmonary disease. *N. Engl. J. Med.* 331:228–233, https://doi.org/10.1056/NEJM199407283310403.

67. McKeever TM et al. (2008) The relation between dietary intake of individual fatty acids, FEV1 and respiratory disease in Dutch adults. *Thorax* 63:208–214, https://doi.org/10.1136/thx.2007.090399.

68. Broekhuizen R et al. (2005) Polyunsaturated fatty acids improve exercise capacity in chronic obstructive pulmonary disease. *Thorax* 60:376–382, https://doi.org/10.1136/thx.2004.030858

69. Lin Y-C et al. (2016) Supplementation of fish oil improves functional capacity and quality of life in patients with chronic obstructive pulmonary disease. *Curr. Topics Nutraceutical Res.* 14:191–198, link.gale.com/apps/doc/A479943049 /HRCA?u=googlescholar&sid=bookmark-HRCA&xid=9e33c5b8.

70. Dirjayanto VJ et al (2020) Evidence on the efficacy of omega-3 polyunsaturated fatty acids as an adjunct therapy for chronic obstructive pulmonary disease. *J Asian Med Stud Assoc.* 9:123–138, https://doi.org/10.52629/jamsa.v9i1.238.

71. Kauppinen A et al. (2016) Inflammation and its role in age-related macular degeneration. *Cell. Mol. Life Sci.* 73:1765–1786, https://doi.org/10.1007/s00018 -016-2147-8.

72. Wong WL et al. (2014) Global prevalence of age-related macular degeneration and disease burden projection for 2020 and 2040: a systematic review and meta-analysis. *Lancet Glob Health* 2: e106–16, https://doi.org/10.1016 /S2214-109X(13)70145-1.

73. Evans J, Wormald R (1996) Is the incidence of registrable age-related macular degeneration increasing? *Brit. J. Ophthalmol.* 80:9–14, https://doi.org/10.1136 /bjo.80.1.9.

74. Chua B et al. (2006) Dietary fatty acids and the 5-year incidence of age-related maculopathy. *Arch. Ophthalmol.* 124:981–986, https://doi.org/10.1001/archopht .124.7.981

75. Tan JSL et al. (2009) Dietary fatty acids and the 10-year incidence of age-related macular degeneration. The Blue Mountains Eye Study. *Arch. Ophthalmol.* 127:656–665, https://doi.org/10.1001/archophthalmol.2009.76.

76. Seddon JM et al. (2006) Cigarette smoking, fish consumption, omega-3 fatty acid intake, and associations with age-related macular degeneration. The US twin study of age-related macular degeneration. *Arch. Ophthalmol.* 124:995–1001, https://doi.org/10.1001/archopht.124.7.995.
77. San Giovanni JP et al. (2007) The relationship of dietary lipid intake and age-related macular degeneration: a case-control study in the Age-Related Eye Disease Study. *Arch. Ophthalmol.* 125:671–679, https://doi.org/10.1001/archopht.125.5.671; San Giovanni JP et al. (2009) ω-3 long-chain polyunsaturated fatty acid intake and 12-y incidence of neovascular age-related macular degeneration and central geographic atrophy. *Am. J. Clin. Nutr.* 90:1601–1607, https://doi.org/10.3945/ajcn.2009.27594; San Giovanni JP et al. (2008) The relationship of dietary ω-3 long-chain polyunsaturated fatty acid intake with incident age-related macular degeneration. *Arch. Ophthalmol.* 126:1274–1279, https://doi.org/10.1001/archopht.126.9.1274.
78. Merle BMJ et al. (2013) High concentrations of plasma n3 fatty acids are associated with decreased risk for late age-related macular degeneration. *J. Nutr.* 143:505–511, https://doi.org/10.3945/jn.112.171033.
79. AREDS2 Research Group (2013) Lutein + zeaxanthin and omega-3 fatty acids for age-related macular degeneration. *JAMA.* 309:2005–2015, https://doi.org/10.1001/jama.2013.4997; Souied EH et al. (2013) Oral docosahexaenoic acid in the prevention of exudative age-related macular degeneration. The nutritional AMD treatment 2 study. *Opthalmol.* 120:1619–1631, https://doi.org/10.1016/j.ophtha.2013.01.005.
80. Korniluk A et al. (2017) From inflammation to cancer. *Ir. J. Med. Sci.* 186:57–62, https://doi.org/10.1007/s11845-016-1464-0.
81. Stidham RW, Higgins PDR (2018) Colorectal cancer in inflammatory bowel disease. *Clinics in Colon and Rectal Surgery* 31:168–178, https://doi.org/10.1055/s-0037-1602237.
82. Crusz SM, Balkwill FR (2015) Inflammation and cancer: advances and new agents. *Nature Rev. Clin. Oncol.* 12:584–596, https://doi.org/10.1038/nrclinonc.2015.105.
83. Condeelis J, Pollard JW (2006) Macrophages: obligate partners for tumor cell migration, invasion, and metastasis. *Cell* 124:263–266, https://doi.org/10.1016/j.cell.2006.01.007.
84. Allin KH et al. (2009) Baseline C-reactive protein is associated with incident cancer and survival in patients with cancer. *J. Clin. Oncol.* 27:2217–2224, https://doi.org/10.1200/JCO.2008.19.8440.
85. Song M et al. (2014) Dietary intake of fish, ω-3 and ω-6 fatty acids and risk of colorectal cancer: a prospective study in U.S. men and women. *Int. J. Cancer* 135:2413–2423, https://doi.org/10.1002/ijc.28878.
86. Carrie R et al. (2009) Dietary intake of w-6 and w-3 fatty acids and risk of colorectal cancer in a prospective cohort of U.S. men and women. *Cancer Epidemiol. Biomarkers Prev.* 18:516–525, https://doi.org/10.1158/1055-9965.EPI-08-0750.

87. Hall MN et al. (2008) A 22-year prospective study of fish, n-3 fatty acid intake, and colorectal cancer risk in men. *Cancer Epidemiol. Biomarkers Prev.* 17:1136–1143, https://doi.org/10.1158/1055-9965.EPI-07-2803.

88. Sasazuki S et al. (2011) Intake of n-3 and n-6 polyunsaturated fatty acids and development of colorectal cancer by subsite: Japan Public Health Center-based prospective study. *Int. J. Cancer* 129:1718–1729, https://doi.org/10.1002/ijc.25802; Sawada N et al. (2012) Consumption of n-3 fatty acids and fish reduces risk of hepatocellular carcinoma. Gastroenterol. 142:1468–1475, https://doi.org/10.1053/j.gastro.2012.02.018.

89. Manson JE et al. (2019) Marine n–3 fatty acids and prevention of cardiovascular disease and cancer. *N. Engl. J. Med.* 380:23–32, https://doi.org/10.1056/NEJMoa1811403.

90. Zheng J-S et al. (2013) Intake of fish and marine n-3 polyunsaturated fatty acids and risk of breast cancer: meta-analysis of data from 21 independent prospective cohort studies. *BMJ* 346:f3706, https://doi.org/10.1136/bmj.f3706.

91. Lovegrove C et al. (2015) Systematic review of prostate cancer risk and association with consumption of fish and fish oils: analysis of 495,321 participants. *Int. J. Clin. Pract.* 69:87–105, https://doi.org/10.1111/ijcp.12514.

Chapter 9. On the Brain and on Pain

1. Stiles J, Jernigan TL (2010) The basics of brain development. *Neuropsychol. Rev.* 20:327–348, https://doi.org/10.1007/s11065-010-9148-4.

2. Wang W-X (2018) Micromanaging memory. *Biol. Psychiat.* 83:390–392, https://doi.org/10.1016/j.biopsych.2017.12.013.

3. Cotman C et al. (1969) Lipid composition of synaptic plasma membranes isolated from rat brain by zonal centrifugation. *Biochemistry* 8:4606–4612, https://doi.org/10.1021/bi00839a056; Breckienridge WC et al. (1973) Adult rat brain synaptic vesicles. II Lipid composition. *Biochim. Biophys. Acta* 320:681–686, https://doi.org/10.1016/0304-4165(73)90148-7.

4. Svennerholm L (1968) Distribution and fatty acid composition of phosphoglycerides in normal human brain. *J. Lipid Res.* 9:570–579; Carver JD et al. (2001) The relationship between age and the fatty acid composition of cerebral cortex and erythrocytes in human subjects. *Brain Res. Bull.* 56:79–85, https://doi.org/10.1016/S0361-9230(01)00551-2.

5. Calderon F, Kim H-Y (2004) Docosahexaenoic acid promotes neurite growth in hippocampal neurons. *J. Neurochem.* 90:979–988, https://doi.org/10.1111/j.1471-4159.2004.02520.x.

6. Suzuki H et al. (1998) Effect of the long-term feeding of dietary lipids on the learning ability, fatty acid composition of brain stem phospholipids and synaptic membrane fluidity in adult mice: a comparison of sardine oil diet with palm oil diet. *Mech. Ageing Develop.* 101:19–128, https://doi.org/10.1016/S0047-6374(97)00169-3; Hajjar T et al. (2012) Omega 3 polyunsaturated fatty acid improves spatial learning and hippocampal Peroxisome Proliferator Activated

Receptors (PPARα and PPARγ) gene expression in rats. *Neuroscience* 13:109, https://doi.org/10.1186/1471-2202-13-109; Bourre J-M et al. (1989) The effects of dietary α-linolenic acid on the composition of nerve membranes, enzymatic activity, amplitude of electrophysiological parameters, resistance to poisons and performance of learning tasks in rats. *J. Nutr.* 119:1880–1892, https://doi .org/10.1093/jn/119.12.1880; Yamamoto N et al. (1987) Effect of dietary α-linolenate/linoleate balance on brain lipid compositions and learning ability of rats. *Lipid Res.* 28:144–151, https://doi.org/10.1016/S0022-2275(20)38713-7; Enslen M et al. (1991) Effect of low intake of n-3 fatty acids during develop-ment on brain phospholipid fatty acid composition and exploratory behavior in rats. *Lipids* 26:203–208, https://doi.org/10.1007/BF02543972.

7. Arien Y et al. (2015) Omega-3 deficiency impairs honey bee learning. *Proc. Nat. Acad. Sci.* 112:15761–15766, https://doi.org/10.1073/pnas.1517375112.

8. Auestad N, Innis SM (2000) Dietary n-3 fatty acid restriction during gestation in rats: neuronal cell body and growth-cone fatty acids. *Am. J. Clin. Nutr.* 71:312S–314S, https://doi.org/10.1093/ajcn/71.1.312s.

9. Cao D et al. (2009) Docosahexaenoic acid promotes hippocampal neuronal development and synaptic function. *J. Neurochem.* 111:510–521, https://doi.org /10.1111/j.1471-4159.2009.06335.x.

10. Hettenlocher PR, Dabholkar AS (1997) Regional differences in synaptogenesis in human cerebral cortex. *J. Comp. Neurol.* 387:167–178, https://doi.org/10.1002 /(sici)1096-9861(19971020)387:2<167::aid-cne1>3.0.co;2-z.

11. Al MDM et al. (1995) Maternal essential fatty acid patterns during normal pregnancy and their relationship to the neonatal essential fatty acid status. *Brit. J. Nutr.* 74:55–68, https://doi.org/10.1079/bjn19950106; Rump P et al. (2001) Leptin and phospholipid-esterifed docosahexaenoic acid concentra-tions in plasma of women: observations during pregnancy and lactation. *Eur. J. Clin. Nutr.* 55:244–251, https://doi.org/10.1038/sj.ejcn.1601151; Otto SJ et al. (2001) Comparison of the peripartum and postpartum phospholipid polyun-saturated fatty acid profiles of lactating and nonlactating women. *Am. J. Clin. Nutr.* 73:1074–1079, https://doi.org/10.1093/ajcn/73.6.1074.

12. Larqué E et al. (2003) In vivo investigation of the placental transfer of 13C-labeled fatty acids in humans. *J. Lipid Res.* 44:49–55, https://doi.org/10 .1194/jlr.M200067-JLR200.

13. Otto SJ et al. (1997) Maternal and neonatal essential fatty acid status in phos-pholipids: an international comparative study. *Eur. J. Clin. Nutr.* 51:232–242, https://doi.org/10.1038/sj.ejcn.1600390.

14. Hibbeln JR et al. (2007) Maternal seafood consumption in pregnancy and neurodevelopmental outcomes in childhood (ALSPAC study): an observational cohort study. *Lancet* 369:578–585, https://doi.org/10.1016/S0140–6736 (07)60277–3; Oken E et al. (2008) Associations of maternal fish intake during pregnancy and breastfeeding duration with attainment of developmental milestones in early childhood: a study from the Danish National Birth Cohort.

Am. J. Clin. Nutr. 88:789–796, https://doi.org/10.1093/ajcn/88.3.789; Oken E et al. (2008) Maternal fish intake during pregnancy, blood mercury levels, and child cognition at age 3 years in a US cohort. *Am. J. Epidemiol.* 167:1171–1181, https://doi.org/10.1093/aje/kwn034.

15. Bernard JY et al. (2016) Early life exposure to polyunsaturated fatty acids and psychomotor development in children from the EDEN mother-child cohort. *OCL* 23: D106, https://doi.org/10.1051/ocl/2015060.
16. Makrides M et al. (2010) Effect of DHA supplementation during pregnancy on maternal depression and neurodevelopment of young children. A randomized controlled trial. *JAMA* 304:1675–1683, https://doi.org/10.1001/jama.2010.1507.
17. Dunstan JA et al. (2008) Cognitive assessment of children at age 2½ years after maternal fish oil supplementation in pregnancy: a randomised controlled trial. *Arch. Dis. Child Fetal Neonatal Ed.* 93:F45–F50, https://doi.org/10.1136/adc.2006 .099085.
18. Helland IB et al. (2003) Maternal supplementation with very-long-chain n-3 fatty acids during pregnancy and lactation augments children's IQ at 4 years of age. *Pediatrics* 111:e39–e44, https://doi.org/10.1542/peds.111.1.e39.
19. Gibson RA, Kneebone GM (1981) Fatty acid composition of human colostrum and mature breast milk. *Am. J. Clin. Nutr.* 34:252–257, https://doi.org/10.1093 /ajcn/34.2.252; Macy IG (1949) Composition of human colostrum and milk. *Am. J. Dis. Child.* 78:589–603, doi:10.1001/archpedi.1949.02030050604009.
20. Makrides M et al. (1995) Changes in the polyunsaturated fatty acids of breast milk from mothers of full-term infants over 30 wk of lactation. *Am. J. Clin. Nutr.* 61:1231–1233, https://doi.org/10.1093/ajcn/61.6.1231.
21. Yuhas R et al. (2006) Human milk fatty acid composition from nine countries varies most in DHA. *Lipids* 41:851–858, https://doi.org/10.1007/s11745-006 -5040-7.
22. Brenna JT et al. (2007) Docosahexaenoic and arachidonic acid concentrations in human breast milk worldwide. *Am. J. Clin. Nutr.* 85:1457–64, https://doi.org /10.1093/ajcn/85.6.1457.
23. Sanders TAB et al. (1978) Studies of vegans: the fatty acid composition of plasma choline phosphoglycerides, erythrocytes, adipose tissue, and breast milk, and some indicators of susceptibility to ischemic heart disease in vegans and omnivore controls. *Am. J. Clin. Nutr.* 31:805–813, https://doi.org/10.1093 /ajcn/31.5.805.
24. Gibson RA, Kneebone GM (1981) Fatty acid composition of infant formulae. *Aust. Paediatr. J.* 17:46–53, https://doi.org/10.1111/j.1440-1754.1981.tb00014.x.
25. Clark KJ et al. (1992) Determination of the optimal ratio of linoleic acid to a-linolenic acid in infant formulas. *J. Pediatr.* 120:S151–S158, https://doi.org /10.1016/s0022-3476(05)81250-8.
26. Makrides M et al. (1994) Fatty acid composition of brain, retina, and erythro-cytes in breast- and formula-fed infants. *Am. J. Clin. Nutr.* 60: 189–194, https:// doi.org/10.1093/ajcn/60.2.189.

27. Farquharson J et al. (1992) Infant cerebral cortex phospholipid fatty-acid composition and diet. *Lancet* 340:810–813, https://doi.org/10.1016/0140-6736 (92)92684-8.

28. Calculation of total synapses in human brain uses synaptic density data from figure 2 of Hettenlocher PR, Dabholkar AS (1997) Regional differences in synaptogenesis in human cerebral cortex. *J. Comp. Neurol.* 387:167–178, https://doi.org/10.1002/(sici)1096-9861(19971020)387:2<167::aid-cne1>3.0.co;2-z.

29. Morley R et al. (1988) Mother's choice to provide breast milk and developmental outcome. *Archives of Disease in Childhood.* 63:1382–1385, https://doi.org/10.1136/adc.63.11.1382.

30. Lucas A et al. (1992) Breast milk and subsequent intelligence quotient in children born preterm. *Lancet* 339:261–264, https://doi.org/10.1016/0140-6736 (92)91329-7.

31. Willatts P et al. (1998) Effect of long-chain polyunsaturated fatty acids in infant formula on problem solving at 10 months of age. *Lancet* 352:688–91, https://doi.org/10.1016/s0140-6736(97)11374-5.

32. Willatts P et al. (2013) Effects of long-chain PUFA supplementation in infant formula on cognitive function in later childhood. *Am. J. Clin. Nutr.* 98:536S–42S, https://doi.org/10.3945/ajcn.112.038612.

33. Shah B, Pattanayak RD, Sagar R (2014) The study of patient Henry Molaison and what it taught us over past 50 years: contributions to neuroscience. *J. Mental Health & Human Behav.* 19:91–93, https://doi.org/10.4103/0971-8990.153719.

34. Wikipedia, s.v. Long-term potentiation, https://en.wikipedia.org/wiki/Long -term_potentiation.

35. Lazarov O, Hollands C (2016) Hippocampal neurogenesis: learning to remember. *Prog. Neurobiol.* 138–140:1–18, https://doi.org/10.1016/j.pneurobio.2015 .12.006.

36. Kawakita E, Hashimoto M, Shido O (2006) Docosahexaenoic acid promotes neurogenesis in vitro and in vivo. *Neuroscience* 139:991–997, https://doi.org/10 .1016/j.neuroscience.2006.01.021.

37. Cao D et al. (2009) Docosahexaenoic acid promotes hippocampal neuronal development and synaptic function. *J. Neurochem.* 111:510–521, https://doi.org /10.1111/j.1471-4159.2009.06335.x; Catalan J et al. (2002) Cognitive deficits in docosahexaenoic acid-deficient rats, *Behav. Neurosci.* 116:1022–1031, https:// doi.org/10.1037//0735-7044.116.6.1022; Moriguchi T et al. (2000) Behavioral deficits associated with dietary induction of decreased brain docosahexaenoic acid concentration. *J. Neurochem.* 75:2563–2573, https://doi.org/10.1046/j.1471 -4159.2000.0752563.x.

38. Andruchow ND et al. (2017) A lower ratio of omega-6 to omega-3 fatty acids predicts better hippocampus-dependent spatial memory and cognitive status in older adults. *Neuropsychol.* 31:724–734, https://doi.org/10.1037/neu0000373.

39. Maurer K et al. (1997) Auguste D and Alzheimer's disease. *Lancet* 349:1546–1549, https://doi.org/10.1016/S0140-6736(96)10203-8; Bullmore E (2018) *The Inflamed Mind.* London: Short Books.

40. Heneka MT et al. . (2015) Neuroinflammation in Alzheimer's disease. *Lancet Neurol* 14:388–405, https://doi.org/10.1016/S1474-4422(15)70016-5.

41. Ransohoff RM (2016) How neuroinflammation contributes to neurodegeneration. *Science* 353:777–783, https://doi.org/10.1126/science.aag2590; Tuppo EE, Arias HR (2005) The role of inflammation in Alzheimer's disease. *Int. J. Biochem. & Cell Biol.* 37:289–305, https://doi.org/10.1016/j.biocel.2004.07.009.

42. In't Veld BA et al. (2001) Nonsteroidal anti-inflammatory drugs and the risk of Alzheimer's disease. *New. Engl. J. Med.* 345:1515–1521, https://doi.org/10.1056/NEJMoa010178.

43. GBD 2016 Dementia Collaborators (2019) Global, regional, and national burden of Alzheimer's disease and other dementias, 1990–2016: a systematic analysis for the Global Burden of Disease Study 2016. *Lancet Neurol.* 18:88–106, https://doi.org/10.1016/S1474-4422(18)30403-4.

44. PopulationPyramid.net, Population pyramids of the world from 1950 to 2100, https://www.populationpyramid.net/world/.

45. Alzheimer's Association (2018) 2018 Alzheimer's Disease Facts and Figures. *Alzheimers Dement.* 14:367–429, https://www.alz.org/media/homeoffice/facts%20and%20figures/facts-and-figures.pdf; Reitz C, Mayeux R (2014) Alzheimer disease: Epidemiology, diagnostic criteria, risk factors and biomarkers. *Biochem. Pharmacol.* 88:640–651, https://doi.org/10.1016/j.bcp.2013.12.024.

46. Graves AB et al. (1996) Prevalence of dementia and its subtypes in the Japanese American population of King County, Washington State: The Kame Project, *Am. J. Epidemiol.* 144:760–71, https://doi.org/10.1093/oxfordjournals.aje.a009000; White L et al. (1996) Prevalence of dementia in older Japanese-American men in Hawaii. The Honolulu-Asia aging study. *JAMA* 276:955–960, https://doi.org/10.1001/jama.1996.03540120033030.

47. Yamada T et al. (2002) Prevalence of dementia in the older Japanese-Brazilian population. *Psychiatr. & Clin. Neurosci.* 56:71–75, https://doi.org/10.1046/j.1440-1819.2002.00931.x.

48. Hendrie HC et al. (1995) Prevalence of Alzheimer's disease and dementia in two communities: Nigerian Africans and African Americans. *Am. J. Psychiatry* 152:1485–1492, https://doi.org/10.1176/ajp.152.10.1485.

49. Kalmijn S et al. (1997) Dietary fat intake and the risk of incident dementia in the Rotterdam study. *Ann. Neurol.* 42:776–782, https://doi.org/10.1002/ana.410420514.

50. Cunnane SC et al. (2009) Fish, docosahexaenoic acid and Alzheimer's disease. *Prog. Lipid Res.* 48:239–256, https://doi.org/10.1016/j.plipres.2009.04.001.

51. Morris MC et al. (2016) Association of seafood consumption, brain mercury level, and APOE ε4 status with brain neuropathology in older adults. *JAMA* 315:489–497, https://doi.org/10.1001/jama.2015.19451.

52. Burckhardt M et al. (2016) Omega-3 fatty acids for the treatment of dementia. *Cochrane Database of Systematic Reviews* issue 4. Art. no. CD009002, https://doi.org/10.1002/14651858.CD009002.pub3.

53. Freund-Levi Y et al. (2006) ω-3 fatty acid treatment in 174 patients with mild to moderate Alzheimer disease: OmegAD study. A randomized double-blind trial. *Arch Neurol.* 63:1402–1408, https://doi.org/10.1001/archneur.63.10.1402.

54. Yehuda S, Carasso RL (1993) Modulation of learning, pain thresholds, and thermoregulation in the rat by preparations of free purified α-linolenic and linoleic acids: Determination of the optimal ω3-to-ω6 ratio. *Proc. Natl. Acad. Sci.* 90:10345–10349, https://doi.org/10.1073/pnas.90.21.10345.

55. Muldoon MF et al. (2010) Serum phospholipid docosahexaenoic acid is associated with cognitive functioning during middle adulthood. *J. Nutr.* 140:848–853, https://doi.org/10.3945/jn.109.119578.

56. Hamazaki-Fujita N et al. (2011) Polyunsaturated fatty acids and blood circulation in the forebrain during a mental arithmetic task. *Brain Res.* 1397:38–45, https://doi.org/10.1016/j.brainres.2011.04.044.

57. Conklin SM et al. (2007) Long-chain omega-3 fatty acid intake is associated positively with corticolimbic gray matter volume in healthy adults. *Neuroscience Letters* 421:209–212, https://doi.org/10.1016/j.neulet.2007.04.086.

58. Kalmijn S et al. (2004) Dietary intake of fatty acids and fish in relation to cognitive performance at middle age. *Neurology* 62:275–280, https://doi.org/10.1212/01.wnl.0000103860.75218.a5.

59. Stonehouse W (2014) Does consumption of LC omega-3 PUFA enhance cognitive performance in healthy school-aged children and throughout adulthood? Evidence from clinical trials. *Nutrients* 6:2730–2758, https://doi.org/10.3390/nu6072730.

60. Fontani G et al. (2005) Cognitive and physiological effects of Omega-3 polyunsaturated fatty acid supplementation in healthy subjects. *Eur. J. Clin. Invest.* 35:691–699, https://doi.org/10.1111/j.1365-2362.2005.01570.x.

61. Montgomery P et al. (2013) Low blood long chain omega-3 fatty acids in UK children are associated with poor cognitive performance and behavior: A cross-sectional analysis from the DOLAB study. *PLoS ONE* 8:e66697, https://doi.org/10.1371/journal.pone.0066697.

62. Richardson AJ et al. (2012) Docosahexaenoic acid for reading, cognition and behavior in children aged 7–9 years: A randomized, controlled trial (the DOLAB study). *PLoS ONE* 7:e43909, https://doi.org/10.1371/journal.pone.0043909.

63. Richardson AJ (2006) Omega-3 fatty acids in ADHD and related neurodevelopmental disorders. *Int. Rev. Psychiat.* 18:155–172, https://doi.org/10.1080/09540260600583031.

64. Chang JP-C et al. (2018) Omega-3 polyunsaturated fatty acids in youths with attention deficit hyperactivity disorder: a systematic review and meta-analysis of clinical trials and biological studies. *Neuropsychopharmacol.* 43:534–545, https://doi.org/10.1038/npp.2017.160.

65. Hadjighassem M et al. (2015) Oral consumption of α-linolenic acid increases serum BDNF levels in healthy adult humans. *Nutr. J.* 14:20, https://doi.org/10.1186/s12937-015-0012-5.

66. Ji R-R et al. (2016) Pain regulation by non-neuronal cells and inflammation. *Science* 354:572–577, https://doi.org/10.1126/science.aaf8924.

67. Shapiro H et al. (2016) Beyond the classic eicosanoids: Peripherally-acting oxygenated metabolites of polyunsaturated fatty acids mediate pain associated with tissue injury and inflammation. *Prost. Leukot. Essent. Fatty Acids* 111:45–61, https://doi.org/10.1016/j.plefa.2016.03.001.

68. Ramsden CE et al. (2017) A systems approach for discovering linoleic acid derivatives that potentially mediate pain and itch. *Sci. Signal.* 10:eaal5241, https://doi.org/10.1126/scisignal.aal5241.

69. Ramsden CE et al. (2012) Lowering dietary linoleic acid reduces bioactive oxidized linoleic acid metabolites in humans. *Prost. Leukot. Essent. Fatty Acids.* 87:135–141, https://doi.org/10.1016/j.plefa.2012.08.004.

70. GBD 2015 Collaborators (2016) Global, regional, and national incidence, prevalence, and years lived with disability for 310 diseases and injuries, 1990–2015: a systematic analysis for the Global Burden of Disease Study 2015. *Lancet* 388:1545–602, https://doi.org/10.1016/S0140-6736(16)31678-6.

71. Sibille KT et al. (2018) Omega-6:omega-3 PUFA ratio, pain, functioning, and distress in adults with knee pain. *Clin. J. Pain* 34:182–189, https://doi.org/10.1097/AJP.0000000000000517.

72. Ramsden CE et al. (2013) Targeted alteration of dietary n-3 and n-6 fatty acids for the treatment of chronic headaches: A randomized trial. *Pain* 154:2441–2451, https://doi.org/10.1016/j.pain.2013.07.028.

73. MacIntosh BA et al. (2013) Low-n-6 and low-n-6 plus high-n-3 diets for use in clinical research. *Br. J. Nutr.* 110:559–568, https://doi.org/10.1017/S0007114512005181.

74. Piomelli D et al. (2014) A lipid gate for the peripheral control of pain. *J. Neurosci.* 34:15184–15191, https://doi.org/10.1523/jneurosci.3475-14.2014.

75. Habib AM et al. (2019) Microdeletion in a FAAH pseudogene identified in a patient with high anandamide concentrations and pain insensitivity. *Brit. J. Anaesthesia* 123: e249–e253, https://doi.org/10.1016/j.bja.2019.02.019; Katz B (2019), A Scottish woman doesn't feel pain or stress: Now researchers think they know why, *Smithsonian*, March 28, 2019, https://www.smithsonianmag.com/smart-news/scottish-woman-doesnt-feel-pain-now-researchers-think-they-know-why-180971822/.

76. Ramsden CE et al. (2015) Diet-induced changes in n-3 and n-6 derived endocannabinoids and reductions in headache pain and psychological distress. *J Pain* 16:707–716, https://doi.org/10.1016/j.jpain.2015.04.007.

77. Ramsden CE et al. (2015) Targeted alterations in dietary n-3 and n-6 fatty acids improve life functioning and reduce psychological distress among chronic headache patients: secondary analysis of a randomized trial. *Pain* 156:587–596, https://doi.org/10.1097/01.j.pain.0000460348.84965.47.

78. Polatin PB et al. (1993) Psychiatric illness and chronic low-back pain. *Spine* 18:66–71, https://doi.org/10.1097/00007632-199301000-00011.

Chapter 10. Mental Health and Happiness

1. Fiennes RNT-W et al. (1973) Essential fatty acid studies in primates. Linolenic acid requirements of Capuchins. *J. Med. Primatol.* 2:155–169, https://doi.org/10.1159/000460319.
2. Raygada M et al. (1998) High maternal intake of polyunsaturated fatty acids during pregnancy in mice alters offsprings' aggressive behavior, immobility in the swim test, locomotor activity and brain protein kinase C activity. *J. Nutr.* 128:2505–2511, https://doi.org/10.1093/jn/128.12.2505; DeMar Jr. JC et al. (2006) One generation of n-3 polyunsaturated fatty acid deprivation increases depression and aggression test scores in rats. *J. Lipid Res.* 47:172–180, https://doi.org/10.1194/jlr.M500362-JLR200.
3. Muldoon MF et al. (1990) Lowering cholesterol concentrations and mortality: a quantitative review of primary prevention trials. *Brit. Med. J.* 301:309–14, https://doi.org/10.1136/bmj.301.6747.309.
4. Virkkunen M (1979) Serum cholesterol in antisocial personality. *Neuropsychobiol.* 5:27–30, https://doi.org/10.1159/000117660; Virkkunen M (1983) Serum cholesterol levels in homicidal offenders. A low cholesterol level is connected with a habitually violent tendency under the influence of alcohol. *Neuropsychobiol.* 10:65–69, https://doi.org/10.1159/000117987.
5. Weidner G et al. (1992) Improvements in hostility and depression in relation to dietary change and cholesterol lowering. The Family Heart Study. *Ann. Intern. Med.* 117:820–823, https://doi.org/10.7326/0003-4819-117-10-820.
6. Hibbeln JR, Salem Jr. N (1995) Dietary polyunsaturated fatty acids and depression: when cholesterol does not satisfy. *Am. J. Clin. Nutr.* 62:1–9, https://doi.org/10.1093/ajcn/62.1.1.
7. Pekkanen J et al. (1989) Serum cholesterol and risk of accidental or violent death in 25-year follow-up. The Finnish cohorts of the Seven Countries Study. *Arch. Intern. Med.* 149:1589–1591, https://doi.org/10.1001/archinte.1989.00390070107016.
8. Iribarren C et al. (2004) Dietary intake of n-3, n-6 fatty acids and fish: Relationship with hostility in young adults—the CARDIA study. *Eur. J. Clin. Nutr.* 58:24–31, https://doi.org/10.1038/sj.ejcn.1601739.
9. Hamazaki T et al. (1996) The effect of docosahexaenoic acid on aggression in young adults. A placebo-controlled double-blind study. *J. Clin. Invest.* 97:1129–1133, https://doi.org/10.1172/JCI118507.
10. Buydens-Branchey L et al. (2003) Polyunsaturated fatty acid status and aggression in cocaine addicts. *Drug and Alcohol Dependence* 71:319–323, https://doi.org/10.1016/s0376-8716(03)00168-6.
11. Buydens-Branchey L et al. (2008) Associations between increases in plasma n-3 polyunsaturated fatty acids following supplementation and decreases in anger and anxiety in substance abusers. *Prog. Neuropsychopharmacol. Biol. Psychiatry* 32:568–575, https://doi.org/10.1016/j.pnpbp.2007.10.020.
12. Meyer BJ et al. (2015) Baseline omega-3 index correlates with aggressive and

attention deficit disorder behaviours in adult prisoners. *PLoS One*, 10:e0120220, https://doi.org/10.1371/journal.pone.0120220.

13. Joseph Hibbeln is a captain in the United States Public Health Service. He graduated MD (University of Illinois at Chicago, 1988), is certified in psychiatry and neurology, and is an important contributor to the role of omega-3 and omega-6 fats in mental health.

14. Hibbeln JR (2001) Seafood consumption and homicide mortality. A crossnational ecological analysis. *World Rev. Nutr. Diet.* 88:41–46, https://doi.org/10.1159/000059747.

15. Hibbeln JR et al. (2004) Increasing homicide rates and linoleic acid consumption among five western countries, 1961–2000. *Lipids* 39:1207–1213, https://doi.org/10.1007/s11745-004-1349-5.

16. Darcey VL et al. (2019) Dietary long-chain omega-3 fatty acids are related to impulse control and anterior cingulate function in adolescents. *Front. Neurosci.* 12:article 1012, https://doi.org/10.3389/fnins.2018.01012.

17. Gow RV et al. (2013) Omega-3 fatty acids are inversely related to callous and unemotional traits in adolescent boys with attention deficit hyperactivity disorder. *Prost. Leukot. Essent. Fatty Acids* 88:411–418, https://doi.org/10.1016/j.plefa.2013.03.009.

18. Gow RV et al. (2013) Omega-3 fatty acids are related to abnormal emotion processing in adolescent boys with attention deficit hyperactivity disorder. *Prost. Leukot. Essent. Fatty Acids.* 88:419–429, https://doi.org/10.1016/j.plefa.2013.03.008.

19. Raine A et al. (2010) Cohort Profile: The Mauritius Child Health Project. *Int. J. Epidemiol.* 39:1441–1451, https://doi.org/10.1093/ije/dyp341.

20. Raine A et al. (2015) Reduction in behavior problems with omega-3 supplementation in children aged 8–16 years: A randomized, double-blind, placebo-controlled, stratified, parallel-group trial. *J. Child Psychol. Psychiatry* 56:509–520, https://doi.org/10.1111/jcpp.12314.

21. Portnoy J et al. (2018) Reductions of intimate partner violence resulting from supplementing children with omega-3 fatty acids: A randomized, doubleblind, placebo-controlled, stratified, parallel-group trial. *Aggressive Behav.* 44:491–500, https://doi.org/10.1002/ab.21769.

22. Wikipedia, s.v. Major depressive disorder, https://en.wikipedia.org/wiki/Major_depressive_disorder.

23. Malhi GS, Mann JJ (2018) Depression. *Lancet* 392:2299–2312, https://doi.org/10.1016/S0140-6736(18)31948-2.

24. Kendler KS et al. (1999) Causal relationship between stressful life events and the onset of major depression. *Am. J. Psychiatry* 156:837–841, https://doi.org/10.1176/ajp.156.6.837.

25. Moussavi S et al. (2007) Depression, chronic diseases, and decrements in health: results from the World Health Surveys. *Lancet* 370:851–858, https://doi.org/10.1016/S0140-6736(07)61415-9.

26. Egede LE (2007) Major depression in individuals with chronic medical disorders: prevalence, correlates and association with health resource utilization, lost productivity and functional disability. *Gen. Hosp. Psychiatry* 29:409–416, https://doi.org/10.1016/j.genhosppsych.2007.06.002.

27. Jokela M et al. (2014) Association of metabolically healthy obesity with depressive symptoms: pooled analysis of eight studies. *Mol. Psychiatry* 19:910–914, https://doi.org/10.1038/mp.2013.162.

28. Hadjighassem M et al. (2015) Oral consumption of α-linolenic acid increases serum BDNF levels in healthy adult humans. *Nutr. J.* 14:20, https://doi.org/10.1186/s12937-015-0012-5.

29. Khandaker GM et al. (2014) Association of serum interleukin 6 and C-reactive protein in childhood with depression and psychosis in young adult life. A population-based longitudinal study. *JAMA Psychiatry* 71:1121–1128, https://doi.org/10.1001/jamapsychiatry.2014.1332.

30. Kivimaki M et al. (2014) Long-term inflammation increases risk of common mental disorder: a cohort study. *Mol. Psychiatry* 19:149–150, https://doi.org/10.1038/mp.2013.35

31. McDonald EM et al. (1987) Interferons as mediators of psychiatric morbidity. An investigation in a trial of recombinant α-interferon in hepatitis-B carriers. *Lancet* 330:1175–1178, https://doi.org/10.1016/s0140-6736(87)91319-5.

32. Niiranen A et al. (1988) Behavioral assessment of patients treated with alpha-interferon. *Acta Psychiatr. Scand.* 78:622–626, https://doi.org/10.1111/j.1600-0447.1988.tb06395.x.

33. Dantzer R et al. (2008) From inflammation to sickness and depression: when the immune system subjugates the brain. *Nat. Rev. Neurosci.* 9:46–56, https://doi.org/10.1038/nrn2297.

34. Kappelmann N et al. (2018) Antidepressant activity of anti-cytokine treatment: a systematic review and meta-analysis of clinical trials of chronic inflammatory conditions. *Mol. Psychiatry* 23:335–343, https://doi.org/10.1038/mp.2016.167.

35. Burton R (1651) *The Anatomy of Melancholy in three volumes.* London: J. M. Dent, 1932 edition (based on 6th edition, 1651) (see page 248 of vol. 2)

36. Maggioni M et al. (1990), Effects of phosphatidylserine therapy in geriatric patients with depressive disorders. *Acta Psychiatr. Scand.* 81:265–270, https://doi.org/10.1111/j.1600-0447.1990.tb06494.x.

37. Conklin SM et al. (2010) Age-related changes of n-3 and n-6 polyunsaturated fatty acids in the anterior cingulate cortex of individuals with major depressive disorder. *Prost. Leukot. Essent. Fatty Acids* 82:111–119, https://doi.org/10.1016/j.plefa.2009.12.002; McNamara RK et al. (2007) Selective deficits in the omega-3 fatty acid docosahexaenoic acid in the postmortem orbitofrontal cortex of patients with major depressive disorder. *Biol. Psychiatry* 62:17–24, https://doi.org/10.1016/j.biopsych.2006.08.026; Tatebayashi Y et al. (2012) Abnormal fatty acid composition in the frontopolar cortex of patients with affective disorders. *Transl. Psychiatry* 2:e204, https://doi.org/10.1038/tp.2012

.132; Hamazaki K et al. (2012) Fatty acid composition in the postmortem amygdala of patients with schizophrenia, bipolar disorder, and major depressive disorder. *J. Psychiatric Res.* 46:1024–1028, https://doi.org/10.1016/j.jpsychires .2012.04.012; Hamazaki K et al. (2013) Abnormalities in the fatty acid composition of the postmortem entorhinal cortex of patients with schizophrenia, bipolar disorder, and major depressive disorder. *Psychiatry Res.* 210:346–350, https://doi.org/10.1016/j.psychres.2013.05.006; Lalovic A et al. (2007), Fatty acid composition in postmortem brains of people who completed suicide *J. Psychiatry Neurosci.* 32:363–370, https://pubmed.ncbi.nlm.nih.gov/17823652/.

38. McNamara RK et al. (2013) Lower docosahexaenoic acid concentrations in the postmortem prefrontal cortex of adult depressed suicide victims compared with controls without cardiovascular disease. *J. Psychiatr. Res.* 47:1187–1191, https://doi.org/10.1016/j.jpsychires.2013.05.007.

39. Lin P-Y et al. (2010) A meta-analytic review of polyunsaturated fatty acid compositions in patients with depression. *Biol. Psychiatry* 68:140–147, https:// doi.org/10.1016/j.biopsych.2010.03.018.

40. McNamara RK et al. (2014) Detection and treatment of long-chain omega-3 fatty acid deficiency in adolescents with SSRI-resistant major depressive disorder. *PharmaNutrition* 2:38–46, https://doi.org/10.1016/j.phanu.2014.02.002.

41. Lotrich FE et al. (2013) Elevated ratio of arachidonic acid to long-chain omega-3 fatty acids predicts depression development following interferon-alpha treatment: Relationship with interleukin-6. *Brain Behav. Immun.* 31:48–53, https:// doi.org/10.1016/j.bbi.2012.08.007.

42. Hibbeln JR (1998) Fish consumption and major depression. *The Lancet* 351:1213, https://doi.org/10.1016/S0140-6736(05)79168-6.

43. Edwards R et al. (1998) Omega-3 polyunsaturated fatty acid levels in the diet and in red blood cell membranes of depressed patients. *J. Affect. Disord.* 48:149–155, https://doi.org/10.1016/s0165-0327(97)00166-3.

44. Grosso G et al. (2016) Dietary n-3 PUFA, fish consumption and depression: A systematic review and meta-analysis of observational studies. *J. Affect. Disord.* 205:269–281, https://doi.org/10.1016/j.jad.2016.08.011.

45. Horikawa C et al. (2018) Longitudinal association between *n*-3 long-chain polyunsaturated fatty acid intake and depressive symptoms: a population-based cohort study in Japan. *Nutrients* 10:1655, https://doi.org/10.3390/nu10111655.

46. Grosso G et al. (2014) Role of omega-3 fatty acids in the treatment of depressive disorders: a comprehensive meta-analysis of randomized clinical trials. *PLoS ONE* 9:e96905, https://doi.org/10.1371/journal.pone.0096905.

47. Hallahan B et al. (2016) Efficacy of omega-3 highly unsaturated fatty acids in the treatment of depression. *Brit. J. Psychiatr.* 209:192–201, https://doi.org /10.1192/bjp.bp.114.160242.

48. Appleton KM et al. (2016) ω-3 fatty acids for major depressive disorder in adults: an abridged Cochrane review. *BMJ Open* 6: e010172, https://doi.org/10.1136 /bmjopen-2015-010172.

49. Amminger GP et al. (2015) Longer-term outcome in the prevention of psychotic disorders by the Vienna omega-3 study. *Nature Comm.* 6:7934, https://doi.org /10.1038/ncomms8934.

50. Berger ME et al. (2017) Omega-6 to omega-3 polyunsaturated fatty acid ratio and subsequent mood disorders in young people with at-risk mental states: a 7-year longitudinal study. *Transl. Psychiatr.* 7:e1220, https://doi.org/10.1038 /tp.2017.190.

51. Su K-P et al. (2014) Omega-3 fatty acids in the prevention of interferon-alpha-induced depression: results from a randomized, controlled trial. *Biol. Psychiatr.* 76:559–566, https://doi.org/10.1016/j.biopsych.2014.01.008.

52. Hibbeln JR (2002) Seafood consumption, the DHA content of mothers' milk and prevalence rates of postpartum depression: a cross-national, ecological analysis. *J. Affect. Disord.* 69:15–29, https://doi.org/10.1016/s0165-0327(01)00374-3.

53. Lin P-Y et al. (2017) Polyunsaturated fatty acids in perinatal depression: a systematic review and meta-analysis. *Biol. Psychiatr.* 82:560–569, https:// doi.org/10.1016/j.biopsych.2017.02.1182.

54. Hoge A et al. (2019) Imbalance between omega-6 and omega-3 polyunsaturated fatty acids in early pregnancy is predictive of postpartum depression in a Belgian cohort. *Nutrients* 11:876, https://doi.org/10.3390/nu11040876.

55. Hsu M-C et al. (2018) Omega-3 polyunsaturated fatty acid supplementation in prevention and treatment of maternal depression: Putative mechanism and recommendation. *J. Affect. Disord.* 238:47–61, https://doi.org/10.1016/j.jad .2018.05.018.

56. Sublette ME et al. (2006) Omega-3 polyunsaturated essential fatty acid status as a predictor of future suicide risk. *Am. J. Psychiatr.* 163:1100–1102, https:// doi.org/10.1176/ajp.2006.163.6.1100.

57. Huan M et al. (2004) Suicide attempt and n-3 fatty acid levels in red blood cells: a case control study in China. *Biol. Psychiatr.* 56:490–496, https://doi.org/10 .1016/j.biopsych.2004.06.028.

58. Lewis MD et al. (2011) Suicide deaths of active duty U.S. military and omega-3 fatty acid status: a case control comparison. *J. Clin. Psychiatr.* 72:1585–1590, https://doi.org/10.4088/JCP.11m06879.

59. Hibbeln JR, Gow RV (2014) The potential for military diets to reduce depression, suicide, and impulsive aggression: a review of current evidence for omega-3 and omega-6 fatty acids. *Military Medicine* 179:117–128, https://doi .org/10.7205/MILMED-D-14-00153.

60. Krogh A, Krogh M (1913) A study of the diet and metabolism of eskimos undertaken in 1908 on an expedition to Greenland. *Medd om Gronland* 51:1–52.

61. Deutch B et al. (2007) Traditional and modern Greenlandic food—Dietary composition, nutrients and contaminants. *Science of the Total Environment* 384:106–119, https://doi.org/10.1016/j.scitotenv.2007.05.042.

62. Bjerregaard P, Jeppesen C (2010) Inuit dietary patterns in modern Greenland. *Int. J. Circumpolar Health* 69:13–24, https://doi.org/10.3402/ijch.v69i1.17387.

63. Bang HO et al. (1976) The composition of food consumed by Greenland Eskimos. *Acta Med. Scand.* 200:69–73, https://doi.org/10.1111/j.0954-6820.1976.tb08198.x.

64. Editorial (1983) Eskimo diets and diseases. *Lancet* 321:1139–1141, https://doi .org/10.1016/S0140-6736(83)92871-4.

65. Bjerregaard P et al. (2004) Indigenous health in the Arctic: an overview of the circumpolar Inuit population. *Scand. J. Public Health* 32:390–395, https://doi .org/10.1080/14034940410028398.

66. Bjerregaard P, Larsen CVL (2018) Three lifestyle-related issues of major sig- nificance for public health among the Inuit in contemporary Greenland: a review of adverse childhood conditions, obesity, and smoking in a period of social transition. *Public Health Reviews* 39:5, https://doi.org/10.1186/s40985 -018-0085-8.

67. Hicks J (2007) The social determinants of elevated rates of suicide among Inuit youth. *Indigenous Affairs* 2007 issue 4:30–37, https://www.suicideinfo .ca/resource/siecno-20080031/.

68. Bjerregaard P, Larsen CVL (2015) Time trend by region of suicides and suicidal thoughts among Greenland Inuit. *Int. J. Circumpolar Health* 74:1–8, https://doi .org/10.3402/ijch.v74.26053.

69. Anctil M (2008) *Nunavik Inuit Health Survey 2004, Qanuippitaa? How are we?* Quebec: Institut national de santé publique du Québec (INSPQ) & Nunavik Regional Board of Health and Social Services (NRBHSS).

70. Boothroyd LJ et al. (2001) Completed suicides among the Inuit of northern Quebec, 1982–1996: a case-control study. *Canadian Med. Assoc. J.* 165:749–755, https://pubmed.ncbi.nlm.nih.gov/11584562/.

71. McGrath-Hanna NK et al. (2003) Diet and mental health in the Arctic: is diet an important risk factor for mental health in circumpolar peoples?—a review. *Int. J. Circumpolar Health* 62:228–241, https://www.tandfonline.com/doi/pdf /10.3402/ijch.v62i3.17560.

72. Lucas M et al. (2009) Plasma omega-3 and psychological distress among Nunavik Inuit (Canada). *Psychiatr. Res.* 167:266–278, https://doi.org/10.1016 /j.psychres.2008.04.012.

73. Lucas M et al. (2010) Erythrocyte n-3 is inversely correlated with serious psy- chological distress among the Inuit: data from the Nunavik Health Survey. *J. Am. Coll. Nutr.* 29:211–221, https://doi.org/10.1080/07315724.2010.10719836.

Chapter 11. Of Mice and Men

1. Kang JX et al. (2004) Fat-1 mice convert n-6 to n-3 fatty acids. *Nature* 427:504, https://doi.org/10.1038/427504a.

2. Kim E-H et al. (2012) Endogenously synthesized n-3 polyunsaturated fatty acids in fat-1 mice ameliorate high-fat diet-induced non-alcoholic fatty liver disease. *Biochem. Pharm.* 84:1359–1365, https://doi.org/10.1016/j.bcp.2012.08.029.

3. Smith BK et al. (2010) A decreased *n*-6/*n*-3 ratio in the fat-1 mouse is associ- ated with improved glucose tolerance. *Appl. Physiol. Nutr. Metab.* 35:699–706,

https://doi.org/10.1139/H10-066; Romanatto T et al. (2014) Elevated tissue omega-3 fatty acid status prevents age-related glucose intolerance in fat-1 transgenic mice. *Biochim. Biophys. Acta* 1842:186–191, https://doi.org/10.1016/j.bbadis.2013.10.017.

4. Bhattacharya A et al. (2006) Inhibition of inflammatory response in transgenic fat-1 mice on a calorie-restricted diet. *Biochem. Biophys. Res. Comm.* 349:925–930, https://doi.org/10.1016/j.bbrc.2006.08.093.

5. Mayer K et al. (2009) Acute lung injury is reduced in fat-1 mice endogenously synthesizing n-3 fatty acids. *Am J Respir Crit Care Med* 179:474–483, https://doi.org/10.1164/rccm.200807-1064OC.

6. Schmocker C et al. (2007) Omega-3 fatty acids alleviate chemically induced acute hepatitis by suppression of cytokines. *Hepatology* 45:864–869, https://doi.org/10.1002/hep.21626.

7. Bilal S et al. (2011) Fat-1 transgenic mice with elevated omega-3 fatty acids are protected from allergic airway responses. *Biochim. Biophys. Acta* 1812:1164–1169, https://doi.org/10.1016/j.bbadis.2011.05.002.

8. Jang H-Y et al. (2018) Atopic dermatitis-like skin lesions are suppressed in fat-1 transgenic mice through the inhibition of inflammasomes. *Exp. & Mol. Med.* 50:73, https://doi.org/10.1038/s12276-018-0104-3.

9. Seong Ji et al. (2015) Endogenous conversion of n-6 to n-3 polyunsaturated fatty acids attenuates K/BxN serum-transfer arthritis in fat-1 mice. *J. Nutr. Biochem.* 26:713–720, https://doi.org/10.1016/j.jnutbio.2015.01.011.

10. Zhang Y-M et al. (2018) Endogenous synthesis of n-3 polyunsaturated fatty acids in fat-1 transgenic mice ameliorates streptozocin-induced diabetic nephropathy. *J. Funct. Foods* 45:427–434, https://doi.org/10.1016/j.jff.2018.04.010; Bellenger J et al. (2011) High pancreatic n-3 fatty acids prevent STZ-induced diabetes in Fat-1 mice: inflammatory pathway inhibition. *Diabetes* 60:1090–1099, https://doi.org/10.2337/db10-0901 Wang J et al. (2015) N-3 polyunsaturated fatty acids protect against pancreatic β-cell damage due to ER stress and prevent diabetes development. *Mol. Nutr. Food Res.* 59:1791–1802, https://doi.org/10.1002/mnfr.201500299, https://doi.org/10.1186/s12868-016-0312-5.

11. Siegert E et al. (2017) The effect of omega-3 fatty acids on central nervous system remyelination in fat-1 mice. *BMC Neurosci.* 18:19, https://doi.org/10.1186/s12868-016-0312-5.

12. Yum H-W et al. (2017) Constitutive ω-3 fatty acid production in fat-1 transgenic mice and docosahexaenoic acid administration to wild type mice protect against 2,4,6-trinitrobenzene sulfonic acid-induced colitis. *Biochem. Biophys. Res. Comm.* 487:847–855, https://doi.org/10.1016/j.bbrc.2017.04.140; Hudert CA et al. (2006) Transgenic mice rich in endogenous omega-3 fatty acids are protected from colitis. *Proc. Natl. Acad. Sci.* 103:11276–11281, https://doi.org/10.1073/pnas.0601280103; Gravaghi C et al. (2011) Cox-2 expression, PGE2 and cytokines production are inhibited by endogenously synthesized n-3 PUFAs in inflamed colon of fat-1 mice. *J. Nutr. Biochem.* 22:360–365, https://doi.org/10

.1016/j.jnutbio.2010.03.003; Monk JM et al. (2012) Th17 cell accumulation is decreased during chronic experimental colitis by (n-3) PUFA in Fat-1 mice. *J. Nutr.* 142:117–124, https://doi.org/10.3945/jn.111.147058.

13. Li X-Y et al. (2017) Protection against fine particle-induced pulmonary and systemic inflammation by omega-3 polyunsaturated fatty acids. *Biochim. Biophys. Acta* 1861:577–584, https://doi.org/10.1016/j.bbagen.2016.12.018.

14. Connor KM et al. (2007) Increased dietary intake of ω-3-polyunsaturated fatty acids reduces pathological retinal angiogenesis. *Nat. Med.* 13:868–873, https://doi.org//10.1038/nm1591.

15. Zou Z et al. (2013) Inhibition of the HER2 pathway by n-3 polyunsaturated fatty acids prevents breast cancer in fat-1 transgenic mice. *J. Lipid Res.* 54:3453–3463, https://doi.org/10.1194/jlr.M042754.

16. Yun E-J et al. (2016) Docosahexaenoic acid suppresses breast cancer cell metastasis by targeting matrix-metalloproteinases. *Oncotarget* 7:49961–49971, https://doi.org/10.18632/oncotarget.10266; MacLennan MB et al. (2013) Mammary tumor development is directly inhibited by lifelong n-3 polyunsaturated fatty acids. *J. Nutr. Biochem.* 24:388–395, https://doi.org/10.1016/j.jnutbio.2012.08.002.

17. Han Y-M et al. (2016) Suppressed Helicobacter pylori-associated gastric tumorigenesis in Fat-1 transgenic mice producing endogenous ω-3 polyunsaturated fatty acids. *Oncotarget* 7:66606–66622, https://doi.org/10.18632/oncotarget.11261; Lee H-J et al. (2018) Role of omega-3 polyunsaturated fatty acids in preventing gastrointestinal cancers: current status and future perspectives. *Expert Review of Anticancer Therapy* 18:1189–1203, https://doi.org/10.1080/14737140.2018.1524299.

18. Han Y-M et al. (2016) The ω-3 polyunsaturated fatty acids prevented colitis-associated carcinogenesis through blocking dissociation of β-catenin complex, inhibiting COX-2 through repressing NF-κB, and inducing 15-prostaglandin dehydrogenase. *Oncotarget* 7:63583–63595, https://doi.org/10.18632/oncotarget.11544; Algamas-Dimantov A et al. (2014) Prevention of diabetes-promoted colorectal cancer by (n-3) polyunsaturated fatty acids and (n-3) PUFA mimetic. *Oncotarget* 5:9851–9863, https://doi.org/10.18632/oncotarget.2453; Liu M et al. (2016) Elevation of n-3/n-6 PUFAs ratio suppresses mTORC1 and prevents colorectal carcinogenesis associated with APC mutation. *Oncotarget* 7:76944–76954, https://doi.org/10.18632/oncotarget.12759; Jia Q et al. (2008) Reduced colitis-associated colon cancer in fat-1 (n-3 fatty acid desaturase) transgenic mice. *Cancer Res.* 68:3985–3991, https://doi.org/10.1158/0008-5472.CAN-07-6251; Yao A-J et al. (2018) Endogenous n-3 polyunsaturated fatty acids prevent azoxymethane-induced T colon tumorigenesis in mice fed a high-fat diet. *J. Funct. Foods* 48:439–447, https://doi.org//10.1016/j.jff.2018.07.042; Nowak J et al. (2007) Colitis-associated colon tumorigenesis is suppressed in transgenic mice rich in endogenous n-3 fatty acids. *Carcinogenesis* 28:1991–1995, https://doi.org/10.1093/carcin/bgm166.

19. Mohammed A et al. (2012) Endogenous n-3 polyunsaturated fatty acids delay progression of pancreatic ductal adenocarcinoma in Fat-1-p48^{Cre}/$^+$– LSL-Kras ^{G12D}/$^+$ mice. *Neoplasia* 14:1249–1259, https://doi.org/10.1593/neo.121508.

20. Griffitts J et al. (2010) Non-mammalian Fat-1 gene prevents neoplasia when introduced to a mouse hepatocarcinogenesis model. *Biochim Biophys Acta.* 1801:1133–1144, https://doi.org/10.1016/j.bbalip.2010.06.008; Weylandt KH et al. (2011) Suppressed liver tumorigenesis in fat-1 mice with elevated omega-3 fatty acids is associated with increased omega-3 derived lipid mediators and reduced TNF-a. *Carcinogenesis* 32:897–903, https://doi.org/10.1093/carcin/bgr049.

21. Xia S et al. (2006) Melanoma growth is reduced in fat-1 transgenic mice: Impact of omega-6 omega-3 essential fatty acids. *Proc. Natl. Acad. Sci. USA* 103:12499–12504, https://doi.org/10.1073/pnas.0605394103; Yini X et al. (2016) Endogenously synthesized n-3 fatty acids in fat-1 transgenic mice prevent melanoma progression by increasing E-cadherin expression and inhibiting β-catenin signalling. *Mol. Med. Reports* 14:3476–3484, https://doi.org/10.3892/mmr.2016.5639; Yum H-W et al. (2017) Endogenous ω-3 fatty acid production by Fat-1 transgene and topically applied docosahexaenoic acid protect against UVB-induced mouse skin carcinogenesis. *Scientific Reports* 7: article11658, https://doi.org/10.1038/s41598-017-11443-2.

22. Lu Y et al. (2008) Expression of the fat-1 gene diminishes prostate cancer growth in vivo through enhancing apoptosis and inhibiting GSK-3B phosphorylation. *Mol. Cancer Therap.* 7:3203–3211, https://doi.org/10.1158/1535-7163.MCT-08-0494.

23. Joffre C et al. (2016) Modulation of brain PUFA content in different experimental models of mice. *Prost. Leukot. Essent. Fatty Acids* 114:1–10, https://doi.org/10.1016/j.plefa.2016.09.003.

24. Sakayori N et al. (2016) Maternal dietary imbalance between omega-6 and omega-3 polyunsaturated fatty acids impairs neocortical development via epoxy metabolites. *Stem Cells* 34:470–482, https://doi.org/10.1038/s42003-020-01209-4.

25. He C et al. (2009) Improved spatial learning performance of fat-1 mice is associated with enhanced neurogenesis and neuritogenesis by docosahexaenoic acid. *Proc. Natl. Acad. Sci. USA* 106:11370–11375, https://doi.org/10.1073/pnas.0904835106.

26. Delpech J-C et al. (2015) Transgenic increase in n-3/n-6 fatty acid ratio protects against cognitive deficits induced by an immune challenge through decrease of neuroinflammation. *Neuropsychopharmacol.* 40:525–536, https://doi.org/10.1038/npp.2014.196.

27. Lebbadi M et al. (2011) Endogenous conversion of omega-6 into omega-3 fatty acids improves neuropathology in an animal model of Alzheimer's disease. *J. Alzheimer's Dis.* 27:853–869, https://doi.org/10.3233/JAD-2011-111010; Wu K et al. (2016) Enriched endogenous n-3 polyunsaturated fatty acids alleviate

cognitive and behavioural deficits in a mice model of Alzheimer's disease. *Neuroscience* 333:345–355, https://doi.org/10.1016/j.neuroscience.2016.07.038.

28. Ren H et al. (2017) Omega-3 polyunsaturated fatty acids promote amyloid-β clearance from the brain through mediating the function of the glymphatic system. *FASEB Journal* 31:282–293, https://doi.org/10.1096/fj.201600896.

29. Zhang E et al. (2017) High omega-3 polyunsaturated fatty acids in *fat-1* mice reduce inflammatory pain. *J. Medicinal Food* 20:1–7, https://doi.org/10.1089/jmf.2016.3871.

Chapter 12. The Omega Story and Solutions

1. Wikipedia, s.v. "Shortening," https://en.wikipedia.org/wiki/Shortening.

2. Spector AA, Kim H-Y (2015) Discovery of essential fatty acids. *J. Lipid Res.* 56:11–21, https://doi.org/10.1194/jlr.R055095.

3. Singer SJ, Nicolson GL (1972) The fluid mosaic model of the structure of cell membranes. *Science* 720–731, https://doi.org/10.1126/science.175.4023.720.

4. Reddy KS, Yusuf S (1998) Emerging epidemic of cardiovascular disease in developing countries. *Circulation* 97:596–601, https://doi.org/10.1161/01.cir.97.6.596.

5. Roth GA et al. (2017) Global, regional, and national burden of cardiovascular diseases for 10 causes, 1990 to 2015. *J. Am. Coll. Cardiol.* 70:1–25, https://doi.org/10.1016/j.jacc.2017.04.052.

6. Steele EM et al (2017) The share of ultra-processed foods and the overall nutritional quality of diets in the US: evidence from a nationally representative cross-sectional study. *Population Health Metrics* 15:6, https://doi.org/10.1186/s12963-017-0119-3.

7. Moubarac J-C et al (2017) Consumption of ultra-processed foods predicts diet quality in Canada. *Appetite* 108:512–520, https://doi.org/10.1016/j.appet.2016.11.006.

8. Rauber F et al (2018) Ultra-processed food consumption and chronic non-communicable diseases-related dietary nutrient profile in the UK (2008–2014). *Nutrients* 10:587 https://doi.org/10.3390/nu10050587.

9. da Costa Louzada ML et al (2015) Ultra-processed foods and the nutritional dietary profile in Brazil. *Rev Saúde Pública* 49:38, https://doi.org/10.1590/S0034-8910.2015049006132.

10. Kim H et al (2019) Ultra-processed food intake and mortality in the United States: results from the Third National Health and Nutrition Examination Survey (NHANES III 1988–1994). *Public Health Nutr.* 22:1777–1785, https://doi.org/10.1017/S1368980018003890.

11. Rico-Campà A et al (2019) Association between consumption of ultra-processed foods and all cause mortality: SUN prospective cohort study. *BMJ* 365:l1949, https://doi.org/10.1136/bmj.l1949.

12. Schnabel L et al (2019) Association between ultraprocessed food consumption and risk of mortality among middle-aged adults in France. *JAMA Intern Med.* 179:490–498, https://doi.org/10.1001/jamainternmed.2018.7289.

13. Srour B et al (2019) Ultra-processed food intake and risk of cardiovascular disease: prospective cohort study (NutriNet-Santé). *BMJ* 365:l1451, https://doi.org/10.1136/bmj.l1451.

14. Fiolet T et al (2018) Consumption of ultra-processed foods and cancer risk: results from NutriNet-Santé prospective cohort. *BMJ* 360:k322, https://doi.org/10.1136/bmj.k322.

15. Hall KD et al. (2019) Ultra-processed diets cause excess calorie intake and weight gain: an inpatient randomized controlled trial of ad libitum food intake. *Cell Metabolism* 30:1–11, https://doi.org/10.1016/j.cmet.2019.05.008.

16. Abbott SK et al (2010) Membrane fatty acid composition of rat skeletal muscle is most responsive to the balance of dietary n-3 and n-6 polyunsaturated fatty acids. *Brit. J. Nutr.* 103:522–529 (see figure 2), https://doi.org/10.1017/S0007114509992133; Hulbert AJ (2021) The under-appreciated fats of life: the two types of polyunsaturated fats. *J. Exp. Biol.* 224:jeb232538 (see figure 3). https://doi.org/10.1242/jeb.232538.

17. Abbott, SK (2011) The influence of dietary fatty acid profile on membrane fatty acid composition in the rat and its metabolic implications. D. Phil. thesis, University of Wollongong, https://ro.uow.edu.au/theses/3260/.

18. Lands WE et al (1982) Selective incorporation of polyunsaturated fatty acids into phosphatidylcholine by rat liver microsomes. *J. Biol. Chem.* 257:14968–14972, https://pubmed.ncbi.nlm.nih.gov/7174678/.

19. Wikipedia, s.v. Trans fat, https://en.wikipedia.org/wiki/Trans_fat.

20. The most common ruminant-derived trans fats are variants of either 18:1 or 18:2. In CLAs (conjugated linoleic acids) one of the double-bonds is a repositioned *trans*-double bond, while the other is a *cis*-double bond.

21. Hunter JE (2006) Dietary trans fatty acids: review of recent human studies and food industry responses. *Lipids* 41:967–992, https://doi.org/10.1007/s11745-006-5049-y.

22. Allison DB et al (1999) Estimated intakes of trans fatty and other fatty acids in the US population. *J Am Diet Assoc* 99:166–174, https://doi.org/10.1016/S0002-8223(99)00041-3.

23. Hulshof KFAM et al (1999) Intake of fatty acids in Western Europe with emphasis on trans fatty acids: The TRANSFAIR study. *Eur. J. Clin. Nutr.* 53:143–157, https://www.nature.com/articles/1600692.

24. Craig-Schmidt MC (2006) World-wide consumption of trans fatty acids. *Atherosclerosis Supplements* 7:1–4, https://doi.org/10.1016/j.atherosclerosissup.2006.04.001.

25. Mozaffarian D et al (2004) Dietary intake of trans fatty acids and systemic inflammation in women. *Am. J. Clin. Nutr.* 79:606–612, https://doi.org/10.1093/ajcn/79.4.606; Mozaffarian D et al (2004) Trans fatty acids and systemic inflammation in heart failure. *Am. J. Clin. Nutr.* 80:1521–1525, https://doi.org/10.1093/ajcn/80.6.1521; Lopez-Garcia E et al (2005) Consumption of trans fatty acids is related to plasma biomarkers of inflammation and endothelial dysfunction. *J. Nutr.* 135:562–566, https://doi.org/10.1093/jn/135.3.562.

26. Mensink RP, Katan MB (1990) Effect of dietary trans fatty acids on high-density and low-density lipoprotein cholesterol levels in healthy subjects. *N. Engl. J. Med.* 323:439–45, https://doi.org/10.1056/NEJM199008163230703; Han SN et al (2002) Effect of hydrogenated and saturated, relative to polyunsaturated, fat on immune and inflammatory responses of adults with moderate hypercholesterolemia. *J. Lipid Res.* 43:445–452 https://pubmed.ncbi.nlm.nih.gov/11893781/

27. Mozaffarian D et al (2006) Trans fatty acids and cardiovascular disease. *N. Engl. J. Med.* 354:1601–1613, https://doi.org/10.1056/NEJMra054035.

28. de Souza RJ et al (2015) Intake of saturated and trans unsaturated fatty acids and risk of all cause mortality, cardiovascular disease, and type 2 diabetes: systematic review and meta-analysis of observational studies. *BMJ* 351:h3978, https://doi.org/10.1136/bmj.h3978.

29. Sargis RM, Subbaiah PV (2003) Trans unsaturated fatty acids are less oxidizable than cis unsaturated fatty acids and protect endogenous lipids from oxidation in lipoproteins and lipid bilayers. *Biochem.* 42:11533–11543, https://doi.org/10.1021/bi034927y.

30. MacDonald HB (2000) Conjugated linoleic acid and disease prevention: a review of current knowledge. *J. Am. Coll. Nutr.* 19 (suppl2):111S-118S, https://doi.org/10.1080/07315724.2000.10718082 ; Viladomiu M et al (2016) Modulation of inflammation and immunity by dietary conjugated linoleic acid. *Eur. J. Pharmacol.* 785:87–95, https://doi.org/10.1016/j.ejphar.2015.03.095; Yang B et al (2015) Review of the roles of conjugated linoleic acid in health and disease. *J. Funct. Foods* 15:314–332, https://doi.org/10.1016/j.jff.2015.03.050.

31. Mensink RP, Katan MB (1990) Effect of dietary trans fatty acids on high-density and low-density lipoprotein cholesterol levels in healthy subjects. *N. Engl. J. Med.* 323:439–445, https://doi.org/10.1056/NEJM199008163230703.

32. McBurney MI et al (2021) Using an erythrocyte fatty acid fingerprint to predict risk of all-cause mortality: the Framingham Offspring Cohort. *Am. J. Clin. Nutr.* 114:1447–1454, https://doi.org/10.1093/ajcn/nqab195.

33. Caprari P et al (1999) Aging and red blood cell membrane: a study of centenarians. *Exp. Gerontol.* 34:47–57, https://doi.org/10.1016/s0531-5565(98)00055-2; Rabini RA et al (2002) Reduced susceptibility to peroxidation of erythrocyte plasma membranes from centenarians. *Exp. Gerontol.* 37:657–663, https://doi.org/10.1016/s0531-5565(02)00006-2.

34. Herskind AM et al (1996) The heritability of human longevity: a population-based study of 2872 Danish twin pairs born 1870–1900. *Hum. Genet.* 97:319–323, https://doi.org/10.1007/BF02185763.

35. Puca AA et al (2008) Fatty acid profile of erythrocyte membranes as possible biomarker of longevity. *Rejuvenation Res.* 11:63–72, https://doi.org/10.1089/rej.2007.0566.

36. Erthal J et al (2019) Hot topic: global trends in the use of opioid analgesics. *Current Addiction Reports* 6:41–48, https://doi.org/10.1007/s40429-019-0234-2.

37. Happiness scores are from https://worldhappiness.report/ed/2020/#appendices-and-data, and are average of 2017–2019 scores. The percent

contribution of vegetable oils to total fat supply are calculated from data from http://www.fao.org/faostat/en/#data/FBS.

38. US Department of Agriculture, FoodData Central, https://fdc.nal.usda.gov /index.html

39. Australian Food Composition Database (January 2022), https://www .foodstandards.gov.au/science/monitoringnutrients/afcd/Pages/default.aspx.

40. Kritchevsky D (1998) History of recommendations to the public about dietary fat. *J. Nutr.* 128:449S–452S, https://doi.org/10.1093/jn/128.2.449S.

41. US Department of Agriculture and US Department of Health and Human Services. December 2020. *Dietary Guidelines for Americans, 2020–2025.* 9th ed., https://www.dietaryguidelines.gov.

42. Teicholz N (2014) *The Big Fat Surprise: Why Butter, Meat, and Cheese Belong in a Healthy Diet.* New York: Simon & Schuster

43. National Health and Medical Research Council (2013) Australian Dietary Guidelines Summary. Canberra, Australia, www.nhmrc.gov.au/guidelines -publications/n55a.

44. Public Health England, *Guidance: The Eatwell Guide,* March 17, 2016, updated September 25, 2018, https://www.gov.uk/government/publications/the -eatwell-guide.

45. International Society for the Study of Fatty Acids and Lipids (June 2004), Report on Dietary Intake of Essential Fatty Acids. https://www.issfal.org /assets/issfal%2003%20pufaintakereccomdfinalreport.pdf I assumed a metabolic rate of 10 MJ/d to calculate daily intakes of 5.1g omega-6 and 2.3g omega-3.

46. Ervin RB et al (2004) Dietary intake of fats and fatty acids for the United States population: 1999–2000. *National Center for Health Statistics CDC*, vol. 348. Hyattsville, Maryland https://stacks.cdc.gov/view/cdc/81893.

47. Meyer BJ et al (2003) Dietary intakes and food sources of omega-6 and omega-3 polyunsaturated fatty acids. *Lipids* 38:391–398, https://doi.org/10.1007/s11745 -003-1074-0.

Postscript. Omega Balance and COVID-19

1. Merad M et al. (2022) The immunology and immunopathology of COVID-19. *Science* 375:1122–1127, https://doi.org/10.1126/science.abm8108.

2. Zaid Y et al. (2021) Chemokines and eicosanoids fuel the hyperinflammation within the lungs of patients with severe COVID-19. *J. Allergy Clin. Immunol.* 148:368–380, https://doi.org/10.1016/j.jaci.2021.05.032; Hammock BD et al. (2020) Eicosanoids. The overlooked storm in Coronavirus disease 2019 (COVID-19)? *Am. J. Pathol.* 190:1782–1788, https://doi.org/10.1016/j.ajpath .2020.06.010.; Moore JB, June CH (2020) Cytokine release syndrome in severe COVID-19. *Science* 368:473–474, https://doi.org/10.1080/08830185 .2021.1884248.

3. Carethers JM (2020) Insights into disparities observed with COVID-19. *J. Intern. Med.* 289:463–473, https://doi.org/10.1111/joim.13199.

4. Mehta J et al. (2022) Role of dexamethasone and methylprednisolone cortico-steroids in Coronavirus disease 2019 hospitalized patients: a review. *Front. Microbiol.* 13:813358, https://doi.org/10.3389/fmicb.2022.813358.

5. Zapata R et al. (2021) Omega-3 index and clinical outcomes of severe COVID-19: preliminary results of a cross-sectional study. *Int. J. Environ. Res. Pub Health* 18:7722, https://pubmed.ncbi.nlm.nih.gov/34360016/.

6. Sun Y et al. (2022) Circulating polyunsaturated fatty acids and COVID-19: a prospective cohort study and Mendelian randomization analysis. https://doi.org/10.1101/2022.02.06.22270562.

7. Asher A et al. (2021) Blood omega-3 fatty acids and death from COVID-19: a pilot study, https://doi.org/10.1101/2021.01.06.21249354.

8. Doaei S et al. (2021) The effect of omega-3 fatty acid supplementation on clinical and biochemical parameters of critically ill patients with COVID-19: a randomized clinical trial. *J. Transl. Med.* 19:128, https://doi.org/10.1186/s12967-021-02795-5.

9. Kim H et al. (2021) Plant-based diets, pescatarian diets and COVID-19 severity: a population-based case-control study in six countries. *BMJ Nutr. Prev. Health* 4:e000272, https://doi.org/10.1136/bmjnph-2021-000272.

10. From Table A "Developed Economies" of World Economic Situation and Prospects https://www.un.org/development/desa/dpad/wp-content/uploads/sites/45/WESP2020_Annex.pdf.

11. (1) fatality rate for each nation calculated as "total deaths" as percentage of "total cases" (as of March 4, 2022) https://www.worldometers.info/coronavirus/; (2) percent vaccination for each nation from https://ourworldindata.org/covid-vaccinations?country=ESP ; (3) percent contribution of vegetable oils to total fat supply are calculated from data from http://www.fao.org/faostat/en/#data/FBS.

Index